# Clinical Anatomy and Embryology

Jonathan Leo

# Clinical Anatomy and Embryology

## A Guide for the Classroom, Boards, and Clinic

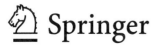 Springer

Jonathan Leo
Alabama College of Osteopathic Medicine
Dothan, AL, USA

ISBN 978-3-031-03809-9          ISBN 978-3-031-03807-5   (eBook)
https://doi.org/10.1007/978-3-031-03807-5

This Springer imprint is published by the registered company Springer Nature Switzerland AG
The registered company address is: Gewerbestrasse 11, 6330 Cham, Switzerland

# Preface

This book is written for medical and other allied health students. Students are stuck in quandary. Since you haven't picked a specialty yet, you need to know a little bit about everything. Once you pick a specialty, say surgery of the inner ear, or evaluation of the lower limb in sport's injuries, or delivering babies, you will obviously go far behind this book in the anatomy of your specialty. And at that point you can be forgiven for not knowing all the anatomy of the body, but in the meantime, all of anatomy is fair game for your gross anatomy course, boards, and for preceptors. At some point, your older self will know a whole lot more detail about your specialty, but conversely 20 years from now you might not remember everything about those regions you don't see every day. If you become an otolaryngologist, the anatomy of the foot will likely be a distant memory. And if you become an orthopedic surgeon, the intricacies of the inner ear might not be on the tip of your tongue.

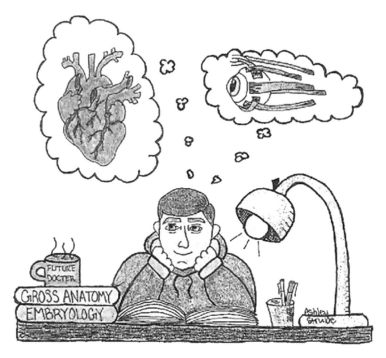

Students might be surprised, but one of the common discussions around the watercooler among anatomy faculty members revolves around what to include in the first-year medical school curriculum. In 1858, when Henry Gray and Henry Carter, both recent graduates of medical school, set out to write their masterpiece, *Gray's Anatomy*, they had first-year medical students in mind as their audience. I imagine they had numerous discussions about what was appropriate to include, and I imagine that 100 years from now, professors will still be having the same discussion. What we anatomists don't always acknowledge is that all our students are going to go on and specialize, so that at some point they can come back and tell us more about the details of their specialty than we know.

Whether or not a particular anatomical factoid should be included in a lecture or not can turn into hours of debate. Should we be teaching it in a first-year course, or leave it to their residency training? There are no "correct" answers to these questions. On the one hand, we don't want to leave out important concepts, but on the other hand, we cannot teach everything. Somewhere in the middle is a happy medium that hopefully this book fills. The figures in the book are not exhaustive diagrams documenting every nook and cranny of a particular region, but instead they are all simple diagrams focusing on one or two anatomical relationships that explain clinical scenarios. The cover image and images used in Figs. 2.9, 2.12, and 2.13 are under license from Shutterstock.com.

The purpose of this text is obviously not an exhaustive deep dive into all of gross anatomy. Rather, it is meant to present each topic with clinical scenarios in mind. Likewise, it is not meant as a clinical text that covers all the clinical scenarios in detail. Hopefully, it will help first-year students with their course, second-year students looking for a refresher before boards, and third- and fourth-year students looking for a refresher before rotations.

I have sat through many clinical lectures, and sitting in these lectures, I always think to myself that I need to get students ready for these lectures. Please keep in mind that I am not teaching clinical procedures or how to make a diagnosis with this text. Instead, I am presenting the anatomy in a clinical format so that when you hear clinical lectures, the anatomy makes sense. For instance, when I mention a test, a diagnosis, or a procedure, I am not teaching all the details, rather I am focusing on the pertinent anatomy that one needs to know to understand those details. For instance, when I discuss inserting lines into arteries or veins, I am focusing on the pertinent anatomical relationships and in no way am I providing a full description of the procedure.

There is no way to learn gross anatomy without dissecting the body. And the medical profession owes an enormous debt to all those donors, or first patients, who have donated their bodies to anatomy departments: you have made the world a better place. I can assure you that your gift has made a tremendous impact on medical students. students. The cover image and Figs. 2.9, 2.12, and 2.13 are under license from Shutterstock.com.

Thank you to Ashley Strube for the picture of the stressed-out student. And thanks to Dr. Ashley Hamati for looking at a first draft from a student's point of view. Last but not least, thanks to all my students for all the questions over the years. You don't realize it but every time you ask a question, the professor learns something also. And as anyone who has written a book knows, the main reason to write a book is to learn something new.

Dothan, AL, USA                                                    Jonathan Leo

# Contents

# Part I

# Gross Anatomy

# The Head and Neck

**1**

## Introduction

The head is the hardest part of gross anatomy. There is more in this small space than either one of the limbs. As an undergraduate student you might have learned a mnemonic for the cranial nerves so that you could answer a question such as: What is the name cranial nerve V? You can forget the mnemonics for the names of the cranial nerves as they will not get you very far in gross anatomy. The pertinent point is not whether you know that cranial nerve V is the trigeminal nerve – that is a given. The question is: How many of the 51 branches of cranial nerve V can you name?

When studying the head, everything is organized around the cranial nerves and the skull. All the cranial nerves are important, but cranial nerves V and VII cover so much territory that when you study the head, think of these two nerves as the scaffold.

## The Skull and Face

Architecture has been said to be the study of how to organize rectangles. The skull is similar to a house with many rooms. When studying the skull, it is helpful to think of the different regions of the skull as individual rooms with floors, ceilings, and walls. And in many cases the ceiling of one room is the floor of the room above it. For instance, the floor of the orbit is the ceiling of the maxillary sinus, and the floor of the maxillary sinus is the ceiling of the oral cavity. And between the various rooms are doorways and hallways transmitting the nerves, arteries, and veins.

The skull is the cranium plus the mandible. There are 22 bones that make up the skull. The neurocranium which holds the brain includes eight bones – the frontal, ethmoid, sphenoid, occipital, plus the two each of temporal and parietal. There are 14 that make up the face (viscerocranium). The *pterion* is the weakest point of the

© The Author(s), under exclusive license to Springer Nature Switzerland AG 2022
J. Leo, *Clinical Anatomy and Embryology*,
https://doi.org/10.1007/978-3-031-03807-5_1

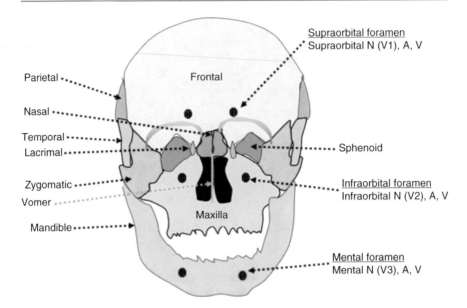

**Fig. 1.1** Anterior view of the skull. Note the three openings lined up in a row. The supraorbital, infraorbital, and mental foramen. Each transmits an artery, nerve, and vein all named after the appropriate foramen. (Leo 2022)

skull and represents the junction of the parietal, temporal, frontal, and sphenoid bones (Fig. 1.1). Fractures here can damage the middle meningeal artery. It is also a neurosurgical landmark. Broca's area is deep to it.

## Skull Foramina

This is just an introduction as the details will be covered in each section. Think of the interior of the skull like a bowl with three sections: The anterior, middle, and posterior cranial fossae. We are going to start with the mnemonic SRO for Standing Room Only. Nestled in on the floor of the middle cranial fossa is the trigeminal ganglion which sits in a space called *Meckel's cave*. Coming out of the ganglion are the three branches of the trigeminal nerve – V1, V2, and V3 – which all exit the skull. V1 goes through the *superior orbital fissure*, V2 through *the foramen rotundum,* and V3 through *foramen ovale* (Fig. 1.2).

1. **S**uperior Orbital Fissure - V1
2. Foramen **R**otundum – V2
3. Foramen **O**vale – V3

We will follow all these along later. But for now, note that next to the foramen ovale is the *foramen spinosum* with the *middle meningeal artery* entering the skull. Along the petrous portion of the temporal bone, we see the *internal acoustic meatus* which

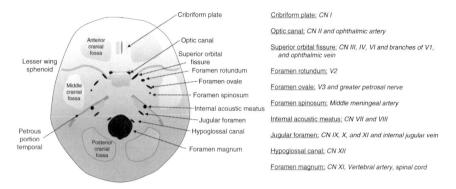

The interior of the skull:

Cribriform plate: *CN I*

Optic canal: *CN II and ophthalmic artery*

Superior orbital fissure: *CN III, IV, VI and branches of V1, and ophthalmic vein*

Foramen rotundum: *V2*

Foramen ovale: *V3 and greater petrosal nerve*

Foramen spinosum: *Middle meningeal artery*

Internal acoustic meatus: *CN VII and VIII*

Jugular foramen: *CN IX, X, and XI and internal jugular vein*

Hypoglossal canal: *CN XII*

Foramen magnum: *CN XI, Vertebral artery, spinal cord*

**Fig. 1.2** The interior of the skull. (Leo 2022)

contains cranial nerves VII and VIII. In the posterior fossa, the *jugular foramen* transmits cranial nerve IX, X, and XI. The *hypoglossal canal* transmits cranial nerve XII. In the center of the posterior fossa is the foramen magnum with the spinal cord, vertebral artery, and cranial nerve XI. Note that at this point cranial nerve XI is *entering* the skull through the foramen magnum, it then *exits* the skull through the jugular foramen. In the anterior cranial fossa, we see the *crista galli* with the olfactory bulbs on either side.

## Jugular Foramen Syndrome

Because cranial nerves IX, X, and XI all travel through the jugular foramen, a mass in the foramen can lead to palsies of all three of these nerves (Vernet's Syndrome). The cranial nerve IX palsy will lead to a loss of sensation from the posterior 1/3 of the tongue and loss of the gag reflex. The cranial nerve X palsy will lead to dysphagia and dysarthria. The cranial nerve XI palsy will lead to paralysis of SCM and trapezius. In addition, if the mass is large enough it can also impinge on CN XII near the hypoglossal canal which would lead to a tongue deficit (Collet Syndrome). And if it expands even more, it can impinge on the sympathetic trunk traveling through the foramen magnum leading to Horner's syndrome (Villaret Syndrome). The internal jugular vein also travels with the nerves through the foramen, so that besides cranial nerve palsies, intracranial pressure can rise. For the nerve palsies given above this is just the short version. Later in this chapter each nerve is discussed in more detail. This is an important region to point out a concept of lesions. While I pointed out the names of the various syndromes above, knowing the exact name of the lesion or syndrome is not as important as knowing the relationships within a given neighborhood. In other words, when there is a lesion of one nerve, there is always a chance that a lesion will expand and comprise the neighboring structures. With lesions to a nerve, it is important to know which neighbors can also be affected. So that if you see a patient with a lesion to CN IX, X, and XI then you think about the jugular foramen, but if a month later there is a tongue deficit, then you know that the lesion has enlarged. It is much more important to understand and have a visual representation of the relationships then to memorize flashcards listing various syndromes.

## Scalp

There is no structure in anatomy better suited to a mnemonic. The mnemonic for the scalp is SCALP (Fig. 1.3).

1. *Skin*. Hair Follicles are located in the skin. Their associated sebaceous glands can become infected which will lead to redness and swelling around the cyst. There are no lymph nodes in the skin. The hair follicles also extend into the layer right below it.
2. *Connective Tissue*. This is layer is made up of dense connective tissue connecting the skin to the underlying aponeurosis. A *caput succedaneum* typically results following a vacuum or forceps assisted vaginal delivery which leads to "molding" of the skull. Because the skull bones are not yet fused, the head can assume a V-shape corresponding to the vacuum shape. This will resolve soon after birth. During this process fluid will drain along the connective tissue layer into the site where the vacuum was attached. The caput will have a soft, boggy feel that can move as the head position is changed. Keep in mind a caput succedaneum occurs *external* to the pericranium.

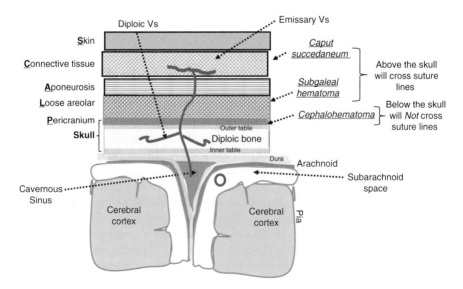

**Fig. 1.3** The layers of the SCALP. Three pathologies, all of which can occur during delivery. Caput Succedaneum is a soft fleshy inflammation in the connective tissue layer. Subgaleal hematomas are found in the loose areolar layer. Cephalohematoma occur below the pericranium. (Leo 2022)

3. *Aponeurosis*. In the front of the head is the frontalis muscle, and posterior is the occipitalis muscle. The *galea aponeurotica* is a strong, tough ligament connecting these two muscles. All these structures together are referred to as the *occipitofrontalis muscle*. Anteriorly the ligament is attached to the upper eyelids. With lacerations, this layer is a landmark for how deep the cut is. If the cut has penetrated this layer, especially in the coronal plane, then the patient will have a gaping wound because the aponeurosis will pull the two flaps apart. When suturing the wound, this will have to be considered. If the wound is only through the skin and connective tissue, it will be "non-gaping" wound.

4. *Loose areolar layer*. Think of this layer as one large continuous space below the aponeurosis. It is sometimes referred to as the *danger area*. If you put your hand on your scalp and move the skin, this is the layer allowing the movement. Traversing this layer are the scalp veins and diploic veins. Bleeding into this space can lead to a *subgaleal hematoma*. Blood in this layer can freely move from one point to another within the layer, and because this layer is still above the skull, the blood flow is not restricted by the suture lines. Subgaleal hematomas are life threatening and much more severe than the above-mentioned caput succedaneum. They can also result from superficial contusions to the scalp. Traumatic deliveries, or even excessive hair pulling can lead to blood pooling in this area. For instance, several hours after a patient receives a fairly minor hit to the top of the head, they might develop racoon eyes. In this case the blood has moved from the site of the contusion to the corners of the eyes – remember the aponeurosis above it is connected to the upper eyelid. Racoon eyes should not be confused with *Battle signs* (or Battle's Sign) which are indicative of major trauma to the skull such as the petrous portion of the temporal bone (basilar skull fracture). In this case blood can pool just posterior to the ear following a basilar skull fracture.

5. *Pericranium*. The pericranium or the periosteum is dense irregular tissue attached to the bone. During a difficult delivery, often with either forceps or a vacuum, shearing forces can lead to blood collecting between the periosteum and the skull bone forming a *cephalohematoma* (subperiosteal hematoma). It will usually take several hours to develop and will typically resolve over time. The most common site is over the parietal bone. The mass will not cross the suture lines and will not put pressure on the brain. A cephalohematoma occurs below the pericranium.

Deep to the periosteum is the bone tissue, made up of inner and outer tables sandwiching the diploic bone. And deep to the bone is the dura mater, which in turn has two layers: the *periosteal* and *endosteal layers*. In several locations these two layers of dura separate from each other to make room for the venous sinuses such as the *superior and inferior sagittal sinuses*. The superficial veins from the scalp, and diploic veins from the skull bone also drain into these sinuses. Adherent to the dura is the arachnoid mater, and deep to the arachnoid mater is the subarachnoid space. The arteries perfusing the brain are found in the subarachnoid space. And just on top of the brain is the pia mater. The pia is tightly adherent to the brain surface, such that if you are touching an embalmed brain, or holding a brain in your hand, you are really touching pia mater. The subarachnoid space is between the pia and arachnoid layers.

## Common, External and Internal Carotid Arteries

The common carotid artery travels in the carotid sheath with the internal jugular vein and the vagus nerve. A landmark for the common carotid artery is the *carotid tubercle* which is the anterior tubercle of the C6 vertebra. The common carotid artery runs anterior to the tubercle and the pulse can be felt here. Posterior to the tubercle is the vertebral artery crossing to enter into the *foramen transversarium* of C6. The carotid artery typically splits at the level of C4 into the internal and external carotid arteries. The internal carotid is strictly intracranial with a few exceptions. The external carotid is strictly extracranial with one exception. The branches of the external carotid are (Fig. 1.4):

1. If you fill the external carotid artery with contrast material, all the branches can be seen ascending towards the head except for the *superior thyroid artery* which will be seen descending towards the thyroid gland. A branch of the superior thyroid artery is the *superior laryngeal artery* which pierces the thyrohyoid membrane with the *internal laryngeal nerve*.
2. The *ascending pharyngeal artery* is a very small artery arising between the internal and external carotid arteries.
3. The *lingual artery* dives deep to the mandible to enter the oral cavity.

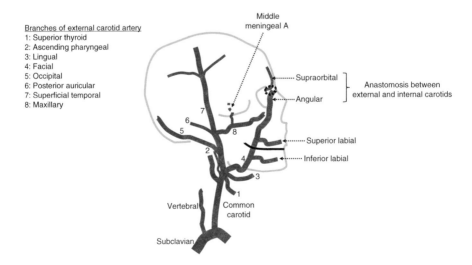

**Fig. 1.4** Branches of the external carotid artery. (Leo 2022)

4. The *facial artery* crosses the mandible just in front of the masseter and heads towards the medial corner of the orbit. Just past its origin, it gives off a tonsillar branch to the palatine tonsils. On the way it gives off the superior and inferior labial arteries going to the superior and inferior lips. As the facial artery crosses the zygomaticus major it becomes the angular artery which travels to the corner of the eye, where it anastomosis with the supraorbital artery which is a branch of the frontal artery. An increased pulse in the corner of the eye could be the result of a blockage of the internal carotid deep in the skull.

5. The *occipital artery* runs across the temporal bone and then runs between the trapezius and sternocleidomastoid. Close to the midline, its terminal branch runs with the greater occipital nerve to reach the posterior skull.

6. The *posterior auricular artery* comes off the external carotid artery in the vicinity of the styloid process and runs between the external ear and the mastoid process.

7. The *superficial temporal artery* runs anterior to the ear where its pulse can be felt. It runs with the auriculotemporal nerve. In cases of giant cell arteritis, biopsies of the superficial temporal artery can be taken. During the procedure the auriculotemporal nerve can be damaged.

8. The *maxillary artery* runs deep to the mandible to enter the infratemporal fossa where it gives of several branches. It then runs through the pterygopalatine fossa to enter the nasal cavity. It will be dealt with in more detail in each of those sections. It is mainly an artery of the deep face, however one of its branches, the middle meningeal artery travels through the foramen spinosum to enter the middle cranial fossa and supply the meninges. Within the skull it divides into anterior and posterior divisions which leave an impression along the inner surface of the skull. In many cases the maxillary artery also gives off an *accessory meningeal artery* which travels through the foramen ovale to also enter the skull and supply the trigeminal ganglion.

## Venous Drainage Superficial Face and Neck

The *superficial temporal vein* drains into the *retromandibular vein*, which in turn divides into the anterior and posterior divisions. The posterior division turns into the *external jugular*, while the anterior division meets with the *facial vein* to form the *common facial vein*. The external jugular vein lies superficial to the sternocleidomastoid muscle. Increased pressure in the veins due to heart or lung pathology, for instance right-sided heart failure, can be seen as *jugular venous distension* (JVD) in the external jugular vein.

If you take a cross section through the mediastinum or the neck, there is a continuous venous channel serving as a landmark. The internal jugular vein travels in the neck where it runs into the right brachiocephalic vein, which in turn runs into the superior vena cava, which then turns into the right atrium of the heart. So, if you start superiorly and a take a cut at the T3 level on the right side will be the right brachiocephalic vein; if you move inferiorly to the superior mediastinum, on the

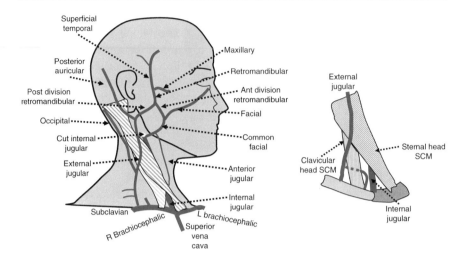

**Fig. 1.5** The venous drainage of the face. The superficial temporal vein turns into the retromandibular vein that in turn divides into an anterior and posterior division. The posterior division goes down through the external jugular, while the anterior division goes down through the internal jugular vein. In the close-up of the neck, you can see the internal jugular between the two heads of the sternocleidomastoid muscle. (Leo 2022)

right side will be the superior vena cava; and if you take a cut through the heart, on the right side is the right atrium. The right atrium forms the right border of the heart (Fig. 1.5).

## Subclavian Vein Line

The subclavian vein passes in front of the anterior scalene muscle, while the subclavian artery passes posterior to the muscle. To access the vein, a needle is passed inferior to the clavicle from lateral to medial. One goal is to avoid piercing the apex of the lung.

## Internal Jugular Vein Line

The *internal jugular vein* lies in a triangle formed by the two heads of the sternocleidomastoid and the clavicle. Within the triangle, the internal jugular vein is lateral to the common carotid artery. With a finger on the pulse of the artery the needle is inserted lateral to the finger and the needle is moved inferolateral. In some cases, the needle will be inserted higher up in the neck (more superior) in which case the access is at the midpoint of the medial border of the sternocleidomastoid. The vein is still lateral to the artery at this point, so again the needle is placed lateral to the pulse of the artery.

## Venous Drainage of the Skull

Within the skull there are two layers of dura and in several regions these two layers separate to allow for venous drainage of blood. The *superior sagittal sinus* lies in the midline within the superior portion of the falx cerebri. Along the inferior portion of the falx cerebri is the *inferior sagittal sinus*, which in turn drains into the *straight sinus* (Fig. 1.6).

The straight sinus and superior sagittal sinus meet posteriorly in the midline at the *confluence of the sinuses*. The single confluence drains laterally to both the right and left sides as the *transverse sinuses*. Each transverse sinus then makes a right turn and descends as the sigmoid sinus to the jugular foramen to turns into the *internal jugular vein*. The cavernous sinus is a space around the sella turcica that receives venous blood from several areas and then drains via the *superior petrosal sinus* to the junction of the transverse sinus, and the *inferior petrosal sinus* to the junction of the sigmoid sinus and the internal jugular vein. It also receives venous drainage from the deep veins of the face.

## Cavernous Sinus

The facial vein is valveless so infections can move in either direction. The danger area of the face is the triangle region around the nose that gets its name because an infection in the danger area of the face can track back along these veins into the cavernous sinus. For instance, take an individual on a walk in the woods who gets a small cut on the face from a tree limb and develops a superficial infection. What could have been just a minor issue can become a life-threatening condition if the infection travels back into the skull where it can lead to increased intracranial pressure.

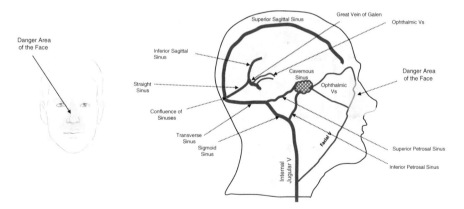

**Fig. 1.6** Venous drainage of skull. The confluence of the sinus receives blood from the superior sagittal sinus and the straight sinus, and then drains into the transverse, sigmoid, and then into the internal jugular vein. The cavernous sinus receives blood from the danger area of the face via the deep veins. The cavernous sinus then drains via the superior and inferior petrosal sinuses. (Leo 2022)

Within the cavernous sinus are several important structures. Entering the sinus is the internal carotid artery which runs forward then does a 180° turn to form the genu of the internal carotid artery. In addition, there are several important cranial nerves. The ophthalmic artery arises at the genu. In the lateral wall of the sinus are cranial nerves III, IV, V1 (ophthalmic nerve), and V2. And deeper in the sinus is CN VI (Abducens Nerve) and the genu of the internal carotid artery. An infection in the sinus will typically first compromise CN VI which will cause a medial strabismus, however as the infection spreads it will also affect the nerves on the lateral wall so that all the eye muscles will be affected, and the patient will have complete ophthalmoplegia. In addition, V1 and V2 will be affected, but _not_ V3 thus the muscles of mastication will be spared (Fig. 1.7).

## Infratemporal Fossa

Where is the infratemporal fossa? The short answer is that it is the space behind the ramus of the mandible. And it contains the majority, but not all, of the muscles of mastication. If you start with your hand on your mandible, you can feel the *masseter muscle*. To dissect the infratemporal fossa, you remove the masseter and then remove the mandible to look into the infratemporal fossa.

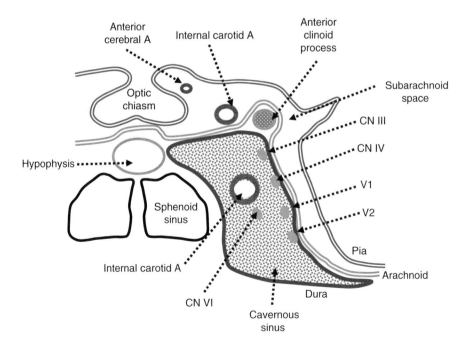

**Fig. 1.7** Cavernous sinus. Running through the cavernous sinus are CNs III, IV, VI, and V1, and V2 – or "all the cranial nerves associated with eye movements plus V1 and V2 but not V3." An infection in the cavernous sinus will typically first lead to a CN VI palsy, followed shortly by ophthalmoplegia. (Leo 2022)

Think of the infratemporal fossa as a room. The ceiling is the greater wing of the sphenoid; the anterior wall is the infratemporal surface of the maxilla; the medial wall is the lateral pterygoid plate; the lateral wall is the mandible; and both the floor and posterior wall are open.

After removing the mandible, which is the lateral wall of the infratemporal fossa, the first muscle that you will notice in the fossa is the *medial pterygoid*. Both the masseter and the medial pterygoid form a sling holding the mandible. Acting together, they are elevators of the mandible (Fig. 1.12).

Just superior to the medial pterygoid is the *lateral pterygoid*, whose fibers run in a anterior to posterior direction. The lateral pterygoid has a superior and inferior head. The lateral pterygoid is the major muscle involved with elevation (closing the mouth) and protrusion of the mandible because via its attachment to the mandibular condyle it pulls the condyle anterior. It also responsible for protrusion. It is innervated by cranial nerve V. If there is an injury to cranial nerve V and the patient is asked to protrude the jaw, then the mandible will deviate towards the weak side. In other words, a lesion to the right trigeminal nerve will lead to the jaw deviating to the right on attempted protrusion. This is because the functioning left lateral pterygoid will pull the jaw towards the right.

Also entering the infratemporal fossa at the anterosuperior corner is the *temporalis muscle,* which inserts onto the *coronoid process* of the mandible. Most of the temporalis muscle belly is found above the infratemporal fossa in the temporal fossa. The superior fibers of temporalis, running in a superior to inferior direction, will elevate the mandible, while the posterior fibers, running in an anterior to posterior direction will retract the mandible.

## Sphenoid Bone (Fig. 1.8)

## Maxillary Artery

Crossing the infratemporal fossa from lateral to medial is the maxillary artery and its branches. For descriptive purposes the artery can be divided into three sections based on their relationship to the lateral pterygoid muscle. The first part of the axillary artery is proximal to lateral pterygoid, the second part is behind the lateral pterygoid, and the third part is distal to lateral pterygoid. As the maxillary artery crosses the infratemporal fossa there are some branches that ascend towards the skull, and other branches that descend towards the mandible, nasal cavity, and the oral cavity (Fig. 1.9).

The first two branches off the maxillary artery are the *middle meningeal* and *accessory meningeal* arteries. The exact branching pattern of these meningeal arteries is variable. In some cases, they emerge as two distinct branches, while in other cases there is a single artery coming off the maxillary that then splits into two branches. Both these arteries ascend towards the skull. The middle meningeal artery travels through the foramen spinosum to enter the middle cranial fossa, while the

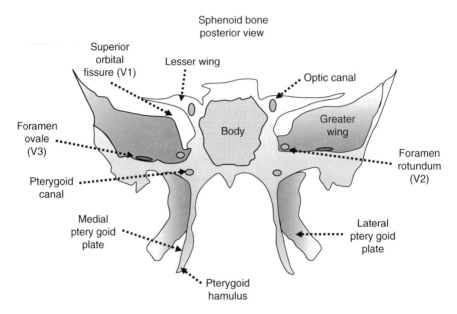

**Fig. 1.8** The sphenoid bone. Note greater and lesser wings with the superior orbital fissure running between them. Foramen rotundum and foramen ovale are also seen on the greater wing. The descending medial and lateral pterygoid plates with the pterygoid hamulus on the medial pterygoid plate. The tensor veli palatini uses the pterygoid hamulus to make a sharp 90° turn as it enters the soft palate. (Leo 2022)

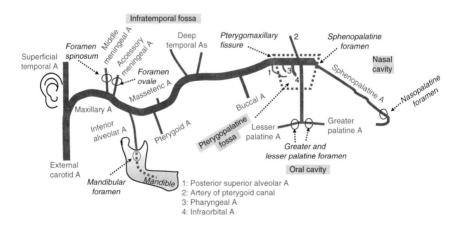

**Fig. 1.9** Maxillary artery. The maxillary artery is seen traveling through the infratemporal fossa and giving off several branches such as infraorbital, middle meningeal, and deep temporal arteries. It then travels through the pterygomaxillary fissure to enter the pterygopalatine fossa. It continues across the pterygopalatine fossa and emerges through the sphenopalatine foramen as the sphenopalatine artery to enter the nasal cavity. It also gives off a descending palatine artery that approaches the palate and splits into a greater palatine artery heading towards the hard palate, and a lesser palatine artery heading to the soft palate. (Leo 2022)

accessory meningeal artery travels through foramen ovale to supply the trigeminal ganglion and then the meninges. The *inferior alveolar artery* is an example of a branch of the maxillary artery that descends. It travels with the inferior alveolar nerve towards to oral cavity to enter the mandible at the mandibular foramen to supply blood to the lower jaw. Right before it enters the mandibular foramen, it gives off a branch to the *mylohyoid muscle*. Likewise, the inferior alveolar nerve gives off a *nerve to mylohyoid* right before the entrance to the mandibular foramen.

Just past the inferior alveolar artery is another descending branch, the *pterygoid artery* which perfuses the pterygoid muscles. Moving along the maxillary are the *masseteric, deep temporal,* and *buccal arteries.* Just before entering the pterygopalatine fossa the maxillary artery gives off the tiny *posterior superior alveolar arteries* which travel through the same named foramina in the maxilla to supply blood to the upper molars. The maxillary artery then passes through the *pterygomaxillary fissure* to enter the pterygopalatine fossa.

## Mandibular Nerve (V3)

The nerve of the infratemporal fossa is the mandibular nerve which enters the fossae by traveling from the middle cranial fossa through the foramen ovale. It comes through foramen ovale as a large nerve trunk, and then right when it enters the fossa it splits into numerous branches. The motor nerves are all named for whichever muscle they are traveling to. For instance, the nerve fibers running to the lateral pterygoid are named the *nerve to lateral pterygoid*. The major sensory branches are as follows (Fig. 1.9):

1. The *auriculotemporal nerve* heads laterally towards the ear. On its way, it splits to go around the middle meningeal artery. As the nerve approaches the ear, it does a 90° turn and heads superiorly in front of the ear. After the nerve comes out of this 90° turn it is now running with the superficial temporal artery. Thus, sensation from just in front of the ear is traveling on the auriculotemporal nerve, and the pulse in front of the ear is the superficial temporal artery.
2. The *inferior alveolar nerve* runs with the inferior alveolar artery to enter the mandibular foramen and is responsible for sensation from the lower teeth. In addition, right before it enters the mandibular foramen, it gives off a motor branch called the nerve to mylohyoid which in addition to mylohyoid supplies the anterior belly of the digastric. The terminal branch of the inferior alveolar nerve exits the mental foramen and carries sensory information from the front of the jaw.
3. The *buccal nerve* is responsible for sensation from the skin on the cheek and buccal mucosa.
4. The *lingual nerve* is travels down to the floor of the mouth and carries general sensory fibers from the anterior 2/3rds of the tongue.

## Temporomandibular Joint

There are two prominent points on the superior surface of the mandible, the *coronoid process*, and the *mandibular condyle*. The mandibular condyle articulates with the *mandibular fossa* on the zygomatic process of the temporal bone. The mandibular fossa is a relatively weak point of the skull. The anterior portion of the condyle also articulates with the posteriorly facing *articular eminence* (Fig. 1.10).

The temporomandibular joint is somewhat unique because it has an articular disk in the middle of the joint. The disk is attached to the superior head of the lateral pterygoid. This articular disk divides the temporomandibular joint into two spaces: a superior space above the articular disk – between the disk and the mandibular fossa, and an inferior space below the disk – between the disk and the condyle. The superior joint allows for protrusion and retraction, while the inferior joint allows for depression and elevation. The disk itself does not have any sensory fibers coming into it, however sensory fibers from the tissue around the joint travel on the auriculotemporal nerve. Lining the bony surfaces abutting the disk is fibrocartilage rather than hyaline cartilage. Hyaline cartilage is present in high stress areas, such as the knee, while fibrocartilage is better for long-term, high use areas.

Opening of the jaw is accomplished by the lateral pterygoid, posterior digastric, and mylohyoid. Closing of the jaw is accomplished by the masseter, temporalis, and

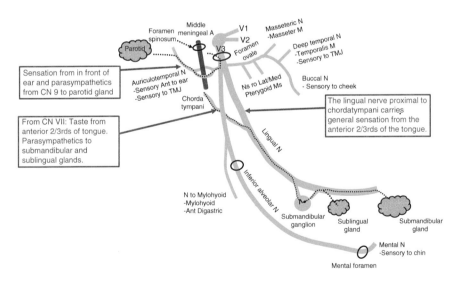

**Fig. 1.10** Mandibular nerve. The mandibular nerve(V3) is seen entering the infratemporal fossa through the foramen ovale. The inferior alveolar nerve is entering the mandibular foramen. The chorda tympani Is a branch of the facial nerve joining the lingual nerve. The chorda tympani carries taste from anterior 2/3rds of the tongue and parasympathetic fibers (dotted black line) to the submandibular ganglion. The parasympathetics from CN IX (dotted black line) travel on the auriculotemporal nerve to reach the parotid gland. (Leo 2022)

medial pterygoid. When the jaw starts to open, the first movement is the hinge movement in the lower part of the joint. As the jaw continues to open, the mandible starts to move forward. This gliding movement now occurs at the upper joint, with the condyle sliding forward and coming to lie just inferior to the articular tubercle with the disk resting between the two structures. Preceding the gliding movement, the lateral pterygoid muscle pulls the disk anterior. Retraction is accomplished by the posterior fibers of the temporalis, while protraction is accomplished by the lateral pterygoid.

During excessive opening of the jaw, such as a big yawn for instance, the condyle can move over the posterior slope and become stuck. The disk then comes to lie between the condyle and the tubercle and the disk acts like a door jamb holding the mandible in place. To reduce this dislocated joint, the mandible is typically pushed down so that the condyle moves away from the tubercle allowing the jaw to close (Fig. 1.11).

## Masticator Space

The mandible is held up by a sling formed by the masseter and the medial pterygoid muscles. The masseter is outside the mandible (superficial), and the medial pterygoid is behind the mandible (deep). They both elevate the mandible. Running down

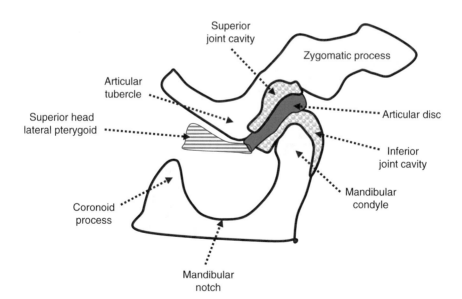

**Fig. 1.11** The temporomandibular joint is a synovial joint between the mandibular condyle and the mandibular fossa. The mandibular fossa is on the zygomatic process of the temporal bone. The anterior surface of the joint, is the posterior slope of the articular tubercle. Between the condyle and the fossa is the articular tubercle. The superior head of the lateral pterygoid is attached to the articular disc. (Leo 2022)

the superficial surface of the masseter and down around the submandibular gland and up the deep side of the medial pterygoid is the *masseteric fascia* surrounding the *masseteric space*. Within this space you can see the lateral pterygoid muscle, plus the various branches of the mandibular nerve (V3), and the maxillary artery. The *buccal nerve* can be seen traveling between the superior and inferior heads of the lateral pterygoid. The inferior alveolar nerve can be seen traveling to the mandible through the mandibular foramen. The *otic ganglion* is found on the medial side of V3 just after it enters the foramen ovale. Infections in the masseteric space can spread to other regions of the head and neck (Fig. 1.12). *Ludwig's Angina* refers to a bacterial infection in the submandibular, sublingual, and submental compartments. It often originates from an infected inferior molar and can lead to difficulty with swallowing, speaking, and breathing.

## The Pterygopalatine Fossa

The pterygopalatine fossa is shaped something like a chicken bucket, but it is about the size of a lifesaver hole. It can also be looked at as something like a train station with numerous train cars coming and going, to and from, all different corners of the city. There are seven doorways in the pterygopalatine fossa which connect the fossa to other rooms in the skull. When you study the pterygopalatine fossa, you are not just studying the skull, but also the nerves, arteries, and veins (Figs. 1.13, 1.14, and 1.15).

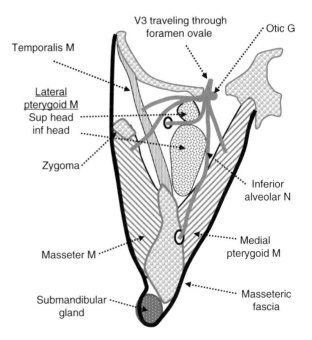

**Fig. 1.12** V3 and foramen ovale. V3 comes through foramen ovale. It has muscular branches going to the muscles of mastication. The medial pterygoid and masseter form a sling to support the mandible. The masseteric fascia covers this sling along with the submandibular gland. The inferior alveolar nerve is seen entering the mandibular foramen. The lateral pterygoid fibers go anterior to posterior, while the medial pterygoids run superior to inferior. (Leo 2022)

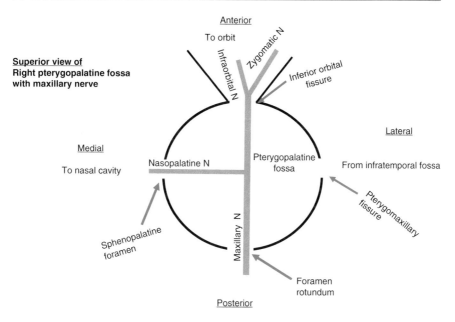

**Fig. 1.13** Pterygopalatine fossa. The maxillary nerve comes through the foramen rotundum and enters the pterygopalatine fossa. It continues through the fossa and emerges into the orbit as the infraorbital nerve, which gives off the zygomatic nerve. In the pterygopalatine fossa you can see the nasopalatine nerve heading through the sphenopalatine foramen to enter the nasal cavity. (Leo 2022)

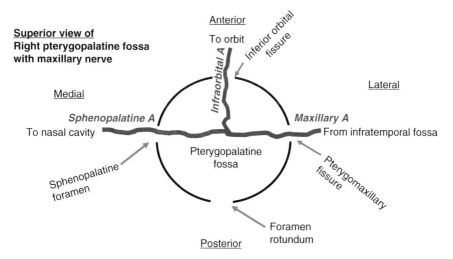

**Fig. 1.14** Maxillary artery. Note the maxillary artery in the infratemporal fossa, coming through the pterygomaxillary fissure and entering the pterygopalatine fossa. It continues through the fossa and emerges into the nasal cavity as the sphenopalatine artery. In the pterygopalatine fossa you can see the infraorbital artery heading through the infraorbital foramen to enter the orbit. There is no artery passing through the foramen rotundum. (Leo 2022)

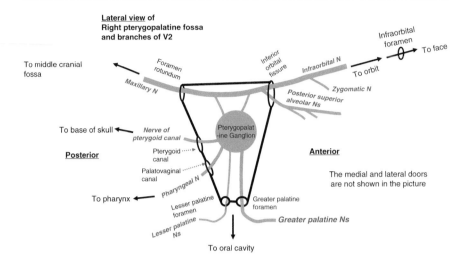

**Fig. 1.15** Maxillary nerve. The maxillary nerve is passing from the middle cranial fossa into pterygopalatine fossa and then moving through the inferior orbital fissure to enter the orbit. Hanging off V2 in the fossa is the pterygopalatine ganglion. Branches of V2 can be seen passing through various foramen into different regions of the skull. The greater and lesser palatine nerves descend and emerge onto the palate in the oral cavity. The nerve of the pterygoid canal is carrying preganglionic fibers from CN VII moving from the base of the skull through the pterygoid canal to enter the pterygopalatine fossa. (Leo 2022)

## Pterygopalatine Fossa Doorways

1. Anterior through the *inferior orbital fissure* to the *orbit*
2. Lateral through the *pterygomaxillary fissure* to the *infratemporal fossa*
3. Medially through the *sphenopalatine foramen* to the *nasal cavity*
4. Inferiorly through the *descending palatine canal* to the *oral cavity*

There are three openings lined up in a column along the posterior wall

5. Posterior through the *foramen rotundum* to the *middle cranial fossa*
6. Posterior through the *pterygoid canal* to the *base of the skull*
7. Posterior through the *palatovaginal canal* to the *pharynx*

As mentioned in the last section, the maxillary artery crosses the infratemporal fossa from lateral to medial. The medial doorway of the infratemporal fossa is the pterygomaxillary fissure. The maxillary artery travels through the pterygomaxillary fissure to enter the pterygopalatine fossa. It then continues across the pterygopalatine fossa and exits the fossa through the sphenopalatine fossa to enter the nasal cavity.

Within the fossa the maxillary artery gives off a descending palatine artery that descends through the *descending palatine canal* and then splits into two branches.

(1) The *greater palatine artery* travels through the *greater palatine canal* to the hard palate, and the (2) *lesser palatine artery* travels through the *lesser palatine canal* to the soft palate. Along the posterior wall, the artery of the pterygoid canal travels back towards the base of the skull. And inferior to the pterygoid canal is the *palato-vaginal canal* with a small artery traveling towards the pharynx.

The infraorbital artery enters the *inferior orbital fissure* to enter the orbit where it runs in the infraorbital grove, to the *infraorbital canal*, and to then emerge onto the face just inferior to the eye through the *infraorbital foramen*.

Coming off V2 within the pterygopalatine fossa, there are typically 2–3 small branches moving anteriorly to enter the very small *posterior superior foramina* in the maxilla. These nerves carry sensory fibers from the posterior superior teeth (the back upper molars).

Just before the *infraorbital nerve* enters the inferior orbital fissure, the *zygomatic nerve* branches off to supply the skin over the zygomatic process via the *zygomaticofacial* and *zygomaticotemporal* branches. Moving medially, through the *sphenopalatine foramen*, is the *nasopalatine nerve* that crosses the superior surface of the nasal cavity to run on the nasal septum forward to the *incisive foramen* (nasopalatine foramen).

## Autonomics of Lacrimal Gland

Preganglionic parasympathetic fibers ultimately destined for the lacrimal gland start off as the *greater petrosal nerve* which is a branch of cranial nerve VII. The greater petrosal nerve leaves cranial CN VII in the vicinity of the geniculate ganglion and enters the pterygoid canal to travel to the pterygopalatine fossa where it synapses in the pterygopalatine ganglion. The post ganglionic fibers then travel on the zygomatic nerve to head towards the lacrimal gland. As they approach the lacrimal gland, they jump on the lacrimal nerve which is a branch of V1 (frontal nerve specifically). Thus, the postganglionic fibers to the lacrimal gland take advantage of the *zygomatic nerve*, which is a branch of V2, and then the *frontal nerve* which is a branch of V1.

## Facial Nerve

The facial nerve comes out of the brainstem and enters the skull by passing through the internal acoustic meatus. It then winds through the skull to eventually emerge onto the face, just posterior to the parotid gland. Within the skull, between the internal acoustic meatus and the stylomastoid foramen the nerve is traveling through the facial canal – think of it as a hallway with several doors. As it travels through the facial canal it gives off three branches. When you look at the nerve in lab, you cannot see the different branches but you cannot "see" the different fibers, but you need to know what types of fibers you find along the different branches. You can't *see* the

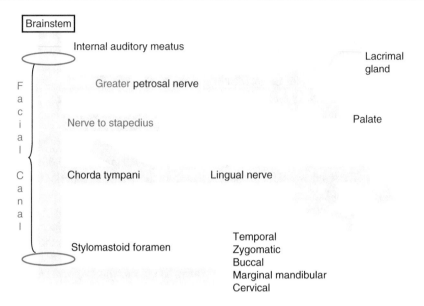

**Fig. 1.16** Facial nerve. The facial nerve comes out of the skull and enters the internal acoustic meatus and then leaves the skull through the stylomastoid foramen. (Leo 2022)

different types of fibers, but you need to *visualize* them. In other words, when you look at the greater petrosal nerve, it looks like any other nerve, but you need to know that it is a parasympathetic nerve (Fig. 1.16).

1. The first branch is the *greater petrosal nerve* which carries preganglionic fibers destined for the pterygopalatine ganglion. The greater petrosal nerve travels through the pterygoid canal to enter the pterygopalatine fossa where the pterygo-palatine ganglion is located.
2. The *nerve to stapedius* carries motor fibers to the stapedius muscle which is involved in sound dampening. Damage to this nerve will result in hyperacusis.
3. The *chorda tympani* carries sensory fibers from the anterior 2/3rds of the tongue and parasympathetic fibers destined for the submandibular ganglion.

## Facial Nerve, Muscles of Facial Expression and Parotid Gland

The facial nerve then exits the stylomastoid foramen and enters the parotid gland. Right as it enters the gland it divides into six branches: Temporal, Zygomatic, Buccal, Mandibular, Cervical, and Posterior auricular. To Zanzibar By Motor Car, Please. A parotid tumor or surgery on the parotid gland can damage branches of the facial nerve here. These branches of the facial nerve innervate the muscles of facial expression which are extremely thin muscles. Without going into all the muscles of facial expression there are several important ones (Figs. 1.17, 1.18, and 1.19).

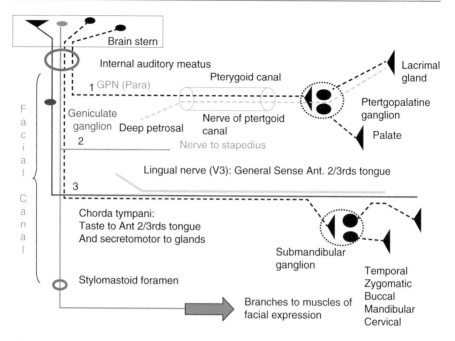

**Fig. 1.17** Facial nerve and its components. Red = sensory, black dotted line = parasympathetic, blue = motor. The green fibers = the lingual nerve from V3. (Leo 2022)

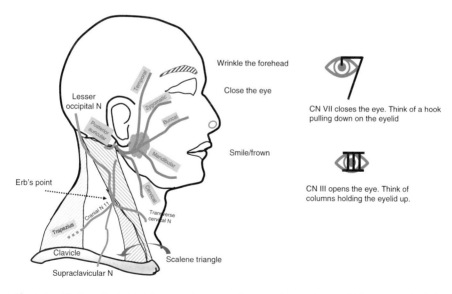

**Fig. 1.18** To Zanzibar By Motor Car Please. Coming out of the stylomastoid foramen and winding through the parotid gland are the branches of the facial nerve: Temporal, Zygomatic, Buccal, Mandibular, Cervical, Posterior auricular. At the posterior border of sternocleidomastoid (Erb's Point) are several nerves: Lesser occipital, great auricular, transverse cervical, supraclavicular. The accessory nerve can also be seen going posterior to trapezius. (Leo 2022)

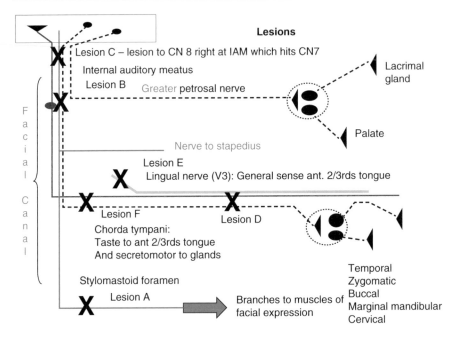

**Fig. 1.19** Lesions to the facial nerve. See the text for a discussion of each lesion. (Leo 2022)

1. The *orbicularis oculi* is the sphincter surrounding the eye. Its primary function is closing the eye. It is also the efferent portion of the blink reflex. The afferent portion is V1 (ophthalmic nerve). For example, dust in the eye would be sensed by V1, and then the closing part of the eye blink would be CN VII acting on the orbicularis oculi.
2. The *orbicularis oris* is the sphincter around the mouth
3. The *zygomaticus major and minor* elevate the corners of the upper lip.
4. The *frontalis* is involved in wrinkling your forehead. It is attached via an aponeurosis to the occipitalis.
5. The *buccinator* plays an important role in eating, drinking and the suckling reflex by keeping the cheek against the teeth. The buccinator is innervated by the *buccal branch of the facial*, while the *buccal nerve* is a branch of V3 in the infratemporal fossa that carries sensory information from the cheek.

There are several potential lesions to the facial nerve. On the diagram the lesions are placed at different parts of the nerve.

**Lesion A**: With a parotid tumor or surgical complications of the parotid gland the facial nerve can be compromised. In this scenario, the patient will lose the muscles of facial expression on one side of the face, but since the nerve in the facial canal is intact there will no deficit in hearing, taste, or glandular secretions from the lacrimal, submandibular, and sublingual glands.

   **Lesion B** represents classic Bell's palsy. In Bell's palsy, an infection of cranial nerve VII is thought to lead to inflammation and subsequent compression of the nerve in the canal. In this scenario, the patient will lose: the muscles of facial expression; taste from the anterior 2/3rds of the tongue; secretions from the lacrimal gland which will lead to a dry eye; the submandibular and sublingual glands. Plus, because of loss of the stapedius, they will complain that loud noises are aggravating. Loss of the submandibular and sublingual glands will not be obvious because the patient still receives secretions from the contralateral glands.

   While Bell's Palsy typically involves all the branches in the facial canal, it is possible for a tumor or other mass to only damage some of the branches. For instance, if there was a lesion to the facial nerve between the nerve to stapedius and the chord tympani, then the stapedius and lacrimal gland would be spared in this patient.

   **Lesion C** is an acoustic neuroma. Because of the proximity of cranial nerves VII and VIII as the enter the internal acoustic meatus, an acoustic neuroma which originates on cranial nerve VIII can also damage cranial nerve VII. This is somewhat rare but worth noting. The patient would have all the signs of the Bell's palsy patient plus a hearing and balance deficit.

   **Lesion D.** Another common injury involves the lingual nerve. The dentist needs to be careful of the lingual nerve when removing a wisdom tooth. If the lingual nerve is severed then the patient will lose: taste to the anterior two-thirds of the tongue; the secretomotor fibers to the submandibular and sublingual glands; and general sense from the anterior two-thirds of the tongue. Remember the chorda tympani joins the lingual nerve, and the lingual nerve is a branch of V3 carrying general sense information from the tongue.

   **Lesion E** is to the lingual nerve before the chorda tympani joins it, so taste and the glands would be spared, but the patient would lose general sensation from the anterior two-thirds of the tongue.

   **Lesion F** is to the chorda tympani before it joins the lingual nerve so only taste and the glands would be affected.

## Temporal Bone

The *petrous portion of the temporal bone* is the strongest portion of the skull. The *internal auditory meatus* (IAM) an opening on the petrous portion which transmits both cranial nerve VII and VIII. They both enter the IAM but quickly head in different directions. Cranial nerve VII does a 90° turn at the genu which is the site of the geniculate ganglion. Coming out of the geniculate ganglion is the greater petrosal nerve which leaves through the hiatus of the greater petrosal nerve and travels in the groove of the greater petrosal nerve to cross the foramen lacerum. The facial nerve then gives off the nerve to stapedius, and then the chorda tympani which crosses the malleus in the middle ear. The facial nerve finally exits the temporal bone at the stylomastoid foramen. Located on the temporal bone is the mastoid process with the mastoid air cells. Infections of the mastoid air cells can lead to inner ear deficits.

**Fig. 1.20** Temporal bone (lateral view). The mandible sits in the mandibular fossa posterior to the articular tubercle. When the Jaw opens the mandible slides forward just inferior to the articular tubercle. The external acoustic meatus is the opening of the auditory tube. The petrotympanic fissure is an opening for the chorda tympani which is traveling on to the lingual nerve. (Leo 2022)

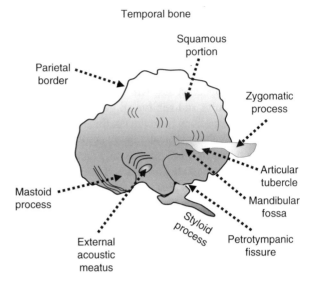

Because of the potential for serious side effects infections in this region are typically quickly treated, but at one point in time this was a significant cause of death in younger patients (Fig. 1.20).

## Nasal Cavity

Before discussing the nasal cavity, it is important to understand the *ethmoid bone*. It is shaped something like a cross. Start with the line running down the middle. Superiorly, this line forms the *crista galli* which projects into the anterior cranial fossa. It serves as an attachment point for the superior sagittal sinus. Running horizontally is another line. On either side of the crista galli is the *cribriform plate* which has a series of small openings for the fibers connecting the olfactory epithelium to the olfactory bulb. Moving inferiorly, the center line continues into the nasal septum as the *perpendicular plate of the ethmoid*. Dropping down laterally, on each side are the labyrinths which house the ethmoid air cells (anterior, middle, and posterior). On the lateral side one also sees the *superior* and *middle concha* which are part of the ethmoid bone. The *inferior concha* is a separate bone.

The ethmoid bone thus contributes to both the nasal septum and lateral nasal wall. The *superior, middle, and inferior concha* form the lateral wall of the nasal cavity. The three conchae are something like bookshelves projecting out into the nasal cavity which are suspended over three spaces. The superior and middle concha are part of the ethmoid while the inferior concha is a separate bone. Underneath the superior concha is the *superior meatus*, underneath the middle concha is the *middle meatus*, and underneath the inferior concha is the *inferior meatus*. There is also a space above the superior meatus which is called the *sphenoethmoidal recess*. Staring superiorly and moving inferior (Fig. 1.21):

**Fig. 1.21** The ethmoid bone contributes to the boundaries of the nasal cavity, the anterior cranial fossa, and the orbit. (Leo 2022)

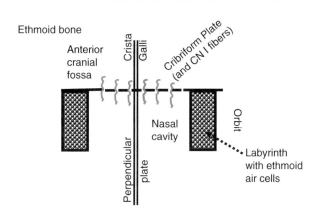

1. the highest opening is the *sphenoethmoidal recess* where the sphenoid sinus drains.
2. In the *superior meatus*, is the opening of the posterior ethmoidal air cells.
3. In the *middle meatus* is a semicircular shaped slit called the semilunar hiatus. On the superior border of the hiatus is the *ethmoidal bulla*, while on the inferior surface, there is a sharp line formed by the *uncinate process* (a projection of the ethmoid bone). Opening into the hiatus is the *ostium of the maxillary sinus*, which drains the maxillary sinus, along with the opening of the *frontonasal duct* which drains the frontal sinus and the anterior ethmoidal air cells. On the ethmoidal bulla are several small openings for the middle ethmoidal air cells.
4. Draining into the *inferior meatus* is the *nasolacrimal duct.*

The opening of the maxillary sinus is relatively high up on the medial wall of the sinus thus a significant amount of fluid can build up in the sinus before draining into the nasal cavity. A fluid filled sinus is a common spot for infections to take hold (sinusitis). If the infection bocks the ostium of the maxillary sinus the fluid can also back up into the frontal sinus via the frontonasal duct.

Nasal polyps can also form in the various sinuses and the ethmoid air cells. When they get large enough, they can herniate the through various openings and then into the various spaces. For instance, a polyp in the maxillary sinus can appear in the middle meatus, while a polyp in the anterior ethmoid air cells can appear in the sphenoethmoidal recess.

On the lateral nasal wall, at the superior posterior corner is the *sphenopalatine foramen* and coming through it is the *sphenopalatine artery* and *nasopalatine nerve* which travel onto the nasal septum and head anterior towards the *incisive foramen* to reach the anterior surface of the hard palate. In addition to the septum, the *sphenopalatine arteries* and *nasopalatine nerves* also send branches to the lateral nasal wall.

Entering superiorly into the nasal cavity are the *anterior* and *posterior ethmoidal arteries* and *nerves* which drop down into the nasal cavity from the orbit. The anterior and posterior ethmoidal arteries come from the *ophthalmic artery*, and the

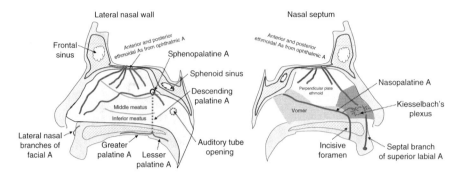

**Fig. 1.22** Nasal Cavity. There are three arteries that contribute to the nasal cavity: (1) Descending from the ophthalmic artery are the anterior and posterior ethmoidal arteries, (2) emerging from the posterior superior corner at the sphenopalatine foramen is the sphenopalatine artery from the maxillary artery, (3) the facial artery sends branches into the vestibule. Kiesselbach's plexus is especially prone to nose bleeds. (Leo 2022)

anterior and posterior ethmoidal nerves come from the *nasociliary nerve* which is a branch of V1 (ophthalmic nerve). And last but not least, coming into the nasal cavity anteriorly at the nose are branches of the facial artery. Just inside the nose, at the vestibule, is *Kiesselbach's plexus* which is an anastomosis of these arteries. Nosebleeds are common in this region.

The nasal septum is composed of the perpendicular plate of the ethmoid, the vomer, and the nasal cartilage. "Broken noses" can lead to a deviated nasal septum.

The floor of the nasal cavity is the hard palate which is made up of the *palatine process of the maxilla* and the *horizontal plate of the palatine bone*. At the inferior border of the horizontal plate are the *greater and lesser palatine foramina*, which are transmitting the greater and lesser palatine nerves and arteries. The greater palatine arteries and nerves travel anterior to supply the hard palate. The lesser palatine arteries and nerves travel posterior along the soft palate and uvula.

The *greater and lesser palatine arteries* are both branches of *the descending palatine artery* which in turn comes from the maxillary artery in the pterygopalatine fossa. The greater and lesser palatine nerves are branches of V2 within the pterygopalatine fossa. Thus, from the pterygopalatine fossa, arteries and nerves descend into the oral cavity. At the superior border of the palatine bone is a notch, which is the *sphenopalatine foramen* (Fig. 1.22).

## Oral Cavity

### Palatine Bone

The *palatine bone* is shaped like a fishhook with a *perpendicular plate* and a *horizontal plate.* The horizontal plates from each side meet in the midline, and these two pieces along with the palatine process of the maxilla form the hard palate. It isn't a

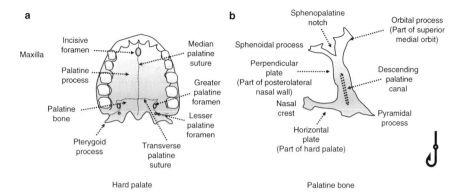

**Fig. 1.23** Panel (**a**) The hard palate is made up of the larger palatine process of the maxilla and the horizontal plate of the palatine bone. The greater and lesser palatine foramina transmit the nerves arteries and veins of the same name which came from the pterygopalatine fossa and descended in the descending palatine canal. Panel (**b**) The palatine bone is shaped somewhat like a fishhook or a "**J**," with a descending perpendicular plate contributing to the lateral nasal wall, and a horizontal plate contributing to the hard palate. (Leo 2022)

perfect fishhook, as the top of the bone really has two pieces: laterally the *orbital process* contributes to the orbit, and medially the *sphenoidal process* contributes to the lateral nasal wall. Descending down through the perpendicular plate are the *descending palatine artery*, the *greater palatine nerve*, and the *lesser palatine nerve*. At the junction of the horizontal plate of the palatine bone and palatine process of the maxilla is the *greater palatine foramen*. Slightly posterior to the greater palatine foramen, but in the palatine bone, is the *lesser palatine foramen* (Figs. 1.22 and 1.23).

## The Tongue

There are many folds, ligaments, and muscles in the head: palatoglossus, palatopharyngeus, stylohyoid, hyoglossus, stylopharyngeus, glossoepiglotic, aryepiglottic, salpingopharyngeus, and the list goes on. When you first hear these names, it can sound overwhelming. But when you look at each one individually, the name makes sense; they are all named for their attachments. The lateral glossoepiglotic ligament, for example, runs from the tongue to the epiglottis.

If you look in the mirror, on each side of your mouth you will see a *palatoglossal arch* and the *palatopharyngeal arch* with the *palatine tonsil* between them. There are numerous arches in this region, which are formed by the mucous membrane of the oral cavity overlying either a muscle or a ligament. Whether it is a muscle or a ligament it will be named for the two structures it connects.

For instance, the palatoglossal arch is made by the underlying palatoglossal muscle which runs from palate to tongue, and the palatopharyngeal arch is made by the underlying palatopharyngeus muscle running from the palate to pharynx.

There are four extrinsic muscles of the tongue: *palatoglossus, styloglossus, genioglossus,* and *hyoglossus.* They are all innervated by the *hypoglossal nerve* (XII) except for palatoglossus which is innervated by the vagus nerve (X). All these muscles are named for where they start and end. The first part of the name is the giveaway. For instance, the styloglossus runs from the styloid process to the tongue. When looking from the lateral side towards the mouth, the styloglossus and hyoglossus muscles resemble a meat cleaver, with the styloglossus being the handle and the hyoglossus being the blade (Fig. 1.24).

The hypoglossal nerve emerges from the hypoglossal canal and wraps around the internal and external carotid arteries to enter the mouth just lateral to the hyoglossus muscle. When it crosses the external carotid artery it is in close proximity to the lingual artery. However, the hypoglossal nerve runs superficial (lateral) to the hyoglossus muscle, while the lingual artery runs deep (medial) to the hyoglossus muscle (Fig. 1.24).

The *submandibular gland* lies in the submandibular triangle and is subdivided into two sections by the mylohyoid muscle. The *submandibular duct* travels anterior and medial to emerge on the *sublingual papilla* on either side of the *frenulum.* As it travels anterior, it crosses the lingual nerve. At the point where the two structures cross, the lingual nerve is lateral. The *sublingual gland* is located more medial and rather than one large duct, it has a network of small ducts that enter on the medial side of the tongue. Both the submandibular and sublingual glands are innervated by postganglionic parasympathetic fibers from the submandibular ganglion, which in turn received preganglionic input from fibers traveling on the lingual nerve.

In the infratemporal fossa the chorda tympani joins the lingual nerve. The lingual nerve is a branch of V3 that travels to the tongue and is responsible for general sense from the anterior 2/3rds of the tongue. Note that the lingual nerve and lingual artery do not run together.

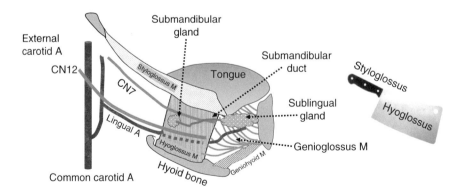

**Fig. 1.24** Tongue. The styloglossus and hyoglossus together resemble a meat cleaver. The hypoglossal nerve runs lateral to the hyoglossus muscle. The lingual artery runs deep to the hyoglossus muscle. The lingual nerve is seen approaching the mouth from above. The submandibular gland is sending its duct to the sublingual caruncle. The geniohyoid runs from the genu of the mandible to the hyoid bone. (Leo 2022)

**Table 1.1** Nerve supply to tongue. In summary there are five cranial nerves involved with the tongue

| Cranial nerve | Modality |
| --- | --- |
| CN V (lingual nerve) | General sense to anterior 2/3rds tongue |
| CN VII (chorda tympani) | Taste to anterior 2/3rds tongue and parasympathetics to submandibular and sublingual glands |
| CN IX (sensory branch) | General sense and taste to posterior 1/3rd of tongue |
| CN X (pharyngeal nerve) | Motor to palatoglossus M. |
| CN XII (motor branch) | Motor to genioglossus, styloglossus, and hyoglossus Ms. |

The glossopharyngeal nerve also comes out of the jugular foramen and travels to the posterior third of the tongue in close proximity to the stylopharyngeus muscle. Besides innervating the stylopharyngeus, it is responsible for general sense and taste to the posterior 1/3rd of the tongue (Table 1.1).

At the back of the mouth, in addition to the pharyngeal tonsils, there are several other locations for tonsillar tissue. The *pharyngeal tonsils* are located in the upper regions of the pharynx, the *lingual tonsils* are on the posterior tongue, and the *tubal tonsils* are near the opening of the auditory tube. Together, this ring of tonsillar tissue is referred to as *Waldeyer's ring* because it forms a ring of tissues between the back of the mouth and the start of the pharynx.

The floor of the mouth is formed by the mylohyoid and geniohyoid muscles. The mylohyoid is like a sheet running between the two sides of the mandible, while the geniohyoid is a strap muscle running from the genu of the mandible to the hyoid bone. The geniohyoid is innervated by a branch of C1 traveling on the hypoglossal nerve, while the mylohyoid is innervated by the nerve to mylohyoid which is a branch of the inferior alveolar nerve.

## Palate

The palate is made up of the hard and soft palate. The hard palate is part of the maxilla. The uvulae is part of the soft palate. Several extrinsic muscles blend in with the soft palate. The *tensor veli palatini* arises from the pterygoid process and descends straight down vertically to wrap around the pterygoid hamulus to then run horizontally and blend in with the soft palate. It is shaped like an "L." Thus, when the muscle contracts it will pull the palate laterally to tense it. The *levator veli palatini* meanwhile runs from the temporal bone diagonally towards the midline to blend in with the soft palate and the levator from the other side, thus the two together are shaped like a "V." The two levators then from a sling so that when they contract, they will elevate the palate. The levator veli palatini also arises from the eustachian tube and is involved in opening the airway to equalize pressure differences (Fig. 1.25).

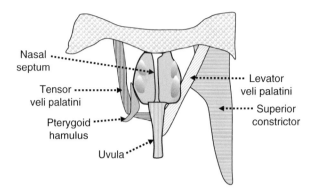

**Fig. 1.25** Tensor and levator veli palatini. Note the levator veli palatine heads diagonally towards the midline to blend in with the soft palate. The tensor veli palatini descends vertically, and then does a 90° turn around the pterygoid hamulus (hook) of the medial pterygoid plate and then heads horizontally to blend into the palate. (Leo 2022)

## Orbit

The eye sits in the orbit but one of the first things to note is that axis of the eye and the orbit are not the same. The orbit is a cone shaped structure pointing laterally. The medial wall of the orbit is more anterior than the lateral wall. Since we need the eye to look straight ahead, the axis of the eye is medially deviated which places the lateral to the location of the optic nerve at the beginning of the optic canal. The axis of the eye runs down through the macula where there is an abundance of cones. Medial to the fovea is the optic disc where the ganglion cells of the retina are converging. As they converge at the optic disc and travel down the optic nerve to the lateral geniculate body, they create a small blind spot in the temporal field of each eye (Fig. 1.26).

The six extraocular muscles are all appropriately named and, except for the inferior oblique, they all originate from a *common tendinous ring* that surrounds the optic nerve at the apex of the orbit. In a superior approach to the orbit, the *levator palpebrae superioris* is the first muscle you encounter. It inserts into the superior eyelid and is responsible for elevating the eyelid – opening the eye. Just deep to the levator palpebrae is the superior rectus.

### Overview of Eye Muscles and Nerves

When you approach a patient with a deficit of an extraocular muscle, think of two parts to the scenario. The first part is when the patient is sitting in your office and you notice, or suspect, that something is amiss with the eyes. The second part of the exam is when you formally test the muscles by asking the patient to follow your

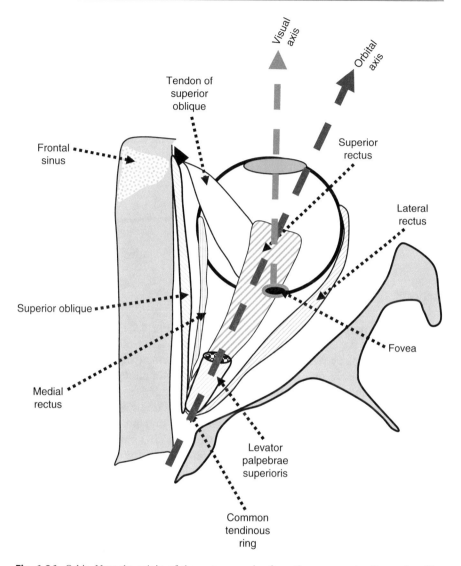

**Fig. 1.26** Orbit. Note the origin of the rectus muscles from the common tendinous ring. The medial wall of the orbital extends farther anteriorly than the lateral wall. The orbital axis is a line straight down the optic nerve to the tendinous ring. However, the eye is medially deviated so that the fovea is pointing straight ahead. (Leo 2022)

finger as you move them through the test. We will first look at the actions of the eye muscles and their respective nerves. We will then look at how you would test the muscle and nerves. To do this we are going to look at two pictures to discuss the eye muscles (Table 1.2).

**Table 1.2** Openings around the orbit

| Structure | Contents |
|---|---|
| Superior orbital fissure | CNs III, IV, V1, V2, and superior ophthalmic vein |
| Inferior orbital fissure | CN V2 |
| Optic canal | CN II, ophthalmic artery |
| Cavernous sinus | CNs III, IV, V1, V2, VI and internal carotid artery |

**Fig. 1.27** Actions of the eye muscles. The arrows show the action of each muscle. For example, the medial rectus pulls the eye in (adducts), and the superior oblique pulls the eye down and out, but it is also does intorsion. (Leo 2022)

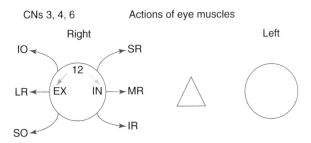

## Actions

The first picture shows the _actions_ of the muscles (Fig. 1.27). This is the picture that you would see in a typical anatomy textbook. After all, anatomists like to talk about actions or function. Note that medial rectus (MR) and lateral rectus (LR) each only have one action. Lateral rectus pulls the eye laterally (abduction), and medial rectus pulls the eyes medially (adduction). However, the other four muscles each have three actions. Superior oblique (SO) pulls the eye down and out, while inferior oblique (IO) pulls the eye up and out. And superior rectus (SR) pulls the eye up and in, while inferior rectus (IR) pulls the down and in. Yet, we also need to pay attention to the oft-ignored intorsion and extortion movements. Intorsion is when the 12 o'clock position of your eye rotates towards your nose, and extortion is when it rotates away from the nose. Superior oblique and superior rectus are intorters. Inferior oblique and inferior rectus are extorters.

Don't confuse intorsion and extorsion with medial and lateral movements. Intorsion and extorsion involve the eyes rotating in the eye socket. While you are reading this, tilt your head to the left. If you did not have intorsion and extorsion your world (the page) would tilt, but you know that the world stays level. This is because your left eye intorted and your right eye extorted. As your walk down the street and your head moves this mechanism allows your eyes to compensate for head movements so that the world does not bob around and make you dizzy. When you look at the picture showing the actions of the muscles you can see that there are two intorters (superior oblique and superior rectus), and two extorters (inferior oblique and inferior rectus).

The action picture for the eyes is important to understand because it explains what happens with the eyes when there is a nerve lesion.

## Cranial Nerve Six Lesion

The eye is a democracy. To look straight ahead you need to have equal tension on medial and lateral rectus. If you have a deficit with the lateral rectus, then medial rectus will then take over and move the eye medially. The patient will have a medial strabismus. If they had a deficit with medial rectus, then lateral rectus takes over and they have a lateral strabismus.

## Cranial Nerve Three Lesion

If you have a lesion to cranial nerve III then you will lose all the muscles except lateral rectus and superior oblique which will lead to the eye projecting down and out – a lateral strabismus. Because cranial nerve III has parasympathetic fibers the patient will also have ptosis (droopy eyelid) and mydriasis (dilated pupil). *Duane Syndrome* is a rare congenital defect of cranial nerve VI (6) that results in a reduced ability to abduct the eye. It is thought that the defect lies with miswiring of cranial nerve VI fibers to the muscle. It is not the muscle that is weak but the nerve. It is typically not present at birth but develops later in childhood. It can affect one eye or both eyes. *Moebius Syndrome* is a rare congenital defect that leads to deficits in the wiring of cranial nerve VII and VI (6). It is present at birth and patients have facial paralysis (CN VII) and an inability to abduct the eye.

## Cranial Nerve Four Lesion

With a lesion to the right CN IV the patient loses the superior oblique, one of the two intorters. With weakened intorsion, the right eye will now be extorted. With the right eye extorted the patient now has two visual fields. To bring the world back to one visual field, the patient will lean away from the lesion side – in this case towards the left. This movement brings the right eye up to level, and since the muscles on the left are working the left eye will intort. Keep in mind that you cannot look at a patient's eyeball and see intorsion and extortion, but you can see their head tilt.

## Testing

The next picture to look at it is the H test which shows how to test the eyes. This is the picture that you would see in a typical clinical-exam textbook. To test the MR and LR you ask the person to look medially or laterally. However, if you want to test the right SO, first you ask the patient to look left, and then once the eye is pulled in, you ask the person to look down. The only way the adducted eye can look inferiorly is with SO. The first part of the test, when the patient looked medially isolated the SO, so that the only way the patient can look down is with SO. The only way they can look up is with IR. Ideally when you test the eyes movements you keep on the H lines, and do not take the diagonal shortcuts (Fig. 1.28).

## Oculomotor Nerve

The *oculomotor nerve* enters the orbit just lateral to the optic nerve and quickly divides into a *superior and inferior division*. The superior division travels between the levator palpebrae superioris and superior rectus. The inferior division travels lateral to the optic nerve and send branches to the medial rectus, inferior rectus, and inferior oblique.

Entering the back of the eye are the *short* and *long ciliary nerves*. There are some commonalities to these nerves and some differences. To explain these two nerves, we need to look at both CN III and CN V1 (ophthalmic nerve) (Fig. 1.29).

1. CN III is a motor nerve or an *eff*erent nerve carrying motor fibers to the muscles mentioned above. Coming out of the brain with CN III are preganglionic parasympathetic fibers that synapse on the ciliary ganglion which is attached to the inferior division of the oculomotor nerve. The *short ciliary nerves* can be seen coming off the ciliary ganglion. These are postganglionic parasympathetic fibers traveling to the constrictor pupillae to constrict the pupil, and to the ciliary muscle for accommodation.

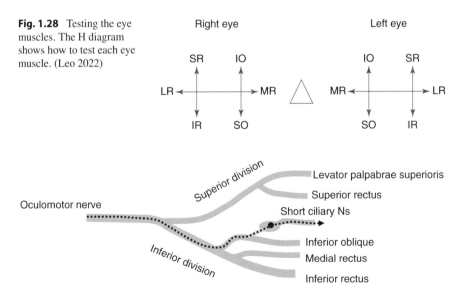

**Fig. 1.28**  Testing the eye muscles. The H diagram shows how to test each eye muscle. (Leo 2022)

Right eye

Left eye

SR   IO       IO   SR
LR ← | → MR    MR ← | → LR
IR   SO       SO   IR

Oculomotor nerve

Superior division

Inferior division

Levator palpabrae superioris
Superior rectus
Short ciliary Ns
Inferior oblique
Medial rectus
Inferior rectus

**Fig. 1.29**  CN III. The oculomotor nerve enters at the superior orbital fissure and splits into a superior and inferior division. The superior division innervates the levator palpebrae superioris and superior rectus. The inferior division innervates the inferior oblique, medial rectus, and inferior rectus. The ciliary ganglion hangs off the inferior division and is the site where the preganglionic fibers of CN III synapse with the postganglionic fibers. The postganglionic fibers innervate the constrictor pupillae, and the ciliary muscle. (Leo 2022)

2. CN V1 (ophthalmic nerve) on the other hand is strictly an *aff*erent or sensory nerve. One of the branches of CN V1 is the nasociliary nerve and coming off of it are the *long ciliary nerves*. Sensation from the eyeball, such as a cotton swab touching the cornea, travels back along the short and long ciliary nerves. It seems logical that the long ciliary nerves would carry sensation, however it does not seem quite as logical for the short ciliary nerves to carry sensory fibers – remember they are coming off of the ciliary ganglion and CN III. What happens is that the sensory information traveling on the short ciliary nerves jumps onto V1 via a communicating branch.

Both the short and long ciliary nerves carry sensory fibers from the cornea. Keep in mind that cranial nerve III is a motor nerve so these sensory fibers in the short ciliary nerves quickly jump onto branches of V1 via the communicating branch. In addition, both sets of nerves carry sympathetic fibers (Fig. 1.30).

## Ophthalmic Artery

The *ophthalmic artery* enters the eye at the optic canal. Within the orbit are several important branches (Fig. 1.31):

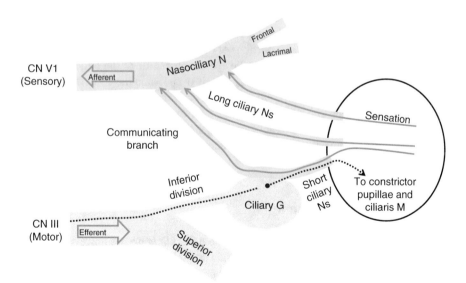

**Fig. 1.30** Short and long ciliary nerves. CN III is a motor (efferent) nerve. The parasympathetic fibers on CN III travel on its inferior division, synapse in the ciliary ganglion and then travel on the short ciliary nerves to the constrictor. V1 is a sensory nerve (afferent). Sensation from the cornea travels on the short and long ciliary nerves to reach the nasociliary nerve. Note the communicating branch from the ciliary ganglion to the nasociliary nerve. Short ciliary nerves carry sensory and parasympathetic fibers. Long ciliary nerves carry sensory fibers. The sympathetic fibers are not shown; they travel on both long and short ciliary nerves. (Leo 2022)

**Fig. 1.31** Orbit. Superior view of the ophthalmic artery in the orbit. The ophthalmic artery is a branch of the internal carotid that enters the orbit at the optic canal, lateral to the optic nerve. The lacrimal artery is a branch that heads to the lacrimal gland. The recurrent branch of the lacrimal anastomoses with the middle meningeal artery. The short posterior ciliary arteries enter the eye lateral to the optic nerve. The supraorbital and supratrochlear emerge onto the face. (Leo 2022)

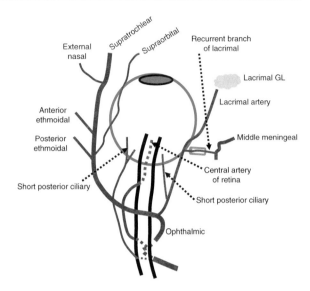

1. The *lacrimal artery* runs laterally and anteriorly to the lacrimal gland. It has a *recurrent branch* that travels through the superior orbital fissure to anastomosis with a branch of the middle meningeal artery. This represents an anastomosis between the internal and external carotid artery.
2. *Anterior and posterior ethmoidal arteries* that travel medially to supply the ethmoid air cells and the superior portions of the nasal septum and lateral nasal wall.
3. *Posterior ciliary arteries* that enter the eye on either side of the optic nerve.
4. The *central artery of the retina* which travels deep inside the optic nerve.
5. The *supraorbital* and *supratrochlear arteries* exit the skull through the foramen of the same names and perfuse the skin over the forehead. Keep in mind that these are branches of the internal carotid that exit the skull. In the medial corner of the eye, they anastomosis with the angular artery which is a branch of the facial artery.

## Blood Supply to the Retina

The blood supply to the retina comes from the *ophthalmic artery,* however it comes from two different branches of the ophthalmic and this branching pattern has important clinical significance. The *central artery of the retina* comes off the ophthalmic artery and travels down the interior of the optic nerve to emerge onto the retina at the optic disc. From the disc region, branches of the central artery then fan out along the inner surface of the retina. Meanwhile, the *posterior ciliary arteries* are also branches of the ophthalmic artery, but these enter the eye at the external surface near the optic nerve and enter the choroid which has a rich blood supply. From the choroid the blood perfuses the outer segments of the retina (Fig. 1.32).

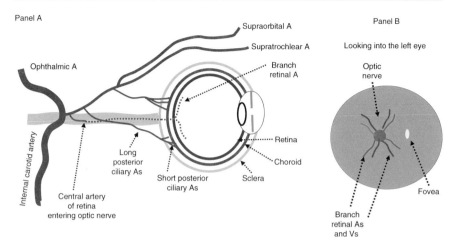

**Fig. 1.32** Arteries to retina. In panel (**a**), the ophthalmic artery is a branch of the internal carotid artery. The blood supply to the inner retina comes from the central artery of the retina which enters the optic nerve and enters the orbit at the optic canal where it divides into retinal artery branches. The outer portions of the retina are supplied by the short ciliary arteries. Panel (**b**) is an anterior view – looking into the eye – showing the central artery of the retina emerging onto the retina and giving off the branch retinal arteries. (Leo 2022)

An occlusion of the central artery of the retina will therefore block the blood to the internal surface of the retina causing the cells to die and the retina to turn cloudy. However, in the vicinity of the optic nerve, the internal surface of the retina is very thin in the region of the fovea because the fibers are pushed to the perimeter of the fovea, and in addition there are no rods and cones in this region. As a practitioner when you look into this patient's eye, you can see the blood perfusing the external retina at the fovea, but not the area around the fovea, leading to the name: "Cherry Red Spot."

## V1 – The Ophthalmic Nerve

The *ophthalmic nerve* (V1) leaves the middle cranial fossa through the superior orbital fissure and enters the orbit where it divides into three branches:

1. The *frontal nerve* travels superior to the levator palpebrae superioris and divides into two branches, the supraorbital and supratrochlear nerves that leave the skull through the same named foramen.
2. The *lacrimal nerve* carries sensory information from the lateral corner of the eye in the region of the lacrimal gland. However, running with it are postganglionic fibers from the pterygopalatine ganglion (CN VII) that innervate the lacrimal gland.

3. The *nasociliary nerve* enters the orbit deep to the tendinous ring and just lateral to the optic nerve. It immediately crosses the optic nerve from lateral to medial to head towards the medial side of the orbit. It gives off the *anterior and posterior ethmoidal nerves* that carry sensory information from the superior nasal cavity. It also gives off the *long ciliary nerves* that carry general sensory information from the cornea. There is also a *communicating branch* running from the oculomotor nerve to the nasociliary to provide a conduit for the sensory information on the short ciliary nerves to jump from cranial nerve III to cranial nerve V1 (ophthalmic nerve) (Figs. 1.32 and 1.33).

## Superior Orbital Fissure

There are three doorways at the back of the orbit for the nerves, arteries, and veins to approach the eye. Because there is overlap between some of the doors, the diagram of this region resembles a Ven diagram. The main door is the *superior orbital fissure* however the *tendinous arch* forms another door that overlays the medial part of the superior orbital fissure, thus there are some structures that come through just the superior orbital fissure – and not the tendinous ring- while there are other structures that come through the tendinous ring and the superior orbital fissure.

1. Coming through just the superior orbital fissure are the **L**acrimal, **F**rontal, and **T**rochlear nerves – think **LFT**. The superior division of the superior ophthalmic vein also comes through here.

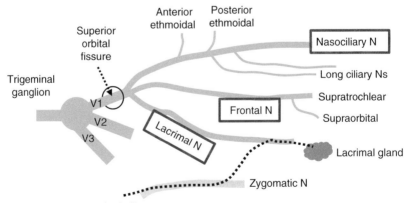

**Fig. 1.33** V1. Ophthalmic nerve (V1). There are three main branches: nasociliary, frontal, and lacrimal. The nasociliary nerve gives off the anterior and posterior ethmoidal nerves and the long ciliary nerves. The frontal nerve gives off the supraorbital and supratrochlear nerves that travel through the same named foramen to reach the skin over the orbit. Parasympathetic fibers from the pterygopalatine ganglion (CN VII) travel on the zygomatic nerve and then the lacrimal nerve to reach the lacrimal gland. (Leo 2022)

2. Coming through the tendinous ring and the superior orbital fissure are the superior and inferior divisions of the oculomotor nerve, the abducens nerve, and the nasociliary nerve – think **36N**.
3. In the medial corner of the superior orbital fissure there is a small space, outside of the tendinous ring that transmits the inferior ophthalmic vein.

In addition to the superior orbital fissure, there is the *optic canal* with the optic nerve and the ophthalmic artery. Note that the ophthalmic artery and ophthalmic vein do not run together.

## Inferior Orbital Fissure

The *inferior orbital fissure* is in the floor of the orbit. The *infraorbital artery* and nerve move from the pterygopalatine fossa through the inferior orbital fissure (the anterior door of the pterygopalatine fossa) to run in the *infraorbital groove*, then the *infraorbital canal*, and to then emerge through the *infraorbital foramen* and onto the face as the infraorbital nerve and artery. Once the nerve and artery come through the infraorbital foramen, they supply the skin between the lower eyelid and the upper lip. The inferior orbital fissure also contains the *zygomatic nerve* (Fig. 1.34).

## Orbit Bones

The roof of the orbit is the *frontal bone* and *lesser wing of the sphenoid*; the floor is the *maxilla, palatine, and zygomatic* bones; the medial wall is the *ethmoid, maxilla, palatine, lacrimal, sphenoid, and zygomatic bones*; the lateral wall is the *zygomatic bone and greater wing of the sphenoid*. It is shaped like an ice cream cone with the optic canal at the apex, and the base opening onto the face. *Blowout fractures* of the orbit result from trauma to the eye that leads to fracture of these walls. The rim surrounding the base is usually spared. Inferior blowout fractures are the most common blowout fractures, and they usually occur in the vicinity of the infraorbital groove with the orbital contents herniating into the maxillary sinus. The "buckling theory" proposes that the pressure on the eye leads to the boney orbit buckling. In many cases the fracture is non-displaced, because while the bone fractures, it returns to its original position. This is referred to as a "trapdoor fracture." Remember all the way back to the discussion about the rooms of the skull, the floor of the orbit is the ceiling of the maxillary sinus (Fig. 1.35).

## The Maxilla

The maxilla is the bone between your lower eyelid and your upper lip. It contributes to the walls of the orbit, the oral cavity, and the nasal cavity, and it houses the maxillary sinus. On the medial side is the nasolacrimal duct running from the medial

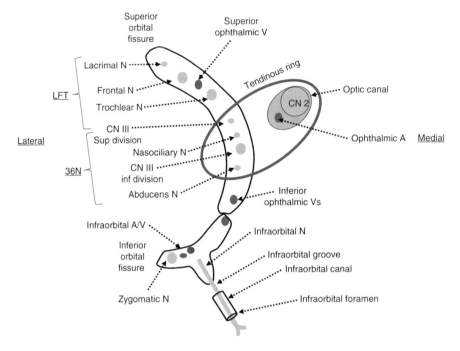

**Fig. 1.34**  <u>L</u>FT, <u>36N</u>. Emerging through the superior orbital fissure are the <u>L</u>acrimal (V1), <u>F</u>rontal (V1), and <u>T</u>rochlear nerves (CN 4), along with the superior ophthalmic vein. Emerging (36N) through the superior orbital fissure <u>***and***</u> the tendinous ring are the two divisions of the oculomotor nerve (CN 3), the abducens nerve (CN 6), and the nasociliary nerve (V1). Emerging through the inferior orbital fissure is the infraorbital nerve (V1), artery, and vein, and the zygomatic nerve (V2). Running through the optic canal are the optic nerve (CN 2) and the ophthalmic artery. Note the ophthalmic arteries and veins do not enter the orbit together. The infraorbital nerve is entering the groove, canal, and then exiting onto the face through the infraorbital foramen. (Leo 2022)

corner of the orbit to the oral cavity. Sinus infections can lead to pain emanating from the upper teeth since they can penetrate into the maxillary sinus. The infraorbital nerve runs through the infraorbital groove, canal, and foramen to enter onto the face. Blowout fractures of the orbit can enter the maxillary sinus (Fig. 1.36).

## Ear

Imagine going to the beach, and with a child's sand shovel you dig two small parallel channels going out to the ocean. The channels stretch to the water's edge and allow water to come into them. On top of each channel, you then lay a piece of paper. With this set up, you have two channels connected to the ocean each with a piece of paper laying on the water's surface. Out on the ocean, are motorboats, canoes, sailboats, fish jumping, and people swimming. All of these activities create a distinct wave pattern. Not only are the patterns different, but the timing of how the

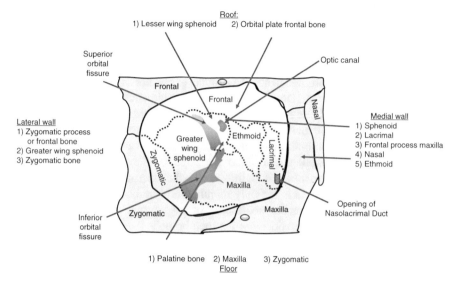

**Fig. 1.35** Bones of the orbit. Note the openings of the superior orbital fissure, inferior orbital fissure, and the optic canal. (Leo 2022)

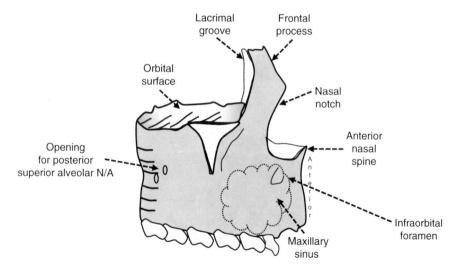

**Fig. 1.36** The maxilla. The maxilla contributes to the orbit and the nasal and oral cavities. It houses the maxillary sinus. (Leo 2022)

waves arrive at each channel varies, unless the vibrations are coming from directly in front in which case they will reach each channel at the same time.

With your eyes closed and your hands on each piece of paper, just by feeling the fluttering of the paper you can interpret all the different activities on the ocean, and you can tell where everything is located. The two pieces of paper represent the basilar membranes inside your inner ear. Even with your eyes closed, the vibrations of the basilar membranes can sense the locations of the motorboat, the sailboat, and the rowboat. All the anatomy around these two membranes is designed to allow them to function properly. I digressed for a moment, but back to the anatomy.

The external ear is designed to act like a funnel to capture and direct sound waves into your external ear canal. Dogs and cats with their big wide ears are really better at this than we are. As the sound waves move into the external ear canal, they eventually reach the tympanic membrane which vibrates. When looking into the external ear at the tympanic membrane with an otoscope, the light creates a *cone of light* stretching from the *umbo* anteriorly to the edge of the tympanic membrane. Swimmer's ear or *otitis externus* is an infection in the external ear canal.

The *tympanic membrane* is the only membrane in humans that is surrounded by air on both sides. It forms the medial wall of the external ear canal, and lateral wall of the middle ear. The majority of the membrane is the *pars tensa*, while the smaller superior portion is the *pars flaccida*. These two regions are separated by the neck of the malleus. The *manubrium* (handle) of the malleus attaches to the pars tensa and ends in the *umbo*. It only takes a miniscule amount of energy to vibrate the tympanic membrane. The amplitudes are in the picometer to nanometer range (smaller than a hydrogen atom). With excess fluid in the middle ear, the most common site to make an incision for drainage is the anterior inferior quadrant of the eardrum. (Fig. 1.37).

On the other side of the tympanic membrane (the medial side) is the middle ear with the three ossicles. The malleus touches the tympanic membrane, and it will vibrate along with the membrane. The malleus then vibrates the incus, and then the stapes. The stapes in turn contacts the oval window, which for the purposes of this

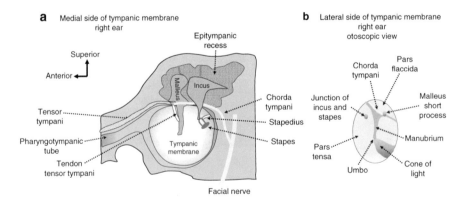

**Fig. 1.37** Two views of the tympanic membrane. Panel (**a**) is from within the middle ear, looking laterally at the medial (interior) surface of membrane. The malleus, incus, and stapes are all in view. The stapedius is attached to the stapes. The tensor tympani is running parallel to the pharyngotympanic tube to attach to the malleus. The chorda tympani can be seen crossing the malleus. Panel (**b**) is looking into the ear at the lateral side of the tympanic membrane. The cone of light is facing anterior. There are several impressions of structures located on the other side of the membrane such as the malleus and the junction of the incus and stapes. (Leo 2022)

book is our stopping point. The joints between the ossicles are hyaline lined synovial joints. The tympanic membrane translates the sound waves into mechanical energy – the movement of the ossicles. The surface area of the tympanic membrane is three times larger than the surface area of the oval window and this differential allows for amplification of the wave between the tympanic membrane and oval window.

At the *oval window* the wave moves from an air-filled cavity into a fluid filled cavity thus the wave is translated from mechanical energy into hydraulic motion. We will leave it to the neuroanatomy, histology, and physiology books to continue with the pathway of vibrations through the inner ear.

However, in the middle ear, we have some important structures.

1. The *chorda tympani* nerve can be seen crossing the handle of the malleus on its way to eventually exit the petrotympanic fissure and enter the infratemporal fossa, where it joins with the lingual nerve. Infections in the middle ear can compromise the chorda tympani.
2. The *tendon of the tensor tympani* can also be seen entering the middle ear and making a 90° turn to insert on the malleus to tense the tympanic membrane during movements such as swallowing, chewing, and talking.
3. The smallest muscle in the body is the *stapedius* which can be seen in the middle ear attaching to the stapes. Its job is to protect the inner ear in the presence of sudden, loud noises.

*Otosclerosis* is an abnormal growth where the stapes joins with the surrounding bone. *Cholesteatoma* is abnormal growth of skin that can erode structures in the middle ear such as the ossicles and tympanic membrane. Surfer's ear come from long term exposure to cold water leads that to the development of a bony protuberance (exostoses) in the external ear.

The malleus and the incus project superiorly into the *epitympanic recess*. The middle ear also connects to the pharynx via the *eustachian tube* or *pharyngotympanic tube* which allows for equalization of pressures between the middle ear and ambient pressure. In adults, the eustachian tube descends from the middle ear to pharynx, which allows drainage to descend into the pharynx. In children the pathway is horizontal which is not as efficient for drainage leaving children more susceptible to infections. Young children with chronic ear infections are candidates for tubes placed in the tympanic membrane to allow the middle ears to drain.

When a snorkeler or a scuba diver is descending, the ambient pressure rises and pushes on the tympanic membrane. Left to its own devices the tympanic membrane would rupture. But by holding their nose and blowing, this raises the pressure in the diver's pharynx, and in turn the middle ear via the eustachian tube. This increased pressure on the medial side of the tympanic membrane pushes the membrane open to allow the pressure to equalize. As the diver descends, they will have to continually equalize. The *tensor veli palatini* and *levator veli palatini* act on the soft palate which in turn acts on the opening of eustachian tube which sits right superior to the soft palate. Some experienced divers can master the movement of the eustachian tube without holding their nose.

The middle and inner ear are housed within the petrous portion of the temporal bone. In the laboratory, with a superior approach to the ear, the roof of the system is typically carefully pried off to look inside the middle and inner ear at the various structures.

There are several nerves that are responsible for sensation of the external ear. The tragus and the medial portion of the ear are supplied by the auriculotemporal nerve. Just posterior to the tragus is the concha bowl, which is supplied by branches of cranial nerves VII, IX, and X. The posteroinferior portion of the external ear is supplied by the great auricular nerve (Fig. 1.38).

## Neck

### Triangles of the Neck

The main divisions of the neck are into the *anterior* and *posterior triangles*. If we start with the neck as a square, there are four sides: the midline of the neck, the mandible, the trapezius, and the clavicle. If we draw a diagonal line on one side from the superior-posterior corner to the anterior-inferior corner. This line represents the sternocleidomastoid and divides the neck up into the anterior and posterior triangles. In addition, each of these two larger triangles can be subdivided into several smaller triangles (Fig. 1.39).

### Anterior Triangle

1. The *muscular triangle* contains the strap muscles of the neck and ansa cervicalis.
2. The *submandibular triangle* is bounded by the mandible and the anterior and posterior belly of the digastric muscle. It contains numerous structures. The

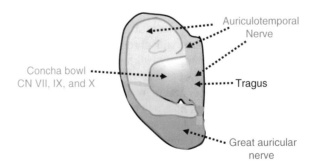

**Fig. 1.38** Nerve supply to external ear. The tragus and superior portion of the ear is innervated by the auriculotemporal nerve. The ear lobe and posteroinferior portion is Innervated by the great auricular nerve. The concha bowl is innervated by branches of CN VII, IX, and X. (Leo 2022)

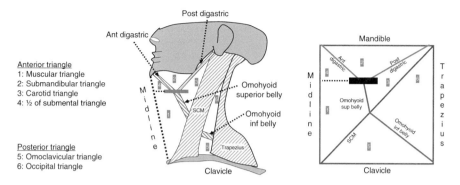

**Fig. 1.39** Neck triangles. The four borders of the square are: anterior, midline; posterior, trapezius; inferior, clavicle; superior, mandible. Drawing a line – the SCM - from corner to corner gives you the anterior and posterior triangles. In the anterior triangle are the muscular, submandibular, carotid, and submental. In the posterior triangle are the omoclavicular (subclavian triangle) and occipital triangles. All of these are paired triangles. The only single or unpaired triangle is the submental bounded by the right and left anterior digastric muscles and the hyoid bone. (Leo 2022)

submandibular gland is located here. The submandibular nodes located here drain the inferior lateral teeth, and the lateral tongue.

3. The *carotid triangle* is bounded by the sternocleidomastoid, the posterior digastric and the superior belly of the omohyoid. It contains the internal carotid artery, the internal jugular vein, and the vagus nerve in the carotid sheath. In addition, the hypoglossal nerve is traveling across the region (Fig. 1.40).

4. There is only one *submental triangle,* located in the midline, which is bounded by the anterior digastric muscles and the hyoid bone. It contains the submental nodes which drain the anterior tongue and the two front teeth.

## Posterior Triangle

5. The *omoclavicular triangle* (AKA: subclavian triangle, or supraclavicular triangle) is bounded by the clavicle, the sternocleidomastoid, and the inferior belly of omohyoid. The anterior corner of the anterior triangle is a danger area meaning that there are important structures in this area.

6. The *occipital triangle* contains the accessory nerve emerging from the posterior border of sternocleidomastoid and traveling to the anterior border of the trapezius.

## Ansa Cervicalis

The *ansa cervicalis* comes from C1, C2, and C3 and forms a loop from which emerge branches to the strap muscles of the neck. It is found in the carotid triangle anterior to the internal jugular vein. Branches of C1 also travel for a moment with the hypoglossal nerve to travel to the geniohyoid and thyrohyoid.

**Fig. 1.40** Branches of the external carotid artery. In the carotid triangle the superior thyroid, ascending pharyngeal (not shown), occipital, lingual, and facial all come off the external carotid. Superior to the posterior digastric muscle, the occipital artery comes off. The two terminal branches of the external carotid are the superficial temporal and maxillary. (Leo 2022)

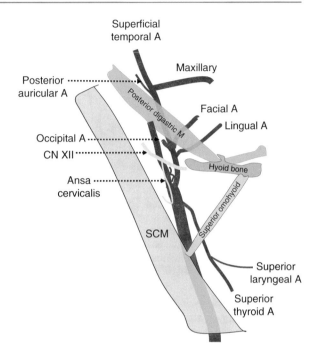

## Fascia of the Neck

When dissecting the anterior neck, the platysma is the first muscle encountered. It is extremely thin and is found within the superficial fascia of the neck. It does not extend into the posterior triangle. It is involved with tensing the skin and is sometimes referred to as the "shaving muscle." Platysmaplasty involves tightening the platysma to remove the creases and wrinkles of the neck. The deep cervical fascia of the neck is divided into investing, prevertebral, and pretracheal fascia.

1. The *investing fascia* is the most superficial layer of the deep cervical fascia, and it surrounds the sternocleidomastoid anteriorly, and the trapezius posteriorly.
2. The *pretracheal fascia* splits into two layers: a muscular layer surrounds the strap muscles of the neck, and a visceral layer surrounds the thyroid gland, trachea, and esophagus. Behind these structures the pretracheal fascia joins with the *buccopharyngeal fascia*. Inferiorly it blends in with the fibrous pericardium of the heart.
3. The *prevertebral layer* surrounds the vertebral vertebrae and the deep muscles.

Anterior to the prevertebral layer is the *retropharyngeal space* which allows movement of the neck structures. However, this space also allows infections to spread. An infection in the retropharyngeal space can spread to the superior mediastinum. The retropharyngeal space is subdivided into two spaces by the alar fascia (Fig. 1.41).

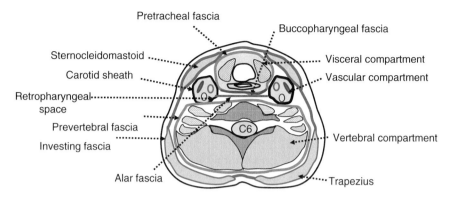

**Fig. 1.41** Fascial compartments of the neck. The trapezius and sternocleidomastoid muscles are surrounded by the investing fascia. The prevertebral fascia surrounds the vertebral muscles and vertebral column. The carotid sheath surrounds the internal carotid artery, internal jugular vein, and the Vagus nerve. The pretracheal and buccopharyngeal fascia surrounds the thyroid gland, trachea, and esophagus. The retropharyngeal space is between the visceral and vertebral compartments. The alar fascia separates the retropharyngeal space into two divisions. (Leo 2022)

## Nerve Point of Neck

The nerve point of the neck is found halfway along a line paralleling the posterior border of the sternocleidomastoid going from the mastoid process to the sternoclavicular head. There are four sensory nerve branches all of which come from the C5–6 roots:

1. The *transverse cervical nerve* crosses laterally in front of the sternocleidomastoid to reach the midline of the neck.
2. The *great auricular nerve* crosses the sternocleidomastoid with the external jugular vein and ascends towards the ear.
3. The *supraclavicular nerve* heads inferiorly towards the clavicle deep to the platysma.
4. The *lesser occipital nerve* runs along the anterior border of the trapezius towards the back of the ear.

While some refer to the nerve point and Erb's point as the same structure they are really different points. Erb's point is a deeper structure that corresponds to the location of the upper trunk of the brachial plexus just before it passes deep to the clavicle. Lesions in this region lead to Erb's palsy, or upper trunk injuries.

## Accessory Nerve

In one sense, it is a misnomer to call the *accessory nerve* a cranial nerve as it arises from spinal cord segments C1-C5. Rootlets coming out of the spinal cord merge together and ascend parallel to the spinal cord to enter the posterior cranial fossa through the *foramen magnum*. The accessory nerve then does a U-turn and leaves the skull through the *jugular foramen*. As it enters the neck it supplies the sterno-cleidomastoid and continues on to cross the posterior triangle on the way to the trapezius. The accessory nerve typically enters the posterior triangle just above the nerve point in the neck found along the posterior border of the sternocleidomastoid muscle. As it crosses the posterior triangle it is deep to the skin and superficial fascia. The platysma does not come back into the posterior triangle, so it does not cover the accessory nerve (Fig. 1.42).

Because of its long and fairly superficial path it is susceptible to trauma during surgery in the posterior triangle. Bilateral action of the sternocleidomastoid elevates the chin by pulling the mastoid processes inferiorly (extension at the atlantooccipi-tal joint). When the sternocleidomastoid on one side is active this will pull the mas-toid process on that side inferiorly which leads to the chin deviating to the opposite side. Thus, if the accessory nerve is injured on one side, for instance the right, when the patient is asked to elevate the chin, it will point towards the right – the left side is working and moves the chin to the right.

## Scalene Triangle and Thoracic Outlet Syndrome

In the anterior corner of the posterior triangle several major structures are emerging from the thorax making this a clinically important region. This is where thoracic outlet syndrome occurs. If we zoom in on this region, we can see how the relation-ships of the various structures dictate the clinical symptoms.

Both the anterior and middle scalene muscles are attached to the first rib. Between the anterior and middle scalene you can see the subclavian artery and the roots of the brachial plexus. Lesions here will lead to a reduced pulse in the upper limb, tingling, and weakness of the hand muscles. The hand muscle weakness is a

**Fig. 1.42** CN IX. The accessory nerve arises from rootlets of the C1-C5 spinal cord and ascends into the foramen magnum to enter the skull with the spinal cord. In the skull, the accessory nerve does a U-turn and exits through the foramen magnum to innervate the sternocleidomastoid and trapezius muscles. (Leo 2022)

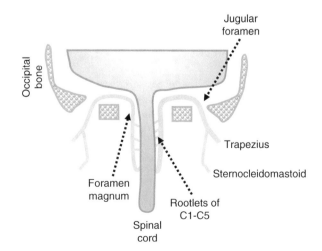

combination of ulnar nerve and median nerve deficits. Note that the subclavian vein is anterior to the anterior scalene (along with the phrenic nerve).

## Subclavian Artery

On the right side, the *subclavian artery* runs from the bifurcation of the brachioce-halic trunk to the lateral border of the first rib. On the left side, the sublclavian artery is a branch from the aortic arch. On both sides, it can be divided into three parts based on the location of the anterior scalane muscle. The first part is proximal to the muscles, the second part is posterior to it, and the third part is distal to the muscle (Fig. 1.43).

### First Part

1. The *vertebral artery* travels superiorly in the foramen transversarium of C1-C6 to enter the skull at the foramen magnum where it will eventually form the basilar artery.
2. The *internal thoracic artery* descends along the posterior border of the sternum where it eventually splits into the *musculophrenic* and *superior epigastric arteries*. Along the way it gives off the *anterior intercostal arteries*.
3. The *thryocervical trunk* gives off *the suprascapular, inferior thyroid, and suprascapular arteries*.

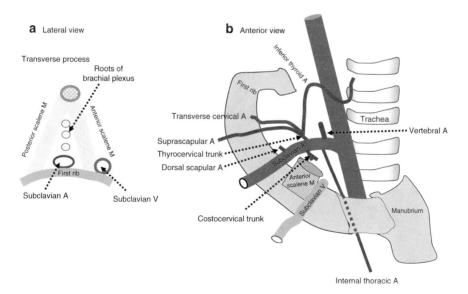

**Fig. 1.43** Scalenes and the neck. In panel (**a**), the lateral view shows the scalene triangle between the anterior and middle scalene triangle. In panel (**b**) the subclavian artery is going over the first rib to become the axillary artery. The branches of the subclavian artery are shown. The anterior scalene is between the subclavian artery and vein. (Leo 2022)

(a) The *suprascapular artery* heads posterior towards the scapula where it runs with the suprascapular nerve. Both these structures approach the *suprascapular notch*. The open superior end of the notch is closed off by the *superior transverse scapular ligament* creating a tunnel. The nerve passes through the tunnel, inferior to the ligament. The artery passes superior to the ligament (Navy under the bridge, army above it). The artery continues deep to the supraspinatus muscle, travels though the supraglenoid notch (the notch connecting the supraspinous and infraspinous fossas) to continue deep to the infraspinatus muscle in the infraspinous fossa.

(b) The *inferior thyroid artery* runs superior between the esophagus and trachea to reach the thyroid gland where it anastomosis with the superior thyroid artery.

(c) The *transverse cervical artery* crosses the phrenic nerve and the anterior scalene muscle to reach the trapezius (Fig. 1.44).

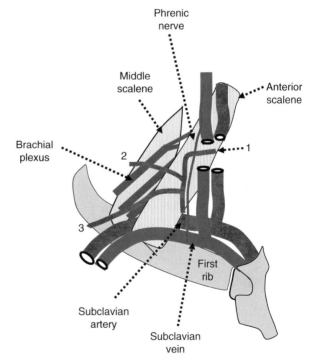

**Fig. 1.44**  Scalene triangle. The scalene triangle is between the first rib and the anterior and middle scalene muscles. The subclavian artery and brachial plexus in it. The subclavian vein and phrenic nerve run in front of the anterior scalene. The three branches of the thyrocervical trunk can be seen. (Leo 2022)

## Second Part

1. The *costocervical trunk* has two branches: (1) *superior intercostal artery* and (2) *deep cervical artery*.
   (a) The *superior intercostal artery* lies just lateral to the stellate ganglion. It runs along the neck of the first rib and gives off branches to the first and second intercostal spaces.
   (b) The *deep cervical artery* ascends posterior to the brachial pexus and between the transverse processes and the spinous processes, superfical to the semi-spinalis cervicis to anastomosis with the descending branch of the occipital artery.

## Third Part

1. The *dorsal scapular artery* runs posterior towards the superior angle of the scapula where it dives deep to the levator scapulae and then descends along the medial border of the scapula to reach the inferior angle. It anastomoses with the *circumflex scapular artery* which comes through the triangular notch, and the *suprascapular artery* which comes through the notch connecting the supraspinous and infraspinous fossae.

---

## Pharynx and Larynx

The pharynx is a muscular tube responsible for transport of air down into the lungs and food down into the esophagus. It has three circular sphincters and two strap muscles. Think of three cups stacked on top of each other with two straws. The constrictors make up the tube, so each starts at a bony prominence on one side and runs in a circular direction to meet the same muscle from the other side at the pterygomandibular raphe in the midline. The superior constrictor is attached to the medial pterygoid plate and the mandible, the middle constrictor to the hyoid bone, and the inferior constrictor to the thyroid cartilage. Running from the torus tuberous and merging into the superior constrictor is the *salpingopharyngeus*. And running from the styloid process and merging into the pharyngeal wall between the middle and inferior constrictor is the *stylopharyngeus*.

The pharynx is subdivided into three divisions, the *nasopharynx* is posterior to the nasal cavity, the *oropharynx* is posterior to the oral cavity, and the *laryngopharynx* is posterior to the larynx.

The *epiglottis* is an oval shaped piece of cartilage extending to the base of the tongue where three ligaments connect the tongue to the epiglottis. In the midline is the single *median glossoepiglotic ligament* and on each side are the *lateral glossoepiglotic ligaments*. Between the median glossoepiglotic ligament and each lateral glossoepiglotic ligament is a space called the *vallecula* (Tables 1.3, 1.4, and 1.5).

**Table 1.3**  Pharyngeal muscles. Three muscles resemble three cups, and two resemble two straws

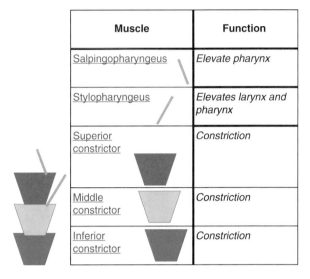

| Muscle | Function |
|---|---|
| Salpingopharyngeus | Elevate pharynx |
| Stylopharyngeus | Elevates larynx and pharynx |
| Superior constrictor | Constriction |
| Middle constrictor | Constriction |
| Inferior constrictor | Constriction |

**Table 1.4**  Intrinsic muscles of larynx. The posterior cricoarytenoid is the only muscle that opens (abducts) the glottis

| Muscle | Action |
|---|---|
| Cricothyroid | Tenses vocal cords |
| Lateral Cricoarytenoid | Adducts vocal cords |
| Posterior Cricoarytenoid | Abducts vocal cords |
| Transverse and Oblique Arytenoids | Adducts vocal cords |
| Thyroarytenoids | Adducts vocal cords |
| Vocalis (Subset of Thyroarytenoids) | Modifies tension on vocal cords |

## Larynx

The two essential pieces of the larynx are the paired vocal cords. When studying the larynx almost everything can be related to the vocal cords. The structures around the vocal cords are mainly designed to either move the cords or to protect them. The space between the vocal cords is the glottis. During inspiration the glottis needs to be open, while during phonation the glottis is closed. All the muscles, cartilage, and nerve innervation can be examined in light of their effects on vocal cord movement.

The *thyroid cartilage* is shaped somewhat like a triangle with one of its points facing anteriorly as the *thyroid prominence*. Thyroid means "shield" and it protects the larynx and serves as an attachment point for various supporting structures and muscles. Flaring out from the midline prominence on each side are the laminae forming two sides of the triangle. The third side of the triangle, which is posterior,

**Table 1.5** Muscles of the pharynx and soft palate

| Muscle | Nerve | Action |
|---|---|---|
| Levator Veli Palatini | CN X | Elevates soft palate, opens auditory tube |
| Tensor Veli Palatini | CN V (V3) | Tenses soft palate, opens auditory Tube |
| Uvulae | CN X Pharyngeal Nerve | Elevates uvula |
| Palatoglossus | CN X | Elevates root of tongue |
| Palatopharyngeus | CN X Pharyngeal nerve | Constricts isthmus |

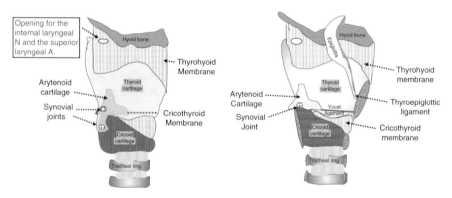

**Fig. 1.45** Larynx. The arytenoid cartilages sit on top of the cricoid cartilages, with a synovial joint between the two structures. The vocal ligament runs from the arytenoid cartilage to the thyroid cartilage. Between the thyroid cartilage and cricoid cartilage is the cricothyroid membrane. Between the thyroid cartilage and cricoid cartilage is the thyrohyoid membrane. The epiglottis runs from the thyroid cartilage and ascends behind the hyoid bone and the tongue. (Leo 2022)

is open. Running from the superior surface of the thyroid up to the hyoid is the *thyrohyoid membrane*. There are four extensions of the thyroid cartilage, two superior horns and two inferior horns. Attached to the inferior border of the thyroid cartilage is the *cricothyroid membrane* (Fig. 1.45).

The *cricoid cartilage* resembles a class ring, with the signet facing posterior. In contrast to the thyroid cartilage, which is open posteriorly, the cricoid is a continuous ring. Sitting on top of the cricoid cartilage are the *arytenoid cartilages*. And where the cricoid and each arytenoid meet, there is a synovial joint that allows

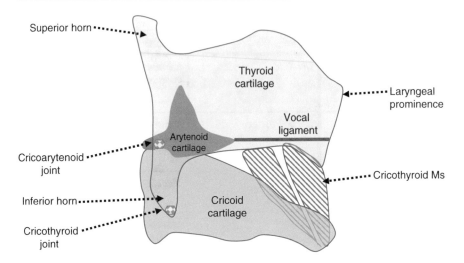

**Fig. 1.46** Larynx. The arytenoid cartilage is sitting on top of the cricoid cartilage. Running from the vocal process of the arytenoid to the thyroid cartilage is the vocal ligament. The cricothyroid muscles are the only extrinsic muscle of the larynx. When they contract, the vocal ligament is stretched, which raises the pitch. There is a synovial joint between the inferior horn of the thyroid cartilage and the cricoid cartilage, and there is another one between the arytenoid and cricoid cartilages. (Leo 2022)

movement of the arytenoid. The arytenoids are shaped like a triangle with their anteriorly facing *vocal processes,* and laterally facing *muscular processes*, serving as attachments for the lateral cricoarytenoid muscles and the posterior cricoarytenoid muscles (Fig. 1.46).

The quadrangular membrane lays down like a sheet running from the epiglottis to the *vestibular folds* (false folds) and covers the laryngeal structures. Inferior to the vestibular folds are the *true vocal folds* housing the vocal ligaments. The true vocal folds appear as thin sharp white line, while the false folds resemble just a loose outpocketing of tissue. Between the true and false folds are the small slit-like *ventricles* which continue laterally into the *saccules.*

1. At the synovial joints between the cricoid and arytenoid cartilages, the *cricoarytenoid joints,* you can see how the *lateral cricoarytenoid* pulls the muscular processes anteromedial, which in turn moves the vocal processes medially to close the glottis.
2. Also attached to the muscular processes are the *posterior cricoarytenoids* which will pull the muscular processes posteromedial which in turn moves the vocal processes laterally to open the glottis. This is the only muscle that opens the glottis.
3. Just behind the arytenoids and running from one arytenoid to another are the *transverse arytenoids* which help to close the glottis.
4. Superficial to the transverse arytenoids are the *oblique arytenoids* which also help to close the glottis.

5. The oblique arytenoids continue superiorly as the *aryepiglotticus* muscles which contribute to closing the laryngeal inlet. The laryngeal membrane overlying the aryepiglotticus muscles make up the *aryepiglottic folds.*
6. Along the sides of the aryepiglottic folds are the *thyroarytenoid muscles* which contribute to opening the laryngeal inlet.

## Cricothyrotomy

An emergency airway opening – *cricothyrotomy* - will be made through the cricothyroid membrane. For instance, if a child swallows a marble or other small toy, it can get stuck in the glottis which would block air from entering the lungs. The emergency opening would be made in the midline through the cricothyroid membrane. Making an opening in the thyrohyoid membrane would not allow air to enter the lungs. During this procedure, to find the incision site, an understanding of the relationships of the thyroid cartilage, hyoid bone, cricoid cartilage, and the cricothyroid membrane is essential. One issue to be wary of is the presence of a *thyroid ima artery*. In approximately 3–4% percent of us, there is a small artery arising from the brachiocephalic trunk and running in the midline to supply the thyroid gland. A midline incision can compromise this thyroid ima artery.

## Tracheotomy

A tracheotomy (tracheostomy) is a surgical procedure that involves placement of a tracheostomy tube between the tracheal rings and into the trachea. It is a short wide tube that can be connected to a ventilator, or it may be left open. Depending on the patient's status, it can be removed, and the hole will heal, or it can remain in place. If it remains in place, a device can be attached to the tube allowing the patient to speak, or they can learn to speak by placing a finger over the hole.

## Cranial Nerve X and the Larynx and Pharynx

Cranial nerve X is the main nerve supply to the larynx and pharynx, and it has motor, sensory, and parasympathetic fibers. During surgery on neck structures, such as a thyroidectomy, these nerves can be damaged (Fig. 1.47).

The first branch of the vagus nerve is the *auricular branch* which carries sensory information from the concha bowl (posterior to tragus).

The next branch of the vagus nerve is the *pharyngeal nerve* which goes to all the muscles of the pharynx and soft palate except for tensor veli palatini (CN V) and stylopharyngeus (CN IX). With lesions to the pharyngeal nerve the uvula will deviate away from the side of the lesion when the patient is asked to say "Aah."

The next branch is the *superior laryngeal nerve* which splits into *internal and external branches (*also known as *internal* and *external laryngeal nerves).* The

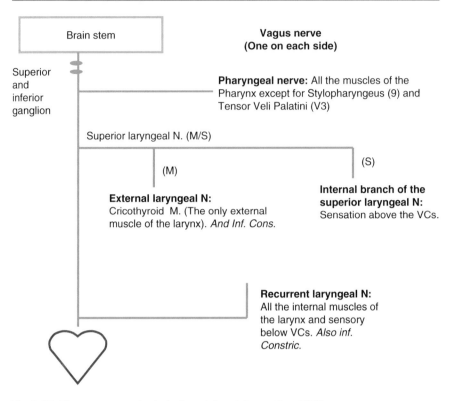

**Fig. 1.47** The vagus nerve. Auricular branch is not shown. (Leo 2022)

internal laryngeal nerve is responsible for sensation above the vocal cords. A fish bone or chicken bone caught in the throat can lodge in the piriform recess and leads to aggravation of the internal laryngeal nerve. The internal laryngeal runs with the superior laryngeal artery (a branch of superior thyroid artery) to pierce the thyrohyoid membrane.

The *external branch* innervates the only external muscle of the larynx – the cricothyroid muscle. It runs with the superior thyroid artery which will be ligated during a thyroidectomy potentially compromising the nerve. A lesion to the external branch will lead to a monotone voice, with a higher pitch than normal and a "breathy" voice.

The *recurrent laryngeal* nerve branches off the vagus nerve in the thorax and ascends in the neck. On the right, it makes a loop around the subclavian artery at the T1-T2 level, and on the left it runs around the aortic arch at the T4 – T5 level. As it travels superiorly in the neck it is found between the trachea and esophagus – the tracheoesophageal space. As the nerve crosses the cricothyroid joint it becomes the inferior laryngeal nerve. As it approaches the inferior constrictor it divides into an anterior branch which is the motor supply to all the laryngeal muscles except for the cricothyroid muscle, and a posterior branch to supply sensation below the vocal cords. One of the muscles the anterior branch supplies is the posterior cricoarytenoid, which is responsible for opening the glottis. It runs with the inferior thyroid artery.

## Arteries to Larynx and Pharynx

The *superior thyroid artery* is the first branch of the external carotid artery, and it is the only branch of the external carotid that descends towards the neck, which can serve as a helpful landmark on an angiogram of the external carotid branches. All the other branches of the external carotid ascend towards the head. On its way to the thyroid gland, the superior thyroid artery gives off a *superior laryngeal artery* which joins the internal branch of the superior laryngeal nerve. Both the superior laryngeal artery and the internal laryngeal nerve then pierce the thyrohyoid membrane.

As the superior thyroid artery continues its descent towards the thyroid gland it is runs with the external laryngeal nerve. As it approaches the thyroid gland it divides into anterior and posterior branches, which form an anastomosis with the *inferior thyroid artery* which is a branch of the thyrocervical trunk (Fig. 1.48).

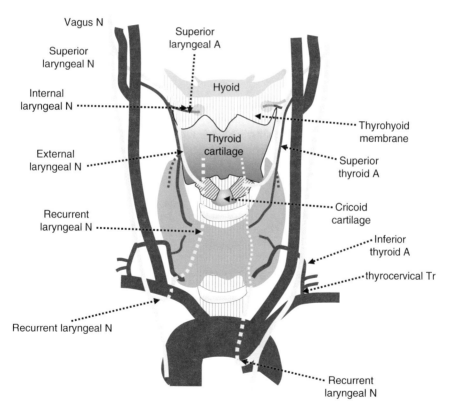

**Fig. 1.48** Larynx nerves and arteries. The superior laryngeal nerve splits into the internal and external branches. The internal branch runs with the superior laryngeal artery and pierces the thyrohyoid membrane. The external branch runs with the superior thyroid artery. The right recurrent laryngeal nerve wraps around the subclavian artery. The left recurrent laryngeal nerve wraps around the aortic arch. The thyrocervical trunk gives off the inferior thyroid artery. (Leo 2022)

As the two recurrent laryngeal nerves run superiorly, they cross the inferior thyroid artery. During their course, the two nerves are very close to each other right behind (posterior to) the trachea. Because of how close they are, they can both be injured at the same time. A horse voice and difficulty with swallowing could be indicative of an aortic aneurysm (Fig. 1.48).

With a unilateral injury to the recurrent laryngeal nerve the affected vocal cord will typically assume a paramedian (off-center) position. This allows the patient to breath, but phonation is compromised. In these individuals, during phonation when you want the vocal cords centered in the midline, the vocal cord on the healthy side will compensate for the injured side and adduct past the midline to meet the damaged vocal cord (Fig. 1.49).

With a bilateral injury, there is variation and as time goes on the position of the cords can change. After the injury, both cords can assume a paramedian position. This will allow the patient to breathe, but speaking is difficult. In some cases, the two cords can move medially and eventually meet in the midline, resulting in a situation where they cannot breathe. Surgery is warranted in this case (Fig. 1.50).

## Parasympathetic Hitchhikers

Cranial nerves III, VII, IX, and X all have a parasympathetic component. Of these four nerves, three of them – III, VII, and IX – all have parasympathetic fibers that hitchhike on branches of CN V to travel to their targets. They have all been discussed with their respective sections earlier in the chapter. The picture below focuses on the

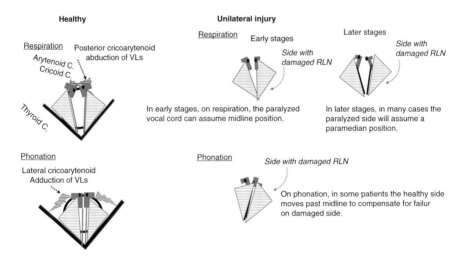

**Fig. 1.49** Recurrent laryngeal nerve injury. In the healthy person, the glottis opens during respiration and closes during phonation. With a unilateral recurrent laryngeal nerve injury, in some patients the vocal cords will assume a median or paramedian position. On phonation the vocal cord on the healthy side will move past the midline. In other patients, the cord can remain adducted on the damaged side. If this happens on both sides then asphyxiation is possible. (Leo 2022)

**Bilateral recurrent laryngeal nerve injury**

Respiration and phonation

Respiration and phonation

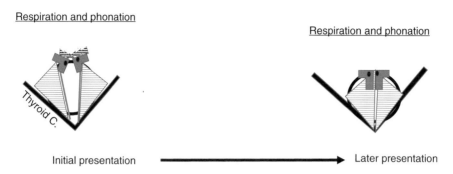

Initial presentation ⟶ Later presentation

**Fig. 1.50** Bilateral recurrent laryngeal nerve injury. In the early stages of bilateral recurrent laryngeal nerve injury, the glottis opens during respiration and phonation. In the later stages, in some patients, the vocal cords will be adducted, leading to a closed glottis, potential asphyxiation, and an emergency. (Leo 2022)

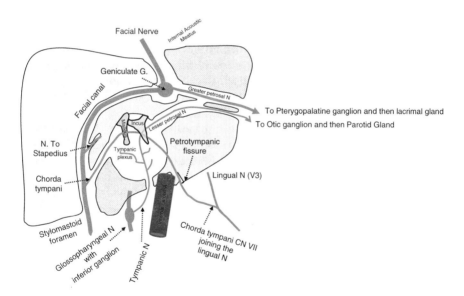

**Fig. 1.51** Parasympathetics of cranial nerves VII and IX. As CN IX leaves the skull through the jugular foramen it gives off the tympanic nerve which enters the middle ear and contributes to the tympanic plexus. It then leaves the middle ear as the lesser petrosal which travels to the parotid gland via the otic ganglion. The greater petrosal is the first branch of cranial nerve VII and travels to the pterygopalatine ganglion and then to the lacrimal gland. (Leo 2022)

greater and lesser petrosal nerves. The greater petrosal nerve is a parasympathetic branch of cranial nerve VII that runs in the groove for the greater petrosal nerve in the temporal bone. It then crosses foramen lacerum to join with the deep petrosal nerve (sympathetic fibers) to form the nerve of the pterygoid canal (Fig. 1.51).

Cranial nerve IX leaves the skull through the jugular foramen. It quickly gives off the tympanic nerve, which enters the middle ear to form the tympanic plexus. From the tympanic plexus the lesser petrosal nerve then leaves the skull through the *hiatus for the lesser petrosal nerve,* runs in the *groove of the lesser petrosal* and travels through the *foramen ovale* to reach the *otic ganglion* in the infratemporal fossa. From the otic ganglion the postganglionic parasympathetic fibers travel to the parotid gland on the auriculotemporal nerve (V3) (Fig. 1.51).

If the auriculotemporal nerve and its parasympathetic fibers are cut during surgery, these fibers can become confused when they regrow and reconnect such that in the presence of food the patient sweats in the region of the parotid gland (Frey Syndrome).

## Aortic Arch, Carotid and Vertebrobasilar Systems

When discussing the major arteries coming out of the aorta it helps to tie them in with the brain and upper limbs. This is an overview of the organization of these arteries. The details of each are addressed within different sections of the book. The three branches arising from the aortic arch are the (1) *brachiocephalic trunk* which goes onto divide into the right common carotid and right subclavian arteries; (2) the *left common carotid artery*; and (3) *the left subclavian artery*. The common carotids travel in the neck to divide into the internal and external carotids. The internal carotid travels through the carotid canal to enter the skull where it will divide into the *middle* and *anterior cerebral arteries* (Fig. 1.52).

The *external carotid artery* goes onto perfuse the face and the skull. The *vertebral arteries* come off the subclavian arteries to enter the skull through the foramen magnum where they come together to form the *basilar artery*. Just before they join, they give off the *posterior inferior cerebellar arteries*. At the top of the basilar artery there are the *right* and *left superior cerebellar arteries* and the *right* and *left posterior cerebral arteries*. Between them is cranial nerve III. The *posterior communicating arteries* connect the posterior cerebral arteries with the internal carotid arteries (Fig. 1.52). Aneurysms of the posterior communicating artery often compress CN III. T*rigeminal neuralgia* is thought to result from compression of the superior cerebellar artery on the trigeminal nerves just as they emerge from the trigeminal ganglion.

## Subclavian Steal Syndrome

*Subclavian steal syndrome* involves the upper limb stealing blood from the brain. To discuss the syndrome, you need to visualize the three main branches off the aorta and know where they are going. In subclavian steal syndrome there is a blockage of the subclavian artery close to its origin which is prior to the start of the vertebral artery. This blockage prevents blood from flowing down to the upper limb, but the vertebral artery comes to the rescue. To keep blood flowing to the upper limb, blood comes down the vertebral artery to move past the blockage. While this benefits the

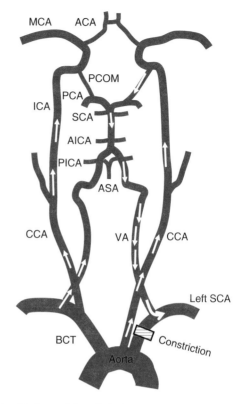

Key to arteries
MCA= Middle cerebral
ACA = Anterior cerebral
AICA = Anterior inferior cerebral
PICA = Posterior inferior cerebral
ICA = Internal carotid
ASA = Anterior spinal
VA = Vertebral
CCA = Common carotid
BCT= Brachiocephalic trunk
PCOM = Posterior communicating
ACOM = Anterior communicating
PCOM = Posterior communicating
SCA = Superior cerebellar

**Fig. 1.52** Subclavian steal syndrome. There is a blockage of the subclavian artery proximal to the vertebral artery. The blood now comes down from the vertebrobasilar system to enter the subclavian artery distal to the constriction – the subclavian "steals" the blood from the brain. (Leo 2022)

upper limb, it causes problems for the brain because the vertebrobasilar system is receiving less blood which leads to syncope and ataxia (Fig. 1.52).

## Lefort Fractures

Lefort fractures are fractures that separate the midface from the skull and can be classified as Type 1, II, or III. All of these subtypes involve a fracture of the pterygoid plate. Without going into all the fine details, the fracture line in Type I is a horizontal line sitting between the oral and nasal cavities just above the palate. This results in a floating palate, malocclusion of the teeth, and difficulty speaking, Type II is slightly higher with the fracture line forming a triangle around the nasal cavity with the apex making its way into the inferior portion of the orbit, Type III is higher and goes through the middle of the orbit and into the base of the skull. One way to remember the different subtypes is: Speak no evil, see no evil, hear no evil. Type I effects speaking, Type II also effects seeing, and Type III also effects hearing.

## Further Reading

Barry BJ, Whitman MC, Hunter DG, Engle EC. Duane syndrome. In: Adam MP, Ardinger HH, Pagon RA, et al., editors. GeneReviews; 2019. Available at https://www.ncbi.nlm.nih.gov/books/NBKX90/.

Chen CE, Liao ZZ, Lee Y, Liu C, Tang C, Chen R. Scalp trauma in an adult. J Emerg Med. 2017;53(5):e85–8.

Coskun Ö, Chatzioglou GN, Öztürk A. Henry Gray (1827–1861): The great author of the most widely used resource in medical education. Childs Nerv Syst. 2020. Available at: https://doi.org/10.1007/s00381-0200047-48-7.

Gray H. Anatomy: descriptive and surgical. Toronto: Strathearn Books; 1858.

Hartl DM. Recurrent laryngeal nerve paralysis: current concepts and treatment: part II causes, diagnosis, and management. Ear Nose Throat J. 2000:918–27.

Hiatt JL, Gartner LP. Textbook of head and neck anatomy. New York: Wolters Kluwer; 2010.

Kirchner JA. Semon's law a century later. J Laryngol Otol. 1981;96:645–57.

Luers JC, Huttenbrink KB. Surgical anatomy and pathology of the middle ear. J Anat. 2015;238:338–53.

Moore K, Dalley AF, Agur A. Clinically oriented anatomy. 7th ed. Baltimore: Lippincott Williams and Wilkin; 2014.

Nicholson L. Caput succedaneum and cephalohematoma: the Cs that leave bumps on the head. Neonatal Netw. 2007;26(5):277–81.

Thiagarajah C, Kersten RC. Medial wall fracture: an update. Craniomaxillofac Trauma Reconstr. 2009;2(3):135–46.

Woodburne RT, Burkel WE. Essentials of human anatomy. 9th ed. New York: Oxford University Press; 1994.

# The Thorax

**2**

## Anterior Thoracic Wall

### Breasts

The *mammary glands* are located anterior to the pectoralis major and serratus anterior muscles. Between the breast tissue and the pectoralis major is the retromammary space. The retromammary space allows movement of the breast on the chest wall. The *suspensory ligaments* (Cooper's Ligaments) of the breast are connective tissue connecting the skin to the deep layer of the superficial fascia. The ligaments are like the spokes of a wheel running from the periphery to the center which results in the formation of compartments housing the ducts and lobules. Carcinoma can lead to the blockage of the lymphatic vessels in one or more compartments which gives a "dimpling" or "orange-peel" appearance to the breast. If one of the compartments is infected and needs to be drained, an incision should remain localized to that segment.

The glands or lobules are housed in these compartments. The smaller glands drain via the small lactiferous ducts to the main lactiferous duct found within a compartment, and then from there to the lactiferous sinus which then emerges as the opening of the lactiferous duct on the nipple at the areola.

Regarding lymphatic drainage of the breast, the lateral side (75%) of the breast drains towards lymph nodes in the vicinity of the armpit, while the medial side (remaining 25%) drains to the parasternal nodes along the sternum.

Now for the details. The nodes around the armpit are subdivided into several different groups, all of which are appropriately named. The *central group* is deep in the arm pit and forms the top of a tripod receiving drainage from the *anterior, posterior, and lateral nodes*. After receiving drainage from these regions, the central group drains to the apical group which is just below the clavicle – not surprisingly this group is sometimes referred to as the *infraclavicular group* (Fig. 2.1).

© The Author(s), under exclusive license to Springer Nature Switzerland AG 2022
J. Leo, *Clinical Anatomy and Embryology*,
https://doi.org/10.1007/978-3-031-03807-5_2

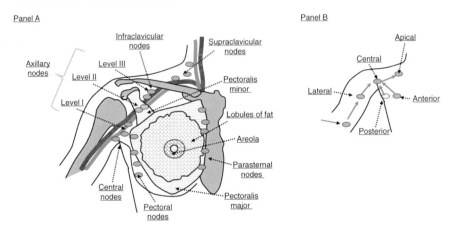

**Fig. 2.1** Lymphatic drainage of breast. Panel (**a**) shows the lateral side of the breast (75%) drains to the axillary nodes which then drain into the infra and supraclavicular nodes. The pectoralis minor is a landmark and divides the axillary nodes into three levels. The remaining medial side (25%) drains into the parasternal nodes. Panel (**b**) shows the lateral, posterior, and anterior nodes all draining into the central nodes which in turn drains into the apical nodes. (Leo 2022)

These axillary nodes can also be organized into three different levels, all based on their location to pectoralis minor. Level 1 is distal to pectoralis minor, level II is posterior to pectoralis minor, and level III is proximal to pectoralis minor. Remember that the axillary artery is also divided into three parts based on the pectoralis minor.

## Neurovascular Supply to the Breast

For clinical scenarios, the most important blood supply to the breast is the *lateral thoracic artery* supplying the lateral side of the breast. This artery runs with the long thoracic nerve, thus radical mastectomies that damage this nerve will paralyze the serratus anterior resulting in a winged scapula and difficulty in abducting the upper limb from 90° to straight over the head. The breast also receives blood from the anterior and posterior intercostal arteries. The nerves to the breast come from the intercostal nerves (T4-T6).

## Anterior Thoracic Wall Muscles

The musculature of the anterior thoracic wall is formed by the three intercostal muscles lying between the ribs and the transversus thoracis. They are all innervated by intercostal nerves.

1. The *external intercostal muscles* pass from the lower border of one rib to upper border of the rib below. Their fibers are oriented as the "hands in the pocket" direction.

2. The *internal intercostal muscles* run from the inferior surface of a costal groove to the superior border of the rib below at right angles to the external intercostal muscles.

3. The *innermost intercostal muscles* run from the superior surface of a costal groove to the superior border of the rib below in the same orientation as the internal intercostal muscles.

4. The origin of the *transverse thoracis* is on the posterior inferior portion of the sternum and the xiphoid process. Its fibers run laterally and ascend to reach ribs 2–6.

## Neurovascular Organization of the Anterior Thoracic Wall

The *costal grooves* are located on the inferior surface of the ribs. Each groove houses a neurovascular bundle containing an intercostal vein, artery, and nerve. These bundles are situated between the internal intercostal and innermost intercostal muscles (Fig. 2.2).

1. The *intercostal nerves* arise from the spinal nerves. They start posteriorly and wrap around to end on the anterior thoracic wall. Note the terminology here, there are no *anterior* or *posterior* intercostal nerves, just intercostal nerves.

2. However, the *intercostal arteries* are given the prefix of either anterior or posterior. For the first two spaces, the posterior intercostal arteries come from the superior intercostal arteries which are branches of the costocervical trunks. The posterior intercostal arteries in the remaining spaces (3–9) arise from the abdominal aorta and wrap around the thoracic wall in the costal groove where they meet with the anterior intercostal arteries. In the first six intercostal spaces the anterior intercostal arteries are branches of the internal thoracic arteries as they descend posterior to the sternum. The internal thoracic eventually gives off a *musculophrenic artery* which in turn gives off the anterior intercostals to enter spaces 7–9.

**Fig. 2.2** Ribs and neurovascular structures. The intercostal veins, arteries and nerves travel in the costal groove on the inferior surface of the ribs. (Leo 2022)

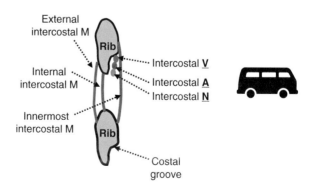

## Chest Tube Placement

Chest tubes are most often placed in the fifth intercostal space in the mid axillary line. To avoid the neurovascular bundle in the costal groove, the line is placed on the superior border of the fifth rib.

## Mediastinum

The dividing line for the *mediastinum* is a horizontal line starting anteriorly at the junction of the second rib with the manubrium and body of the sternum (sternal angle) and running posterior to the junction of the T4 and T5 vertebra. Above the line is the *superior mediastinum*, and below the line are the *anterior, middle, and posterior mediastinum* (Fig. 2.3).

1. The superior border of the *superior mediastinum* is an ascending diagonal line running from the sternal notch upwards to the T1 vertebra. Within the superior mediastinum is the aorta, superior vena cava, trachea, esophagus, vagus nerve, and left recurrent laryngeal nerve. The thoracic duct drains into the venous circulation at the angle between the left internal jugular and left subclavian vein thus is found within the superior mediastinum.

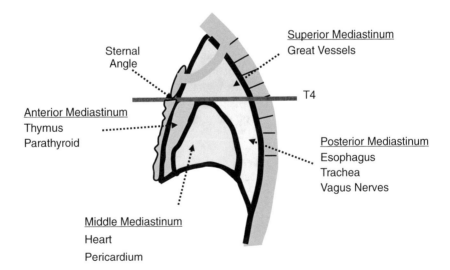

**Fig. 2.3** The important dividing line for the mediastinum runs from the sternal angle to the junction of the T4 and T5 vertebra. The superior mediastinum is Above the line, and the anterior middle, and posterior mediastinum are below the line. The anterior mediastinum includes the thymus and parathyroid. The middle mediastinum includes the heart, pericardium, and phrenic nerve. The posterior mediastinum Includes the esophagus, trachea, and vagus nerves. (Leo 2022)

2. The *anterior mediastinum* is between the body of the sternum and the fibrous pericardium. It contains the thymus in children. During adolescence it is replaced by adipose tissue. However, in adults the anterior mediastinum is a site for tumors – either thymomas or lymphomas. In addition, a thyroid goiter can expand inferiorly and enter the anterior mediastinum. Teratomas can also be found in the anterior mediastinum.

3. The *middle mediastinum* contains the heart and the pericardium, the ascending aorta, the superior vena cava, azygos vein, the pulmonary trunk, pulmonary veins, phrenic nerves, vagus nerves, and the inferior vena cava. Also in middle mediastinum is the trachea which bifurcates at the level of T6.

4. The *posterior mediastinum* contains the esophagus, thoracic aorta, azygous vein, hemiazygos vein, thoracic duct, splanchnic nerves, and vagus nerves. The sympathetic trunk is posterior to the pleura and the mediastinum, but the thoracic splanchnic nerves emerge from the sympathetic trunk and move anteriorly into the posterior mediastinum.

## The Pericardium and Sinuses

There are three layers of *pericardium*. The thick, tough outermost layer is the fibrous pericardium. It is a cone shaped structure attached to the diaphragm inferiorly via the *pericardiophrenic ligaments*, and the adventitia of the great vessels superiorly. The *phrenic nerve* and *pericardiacophrenic vessels* are located just lateral to the fibrous pericardium.

Deep to the fibrous pericardium is the serous pericardium which is subdivided into two layers, the parietal and visceral layers. The parietal and layers are continuous and encase the pericardial space. The visceral layer is attached to the heart and is reflected onto the parietal layer which is attached to the fibrous layer. The parietal layers is reflected around the great vessels to create two compartments. In one compartment is the aorta and pulmonary trunk, and in the second compartment is the superior vena cava, the inferior vena cava, and the four pulmonary veins. This in turn makes two spaces. The *transverse pericardial sinus* is posterior to the aorta and pulmonary trunk, and anterior to the superior vena cava. The *oblique sinus* is posterior to the heart and bound by the four pulmonary veins (Fig. 2.3).

Accumulation of fluid in the pericardial space – between the visceral and parietal layers – can lead to *cardiac tamponade*. Patients will typically present with bulging neck veins, hypotension and distant heart sounds.

## The Heart

The right atrium receives oxygen poor blood from both the superior and inferior vena cava. The coronary sinus also delivers oxygen poor blood from the heart muscle itself to the right atrium. From the right atrium, the blood travels through the

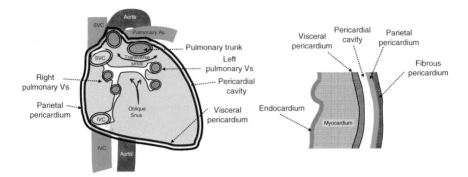

**Fig. 2.4**  Pericardial cavity and sinuses. The visceral pericardium is adherent to the heart. It connects and folds back on the parietal pericardium to form the pericardial cavity. The fibrous pericardium is a thick layer outside the heart attaching to the diaphragm inferiorly. The oblique pericardial sinus is bounded by the pulmonary arteries. The transverse pericardial sinus is anterior to the SVC, but posterior to the aorta and pulmonary trunk. (Leo 2022)

tricuspid valve into the right ventricle. The tricuspid valve is composed of three cusps which are connected via *chorda tendineae* to the papillary muscles. The combination of chorda tendineae and papillary muscles prevent the valve cusps from backflowing into the right atrium during contraction. From the right ventricle, blood moves through the semilunar valve into the coronary trunk on its way to the lungs to pick up oxygen, and it then returns to the left atrium. From the left atrium blood moves through the mitral valve into the left ventricle. From the left ventricle, blood moves from through the aortic semilunar valve to the ascending aorta (Fig. 2.4).

The great vessels emerge from the heart and enter the superior mediastinum. There are several important relationships in this area.

1. The *right brachiocephalic vein* enters the superior vena cava heading towards the right border of the heart.
2. The *left brachiocephalic vein* crosses anterior to the aorta and its three large branches. This is at the T3 level.
3. The *ascending aorta* comes out of the heart at the T4 level just to the left of the superior vena cava. The right pulmonary artery passes deep to the aorta.
4. The *right and left internal jugular veins* are medial to the common carotid arteries. A central line is placed into the internal jugular vein by going lateral to a finger on the pulse of the common carotid (Fig. 2.5).

## Blood Supply to the Heart

The blood supply to the heart comes from the right and left coronary arteries which are the first branches off the aorta. The openings of the right and left coronary arteries are below the cusps of the aortic valve. The right coronary descends in the atrioventricular groove towards the inferior border of the heart where is turns around to

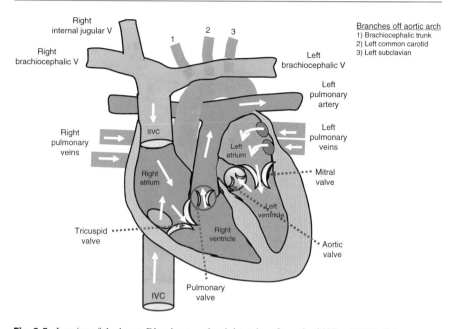

**Fig. 2.5** Interior of the heart. Blood enters the right atrium from the SVC and IVC. It then passes through the tricuspid valve to enter the right ventricle. From the right ventricle it moves through the pulmonic valve into the pulmonary trunk to pulmonary arteries to lungs. After picking up O² in the lungs it comes back to the left atrium. Then through the mitral valve into left ventricle. Then out the left ventricle through the aortic valve to aorta. Note the left brachiocephalic vein crosses the midline from left to right to reach the SVC. The right brachiocephalic vein does not cross the midline. The three branches off the aortic arise behind the left brachiocephalic vein. (Leo 2022)

travel posteriorly to the crux of the heart (the intersection between the atrioventricular and interatrial grooves) (Fig. 2.6).

1. The first branch of the right coronary artery is the *sinoatrial nodal branch* which travels posterior to the superior vena cava to reach the sinoatrial node. In some cases, it can arise from the left coronary artery.
2. As the right coronary artery reaches the inferior border it gives off a *marginal branch.* The right coronary artery supplies most of the right ventricle, a small portion of the left ventricle, and the posterior one third of the interventricular septum.
3. As the right coronary artery reaches the posterior surface of the heart it gives off the *posterior interventricular artery.* Often coming off from the posterior interventricular is the *atrioventricular nodal artery.*

The *left coronary artery* is relatively short and quickly splits into:

1. The *circumflex branch* runs towards the left side in the atrioventricular groove and eventually meets up with the right coronary artery at the crux.

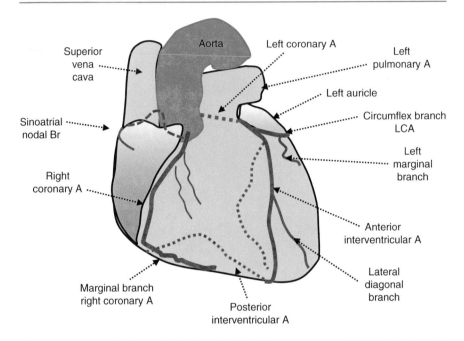

**Fig. 2.6**  Blood supply to heart. The first branch of the right coronary artery (RCA) is the sinoatrial nodal branch which supplies the sinoatrial node. The RCA then descends in the coronary sulcus. It gives off the marginal branch which supplies the inferior border. The RCA continues posterior. The posterior interventricular artery typically arises from the RCA. The left coronary artery is much shorter than the RCA as it quickly divides into the circumflex and the anterior interventricular artery. The circumflex gives off a left marginal branch. (Leo 2022)

The circumflex gives off the *left marginal artery* and the *posterior left ventricular branch of left coronary artery*.

2. The *anterior interventricular branch*, also known as either the left anterior descending, LAD, or widow maker descends towards the apex and supplies most of the left ventricle and left atrium. It also supplies most of the interventricular septum (anterior 2/3rds). As it passes down the anterior surface of the heart it gives off several diagonal branches of the anterior interventricular artery.

Heart dominance refers to whether an individual heart receives most of its blood from either the right or left coronary arteries. The most common distribution of the coronary arteries was presented in the section above. To determine whether the individual is right or left dominant the pertinent question is: Where does the posterior interventricular artery come from? Most individuals are right dominant, in which case the posterior interventricular artery arises from the right coronary artery. However, in some individuals, the circumflex artery which is a branch of the left coronary artery gives off the posterior interventricular artery, making this an example of a left dominant heart. And in some cases, the anterior interventricular artery continues around the apex, turns, and ascends up the interventricular groove as the posterior interventricular artery, which is also an example of a left dominant individual.

## Venous Drainage of the Heart

Most of the venous drainage of the heart enters the *coronary sinus* which then drains into the right atrium. The coronary sinus is found on the posterior surface of the heart and runs with the circumflex artery. Running on the anterior surface, with the anterior interventricular artery is the *great cardiac vein* which turns posterior to turn into the coronary sulcus to meet the coronary sinus. Running with the posterior interventricular artery in the posterior interventricular sulcus is the *middle cardiac vein* which also drains into the coronary sinus. And running on the right border of the heart with the right marginal artery and also draining into the coronary sinus is the *small cardiac vein*. The coronary sinus in turn drains into the right atrium. In addition, besides the vessels mentioned above which all drain into the coronary sinus, there are several small *anterior cardiac veins* which drain directly into the right atrium. At the opening of the coronary sinus, there is a small valve, the valve of the coronary sinus. Also draining into the coronary sinus, close to its origin, is the *oblique vein of the left atrium* (Fig. 2.7).

## Nerves to the Heart

The internal conducting system of the heart starts at the *sinoatrial node* which is found in the vicinity of the opening of the superior vena cava. Impulses then travel to the *atrioventricular node* (AV node) which is found near the septal leaflet of the tricuspid valve and the opening of the coronary sinus. At the AV node there is a slight delay of the impulse to allow the atria to completely empty before the contractions are over. From the AV node the impulses then travel down through the bundle of His fibers in the *interventricular septum* towards the apex. There are two branches of the bundle of His, the *right and left bundle branches*. From the apex the impulse then travels along *Purkinje fibers* on the ventricular walls.

The right and left vagus nerves provide the parasympathetic nerve supply to the heart. They both travel in the carotid sheath with the common carotid and internal

**Fig. 2.7** Venous drainage of the heart. The great cardiac vein, middle cardiac vein, and small cardiac veins all drain into the posteriorly located coronary sinus. The anterior cardiac veins drain directly into the right atrium. (Leo 2022)

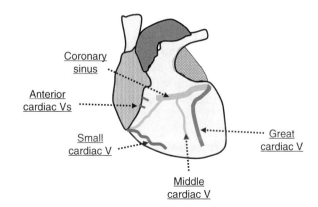

jugular vein to enter the thorax. The left vagus nerve travels over the aortic arch, where it gives off the recurrent laryngeal, and then continues towards the heart. The right vagus nerve gives off the recurrent laryngeal which travels around the subclavian artery.

The sympathetic efferent nerves to the heart come from the inferior and middle cervical ganglion. The superficial cardiac plexus is situated on the aortic arch, while the deep cardiac plexus is under the aortic arch. These plexuses are a combination of parasympathetic and sympathetic fibers. Afferent sensations from the heart travel on the sympathetic nerves to the T1–4 levels which are the same levels responsible for should pain. This is why a patient in the midst of a heart attack will complain about pain in the left shoulder.

## Borders of the Heart

A good place to start with a discussion of the borders of the heart is the right side. If you look at the right side of the heart along with the structures above it, and you draw line straight down the right side you can the progression of the right internal jugular vein draining into the *right subclavian vein*, which then drains into the right brachiocephalic vein, which then drains into the *superior vena cava*, and then down into the right atrium. When you look at a cross section through any of these structures think of this line running down from the neck into the thorax (Fig. 2.8).

The borders of the heart are represented by a trapezoid with horizontal lines running from the costal cartilages of rib 3–6 on the right and ribs 2 to the fifth intercostal space on the left. Horizontal lines then connect the corners to outline the superior and inferior borders. The inferior border of the heart runs from rib 3 to rib 5, crossing behind the sternum. The superior border closes the trapezoid running from rib 2 on the left to rib 3 on the right.

The right border of the heart is the right atrium just to the right of the sternum. The anatomic base of the heart is the posterior surface (not the diaphragmatic surface) and is the left atrium. Just posterior to the base is the esophagus, thus a transesophageal echocardiogram involves an endoscope placed in the esophagus to visualize the heart (Figs. 2.9 and 2.10).

The anterior surface of the heart is mostly formed by the right ventricle, so a stab wound to the left of the sternum, between ribs 2–5 would likely penetrate the right ventricle. Moving left from the sternum across the right ventricle, at the left border of the heart one can see the edge of the left ventricle. Thus, while the majority of the anterior surface is the right ventricle, all the way on the left side, at the left border, the left ventricle makes an appearance.

## Heart Valve Projections and Auscultation Sites

The atrioventricular valves are located between the atria and ventricles. The mitral valve is located on the left side between the left atria and left ventricle, and tricuspid

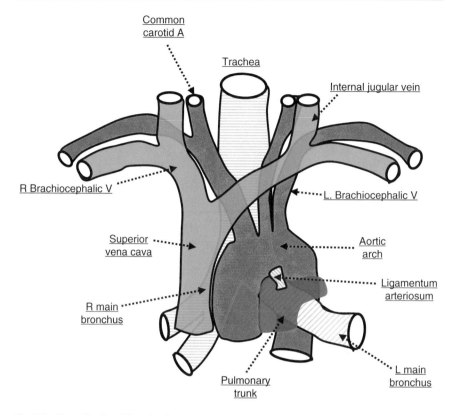

**Fig. 2.8** Heart Outflow. Note the three great vessels lined up in a row: (1) aorta, (2) superior vena cava, and (3) pulmonary trunk. The right and left brachiocephalic veins join to form the superior vena cava. The left βbrachiocephalic vein crosses in front of the three branches coming off the aorta. (Leo 2022)

valve on the right side. During ventricular systole they prevent blood from the ventricle from moving back into the atria – during systole or contraction of the ventricles these doors should remain closed. During diastole they will be open.

The semilunar valves, which are the aortic and pulmonic valves, are between the ventricles and the outflow tracts. Both the aortic and pulmonic valves each have three cusps. Due to the development of these structures during the rotation of the truncus arteriosus, the cusps are situated such that in the pulmonic valve there is an anterior cusp, while the aortic valve has a posterior cusp. Each valve then has a right and left cusp. The tricuspid valve is on the right side, while the mitral valve is on the left. The heart valves are located posterior to the sternum (Fig. 2.11).

The aortic and pulmonic valves are situated close to each other at the third costal cartilage. The aortic valve is slightly lower and to the right of the pulmonic. The tricuspid and mitral valves are lower down, near where the fourth costal cartilage meets the body of the sternum. However, when auscultating the valves, the sounds for each are not heard directly over the valve. For example, the aortic valve is located

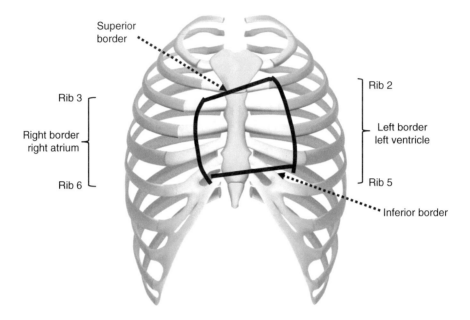

**Fig. 2.9** Borders of the heart. The right border runs from the costal cartilages of rib 3 to rib 6 just to the right of the sternum. The left border runs from rib 2 to the fifth intercostal space on the left side. The right border is the right atrium, the left border is the left ventricle. Hidden from this view is the base of the heart (posterior) which is the left atrium. The inferior border is the right ventricle and apex of left ventricle. The superior border is the right and left atria. (Leo 2022)

just to the right of the sternum, but the sound of the aortic valve is heard at the second intercostal space.

The sound of the aortic valve is heard on the right at the second intercostal space. The pulmonic valve is heard to the left at the second intercostal space. The tricuspid valve is heard just to the left of the sternum at the fifth costal cartilage. The mitral valve is heard at the apex of the heart at the fifth intercostal space on the left in the midclavicular line (Fig. 2.12).

At the beginning of systole, as pressure in the ventricles rises, the AV valves close producing the first heart sound S1. As the pressure in the ventricles rises, the aortic and pulmonic valves open allowing blood to enter the aorta and pulmonary trunk. As the pressure rises in the great vessels, it will eventually be greater than the pressure in the ventricles at which point the aortic and pulmonic valves close producing the second heart sound S2.

Disruptions of blood flow through the various valves can lead to murmurs that can be heard in either systole or diastole. The location of the murmur and whether it is heard at systole or diastole are both important in determining which valve is affected. This disrupted flow typically results from either stenosis of the valve or regurgitation of the valve. Think of the valves like doors, a stenotic valve indicates

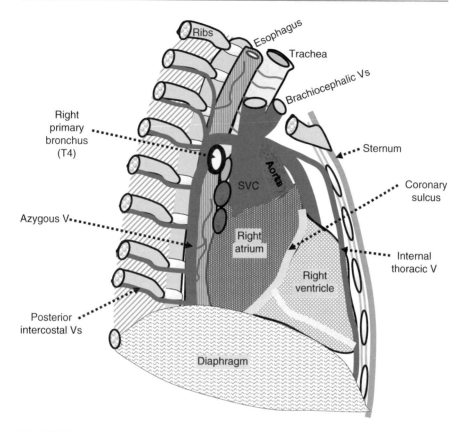

**Fig. 2.10** Posterior mediastinum. The azygous vein is ascending behind the esophagus, arches over the right primary bronchus and enters the superior vena cava (SVC). The posterior intercostal veins drain into the azygous vein. The base of the heart is the right atrium, just anterior to the esophagus. The anterior border of the heart is the right ventricle. The internal thoracic vein drains just posterior to the sternum. The trachea is bifurcating at T4. (Leo 2022)

a problem with opening the door – it doesn't open wide enough. And conversely, regurgitation is a problem with closing the door – it doesn't close all the way.

When a chamber, such as the left ventricle, is contracting and trying to push blood downstream, the outflow or downstream valve wants to remain open, while the valve on the upstream side wants to be closed so that blood does not go in the reverse direction. If the outflow valve is stenotic then blood is being ejected through a much smaller opening which will lead to a sound heard downstream of the valve. In contrast, if the upstream valve is not closed all the way – it is incompetent – then the valve will allow blood to flow in the reverse or retrograde direction. As the sound moves in a retrograde direction the sound will be heard outside the chamber (Fig. 2.13).

On the other hand, when a chamber is filling, it is the upstream valve that wants to be open, to allow blood to flow into the heart, while the downstream valve wants

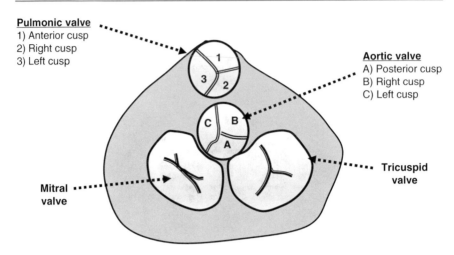

**Pulmonic valve**
1) Anterior cusp
2) Right cusp
3) Left cusp

**Aortic valve**
A) Posterior cusp
B) Right cusp
C) Left cusp

Mitral valve

Tricuspid valve

**Fig. 2.11** Heart valves. There are three cusps each in the aortic and pulmonic valves. Both have right and left cusps, while the pulmonic has an anterior cusp, and the aortic valve has a posterior cusp. The pulmonic valve's anterior cusp is across from the pulmonic valve's posterior cusp. (Leo 2022)

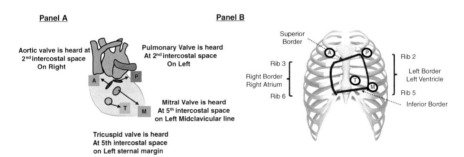

**Panel A**                        **Panel B**

Aortic valve is heard at 2nd intercostal space On Right

Pulmonary Valve is heard At 2nd intercostal space On Left

Mitral Valve is heard At 5th intercostal space on Left Midclavicular line

Tricuspid valve is heard At 5th intercostal space on Left sternal margin

Superior Border

Rib 3

Right Border Right Atrium

Rib 6

Rib 2

Left Border Left Ventricle

Rib 5

Inferior Border

**Fig. 2.12** Two representations of heart sound locations. Panel (**a**) shows the locations of the valves. The arrows show the locations of where the sounds are heard. Panel (**b**) shows the borders of the heart and the locations of the heart sounds relative to the ribs and sternum. (Leo 2022)

to be closed to allow the chamber to fill. If the upstream valve is stenotic this will lead to blood coming through the valve at a higher pressure with the sound also heard in the chamber. In the specific examples below, we are going to focus on the left ventricle, with the mitral valve being the upstream valve, and the aortic valve being the downstream valve. Keep in mind we are focusing on the blood flow and the murmurs, in other words, the anatomy, to simply understand the basics. We are not focusing on all the details about different heart murmurs. The purpose of the following discussion is to make it easier to understand the advanced physiology of heart murmurs.

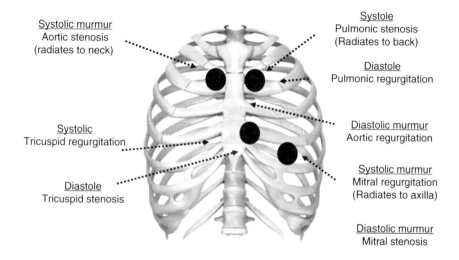

**Fig. 2.13** Common locations for hearing heart murmurs. (Leo 2022)

## Systolic Murmurs

### Mitral Valve Regurgitation

Take a systolic murmur resulting from mitral valve regurgitation as an example. In a healthy individual, during systole, the mitral valve will be closed, and the aortic valve will be open so that blood goes out the aortic valve but not the mitral valve. With mitral valve regurgitation, during systole, there is an incomplete closure of the mitral valve, which allows a small amount of blood to move through the mitral valve in a retrograde direction. The sound will then radiate to the left axilla and be heard throughout systole (pan systolic) (Fig. 2.14).

### Aortic Stenosis

With aortic stenosis, blood flow through the aortic valve is impeded in systole which leads to a sharper faster flow through the aorta resulting in the high-pitched sound radiating to the carotid arteries in the right neck (Fig. 2.15).

## Diastolic Murmurs

### Mitral Valve Stenosis

In a healthy individual, during diastole, the mitral valve remains open, while the aortic valve is closed. This allows filling of the ventricle. With mitral stenosis the blood coming through the mitral valve is impeded and comes through the smaller opening faster and sharper which leads to a murmur heard at the apex – near the left fifth space in the mid-clavicular line (Fig. 2.16).

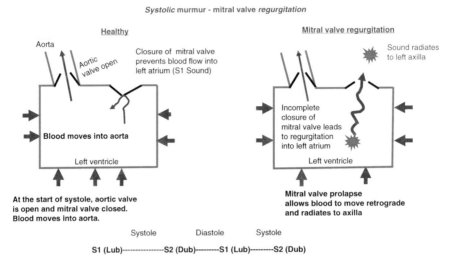

Fig. 2.14   Systolic murmur. (Leo 2022)

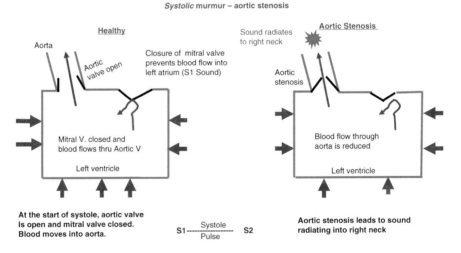

Fig. 2.15   Systolic murmur. Aortic Stenosis . (Leo 2022)

## Aortic Regurgitation

With aortic regurgitation, the aortic valve is incompetent which allows blood to flow back from the aorta into the left ventricle with the sound radiating to the left sternal border near ribs 3–4 (Fig. 2.17).

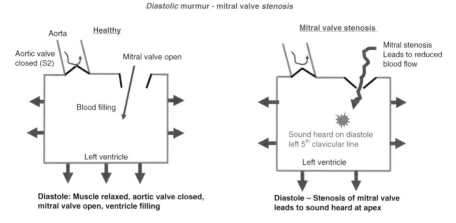

**Fig. 2.16** Diastolic murmur. Mitral valve stenosis. (Leo 2022)

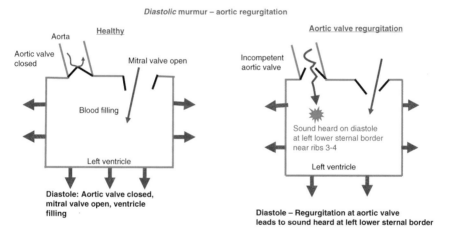

**Fig. 2.17** Diastolic murmur. Aortic Regurgitation. (Leo 2022)

## Mitral Valve Stenosis During Systole Versus Regurgitation During Diastole

With mitral valve regurgitation, the sound will be heard outside the heart – at the right neck during systole. With mitral stenosis, the sound will be heard inside the heart during diastole (Fig. 2.18).

Putting all this together there are two steps to determine the nature of the murmur.

1. In step #1 ask if the murmur is above or below the midsternal line. If the murmur is above the line, then the murmur is either the aortic valve, or pulmonic valve.
2. In step #2 ask if the sound is heard during systole or diastole. If it is above the line and heard during systole then it must be stenosis of the either the aortic or

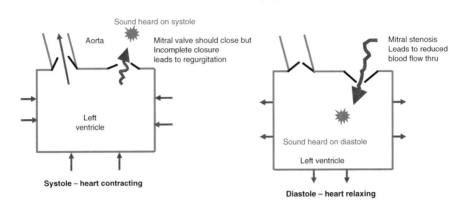

**Fig. 2.18**  Mitral valve: stenosis versus regurgitation. (Leo 2022)

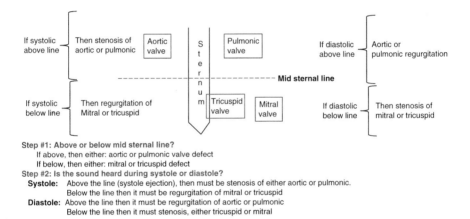

**Fig. 2.19**  Murmur Detection (Leo 2022)

pulmonic valve. If it is below the line during systole then it must be regurgitation of the mitral or tricuspid valve. If it is heard during diastole, and above the line then it must be regurgitation of the aortic or pulmonic. And if it is heard below the line during diastole then it must be stenosis of either the tricuspid or mitral valve (Fig. 2.19).

## Esophagus

The esophagus transmits food from the oral cavity to the stomach and can be divided into thirds. The proximal one-third is made up of skeletal muscle, while the distal one-third is made up of smooth muscle, leaving the middle one-third composed of a combination of skeletal and smooth muscle. In the neck the esophagus passes behind the trachea. Once the trachea bifurcates at T6, the esophagus comes to lie posterior to the left atrium of the heart. It then travels through the diaphragm at the esophageal hiatus accompanying the right and left vagus nerves. Posterior to the esophagus is the thoracic aorta (Fig. 2.20).

There are several points along the esophagus as it travels from the mouth to the diaphragm where structures press on it and lead to constrictions.

1. The *cricopharyngeus* is the thickened inferior end of the inferior constrictor and forms the *pharyngoesophageal constriction*.
2. The aortic arch and the left main bronchus also cross the esophagus very close to each other and from the *aortobronchial constriction*.
3. The last constriction is the *diaphragmatic constriction* at the esophageal hiatus that marks the entrance to the stomach.

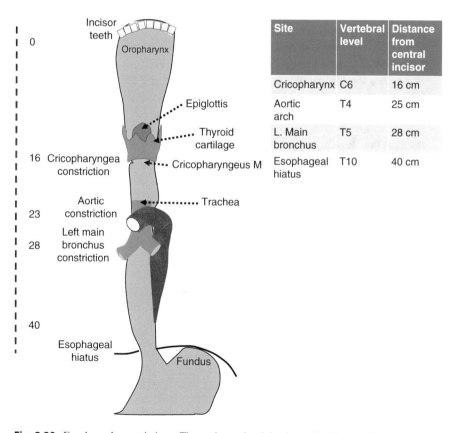

| Site | Vertebral level | Distance from central incisor |
|------|-----------------|-------------------------------|
| Cricopharynx | C6 | 16 cm |
| Aortic arch | T4 | 25 cm |
| L. Main bronchus | T5 | 28 cm |
| Esophageal hiatus | T10 | 40 cm |

**Fig. 2.20** Esophageal constrictions. The scale on the right shows the distance from the middle incisors. The first constriction is at the cricopharyngeus muscle. The next is where the aorta crosses in front of esophagus, and right below the aorta is the left main bronchus. The last constriction is the esophageal hiatus. (Leo 2022)

At the junction with the stomach the phrenoesophageal ligament runs from the esophagus to the diaphragm and is involved in the coordinated movements that allow a bolus to move from esophagus into the stomach.

## Ribs and Sternum

There are three parts to the sternum:

1. the *manubrium* is the widest part of the sternum and has a facet for articulation with the first rib laterally. The manubrium is slanted posteriorly and is located behind the clavicle which makes it impossible to palpate the first rib.
   The clavicle articulates with the superior portion of the manubrium at the *sterno-clavicular joint*. This joint connects the upper limb to the sternum and supports the shoulder. Within the joint cavity is a thick fibrous articular disc dividing the joint into two spaces. The anterior and posterior sternoclavicular ligaments strengthen the joint anterior and inferiorly. The *interclavicular ligament* runs superiorly across the sternal notch and connects the two clavicles. Moving later-ally across the first rib the *costoclavicular ligament* (rhomboid ligament) runs from the costal cartilage of the first rib to the clavicle. Injuries to the joint are rare, but it can be injured in car accidents or sporting injuries. The posterior liga-ments are much stronger than the anterior ligaments thus dislocations usually result in the clavicle being displaced anteriorly.
   The right and left brachiocephalic veins pass posterior to the sternoclavicular joint and then form the brachiocephalic vein, also posterior to the manubrium.
2. The manubrium meets the *body of the sternum* at the *manubriosternal joint* forming the *sternal angle* which is easily palpated. The second rib forms a syno-vial joint via demifacets with the manubrium and sternum also at the sternal angle. The superior most portion of the manubrium is the sternal notch (jugular notch). Using the sternal angle and the second rib as a landmark, the examiner can then move their hands inferiorly to palpate and count ribs 3–7 which attach to the body of the sternum.
3. The inferior portion of the sternum articulates with the *xiphoid process.*

Rib 1 articulates with the manubrium. Anteriorly ribs 2–10 end in costal cartilages which in turn articulate with the sternum. Ribs 1–7 are referred to as true ribs because their costal cartilage attach directly to the sternum. Ribs 8–10 do not attach directly to the sternum and are referred to as false ribs. The costal cartilage of ribs 8–10 attach to the cartilage of the rib above. And ribs 11 and 12 are floating ribs as they do not attach to the sternum but instead end within the musculature of the pos-terior abdominal wall.

## The Pleura

The lungs are surround by the pleura. The *visceral pleura* is adherent to the lungs and is reflected back onto the surrounding structures as the *parietal pleura*. Between the visceral and parietal layers is the *pleural space*. As the parietal pleura passes over various regions it is given a name appropriate to that region. The pleura along the thoracic wall is termed the *costal pleura*, which in turn is divided into anterior, posterior, and lateral divisions. Above the first rib, the *superior costal pleura* meets with the *cupula* of the pleura. At the diaphragm the costal pleura meets with the *diaphragmatic pleura*. And medially, the costal pleura meets with the *mediastinal pleura*. At the root of the lung, the pleura extends inferiorly as the *pulmonary ligament*. On the left side, the pleura is reflected laterally at the fourth costal cartilage and then continues inferiorly and lateral to the sternum past ribs 5 and 6. At the seventh rib, the pleura comes back medially. This diversion creates the *cardiac notch* which leaves a space just lateral to the sternum on the left where a needle can be inserted without going through the pleural space. Where the costal pleura meets the mediastinal and diaphragmatic pleura there are sharp lines of reflection. These lines are important landmarks and can be mapped onto the thoracic wall.

|        | Mid-clavicular line | Mid-axillary line | Paravertebral line |
| ------ | ------------------- | ----------------- | ------------------ |
| Lungs  | Rib 6               | Rib 8             | Rib 10             |
| Pleura | Rib 8               | Rib 10            | Rib 12             |

In the midclavicular line the pleural reflection is at the eighth rib; at the midaxillary line at the tenth rib; and at the paravertebral line at the 12th rib. At each of these locations, the lungs (during normal respiration) are located two levels higher. In other words, lungs are at 6, 8, and 10, while the pleura is at 8, 10, and 12.

In the mid-axillary line this space between ribs 8 and 10 is the *costodiaphragmatic space*. Effusions can collect here. A pleural tap or *thoracocentesis* can be performed here with the needle passing just superior to a rib (which is on the inferior border of the intercostal space) to avoid the neurovascular bundle within the costal groove on the inferior surface of the rib.

Where the costal parietal pleura meets the mediastinal parietal pleura the line of reflection creates the *sternocostal recess*. There are no spaces superiorly.

## The Lungs

The lungs assume the shape of the thorax. On the superior surface they resemble a cone and rise above the first rib and middle of the clavicle to the T1 vertebral body. Structures passing next to the lungs leave impressions on the lung tissue (Fig. 2.21).

1. On the right lung the trachea and esophagus leave distinct impressions on the medial surface. There is a prominent impression of the azygos vein which can be seen arching over the root of the lung. Anterior to the groove for the trachea is

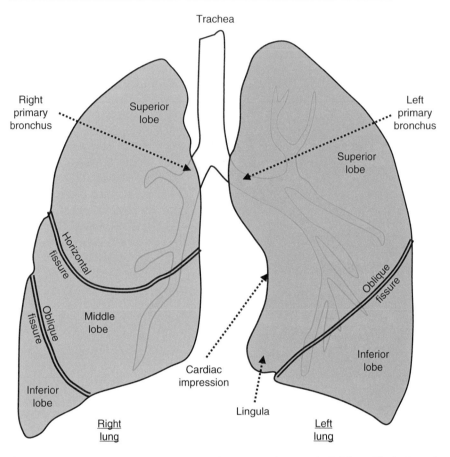

**Fig. 2.21** Lungs. There are three lobes in the right lung and two on the left lung. The horizontal fissure runs parallel to the fourth rib. The oblique fissures intersect the inferior borders of the lung at the sixth rib. Thus, a stab wound in the right midclavicular line between ribs four and six would be in the middle lobe. The cardiac impression is formed by the impression of the heart. The lingula is part of the superior lobe of the left lung. (Leo 2022)

the impression made by the right brachiocephalic vein, which turns into the impression of the superior vena cava.

2. On the left lung the trachea and esophagus together form one impression rather than two distinct impressions that one sees on the right. Anterior to this impression are the impressions of the subclavian artery and brachiocephalic vein. Just inferior to the root of the lung is a distinct impression of the esophagus – remember by this point the trachea has gone into the lungs.

The right lung has three lobes, and the left lung has two lobes. On the right the *horizontal fissure* parallels rib 4 and separates the superior and middle lobes. The *oblique fissure* is found on both lobes and intersects the mid-clavicular line at rib 6. On the

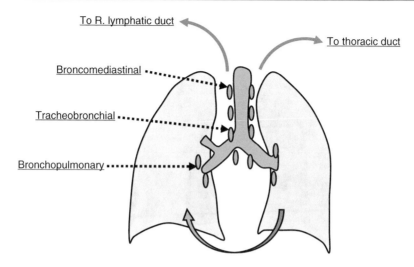

**Fig. 2.22** Lymphatic drainage of the lung. The deep areas of the lung drain into the bronchopulmonary nodes, then into the tracheobronchial nodes, and then into the broncomediastinal nodes. From there on the right the drainage is into the right lymphatic duct, and on the left into the thoracic duct. The lower left lung can drain across the midline to the right side. (Leo 2022)

right, the oblique fissure separates the middle lobe from the inferior lobe. On the left, the oblique fissure separates the superior from inferior lobes. The lingual of the left lung is equivalent to the middle lobe of the right lung.

A stab wound on the right, in the mid-clavicular line, above rib 4, would go through the superior lobe; and between ribs 4–6 in the mid-clavicular line would go through the middle lobe. Keep in mind that most of the inferior lobe lies posterior, so to listen to the inferior lobe one would typically place the stethoscope on the posterior surface. Likewise, the superior lobe faces anterior.

The bronchial arteries which are branches of the thoracic aorta supply the lungs.

The deep regions of the lung drain to the *bronchopulmonary nodes*, then into the *tracheobronchial nodes*, then into the *broncomediastinal nodes*. All of the right lung then drains into the *right lymphatic duct*. On the left, the superior and middle portions of the lung drain into the *thoracic duct*. However, the inferior portion of the left lung drains to the right and left side. Thus, some portion of the left lower lung can cross over to the right side and then drain into the right lymphatic duct.

The superficial surface of the lung – corresponding to the visceral pleura drain to the hilar nodes which in turn drain into the tracheobronchial nodes (Fig. 2.22).

## Pneumothorax

*Pneumothoraxe*s or collapsed lungs can be broken down into several different categories. For example, a stab wound or other penetrating injury of the chest wall that opens the wall is referred to as an *open pneumothorax* because it allows air from

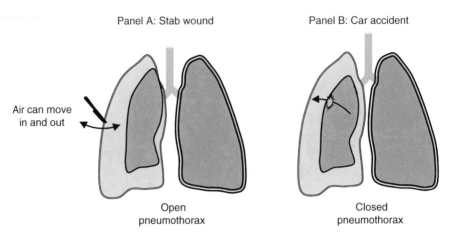

**Fig. 2.23**  Traumatic Pneumothorax. Panel A shows an open pneumothorax (chest wall is open) from a stab wound. The enters the pleural space from outside the body. Panel B shows a closed pneumothorax (chest wall is not compromised) resulting from a car injury which resulted in the lung tissue rupturing and air moving from the lungs into the pleural space. In both cases the lung has collapsed. Not shown is a spontaneous closed pneumothorax which can result from a piece of lung tissue rupturing. A tension pneumothorax occurs when the air in the pleural cavity cannot escape and the pressure pushed the heart to the opposite side. (Leo 2022)

outside the wall to move into and out of the pleural cavity through the opening. However, injuries to the lung wall itself such as a car accident where the lung wall is damaged leads to a *closed pneumothorax*. With a closed scenario the abdominal wall itself is not damaged. The air then moves from the lung into the pleural cavity. A *spontaneous pneumothorax* is a type of closed pneumothorax that does not involve trauma. Instead, a bleb of lung tissue bursts allowing air to move from the lungs into the pleural space (Figs. 2.23 and 2.24).

A *tension pneumothorax* is an emergency situation. Take a penetrating injury to the thoracic wall that creates a skin flap acing as a one-way valve. Air can enter into the pleural cavity through the opening on inspiration, but it cannot exit through the flap on expiration. The pressure then builds up in the pleural space and pushes the heart towards the opposite side. The heart will not move back and forth with each breath but will instead remain on the opposite side.

## Thoracostomy – Chest Tube Placement

To drain air from the pleural space a chest tube can be placed in the T4 space in the anterior axillary line (sometimes T5 depending on the pathology). To find this location, the nipple is the major landmark. A line is drawn from the nipple to the anterior axillary line. This location is within the triangle of safety which is bounded on two

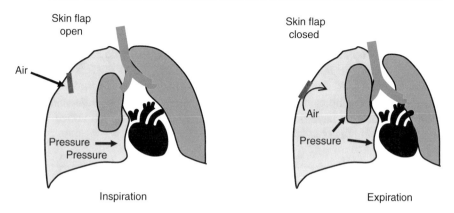

**Fig. 2.24** Tension pneumothorax. There is a penetrating injury that allows air to move through the flap and into the lung. On expiration the flap is closed, and air cannot escape the pleura cavity. Pressure in the cavity increases and with each successive breath the lung moves further towards the opposite side and compresses the heart. (Leo 2022)

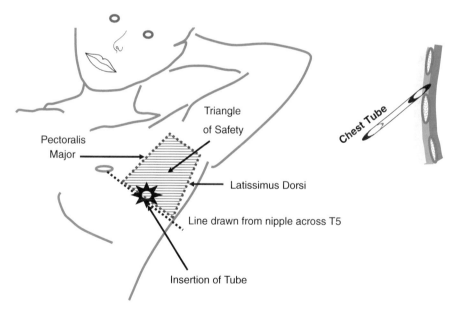

**Fig. 2.25** Triangle of Safety and Intercostal Chest Drain. The triangle is bounded by the lateral borders of pectoralis major and latissimus dorsi muscles. The apex is the axilla. The base is a line drawn laterally from the nipple. (Leo 2022)

sides by the lateral edges of the pectoralis major and the latissimus dorsi muscles. The needle is placed on the superior portion of rib five. This is to avoid the neurovascular bundle (VAN) in the costal groove on the inferior surface of each rib. A needle is used to make an incision and the chest tube is then placed in the opening. A suture is then used to secure the chest tube in the opening (Fig. 2.25).

## Pericardiocentesis

If fluid builds up around the heart (cardiac tamponade) a needle aspiration can be used to remove the fluid. The needle is typically inserted at the left infrasternal angle and is directed towards the left shoulder – specifically the left mid-clavicular line. There is a significant risk with this blind approach to *pericardiocentesis*. As imaging modalities have become more advanced it is common to utilize various types of imaging to assist with the procedure.

## Further Reading

Gittenberger-De Groot AC, Bartelings MM, Deruiter MC, Poelmann RE. Basics of cardiac development for the understanding of congenital heart malformations. Pediatr Res. 2005;57(2): 169–76.

Hanifin C. Cardiac auscultation 101: a basic science approach to heart murmurs. JAAPA. 2010;23(4):44–8.

Hanna IR, Silverman ME. A history of auscultation and some of its contributors. Am J Cardiology. 2002;90:259–67.

Moore K, Dalley AF, Agur A. Clinically oriented anatomy. 7th ed. Baltimore: Lippincott Williams and Wilkin; 2014.

Peigh G, Majdani J. A novel approach to teaching cardiac auscultation. MedEdPublish. 2017. Available at https://doi.org/10.15694/mep.2017.000095.

Tubbs RS, Shah NA, Sullivan BP, Marchase ND, Cömert A, Acar HI, Tekdemir I, Loukas M, Shoja MM. The Costoclavicular ligament revisited: a functional and anatomical study. Rom J Morphol Embryol. 2009;50(3):475–9.

# The Abdominal Cavity

**3**

## Anterior Abdominal Wall

The job of the anterior abdominal wall is to keep the gastrointestinal tract and related organs inside the abdomen but also remain pliable enough to allow for the various trunk movements. When pressure in the abdominal cavity goes up, abdominal contents will look for a way out of the abdominal cavity at weak points in the wall.

The fascia is divided into two layers. *Camper's fascia* is the fatty layer of fascia and *Scarpa's* is the deeper tough membranous layer (Fig. 1.1). Camper's fascia does not continue into the perineum. Scarpa's is continuous with Colle's fascia in the perineum, and with the *fascia lata* of the thigh (Fig. 3.1).

1) Skin
2) Camper's fascia
3) Scarpa's fascia
4) External abdominal oblique M.
5) Internal abdominal oblique M.
6) Transversus abdominus M.
7) Fascia transversalis
8) Extraperitoneal fat
9) Parietal peritoneum

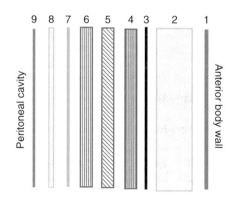

**Fig. 3.1** Layers of anterior abdominal wall. (Leo 2022)

The majority of the wall is made up of four muscles. There are three layers of circular muscles running from posterior to anterior; plus, a long bilateral strap muscle running longitudinally in the midline. The three circumferential muscles are:

1. The *external abdominal oblique* runs from the external surface of ribs 5–12 and circles around the abdominal wall anteriorly to insert into the linea alba, pubic tubercle, and iliac crest. The orientation of the fibers can be mimicked by putting your hands in your pockets. The testes and spermatic cord pierce the external abdominal oblique at the *superficial inguinal ring*, which is superior to the inguinal ligament. The *inguinal ligament* is the curled-under edge of the external abdominal oblique. The *lacunar ligament* is a small, thickened piece that forms the medial wall of the femoral ring.
2. Deep to the external oblique is the *internal abdominal oblique* whose fibers run from the iliac crest, thoracolumbar fascia and ASIS to the linea alba. At the most anteromedial corner of the muscle, the fibers run posterior to the spermatic cord to contribute to the conjoint tendon which inserts into the *pecten pubis*.
3. Deep to the internal oblique is the *transversus abdominis* running from the internal surfaces of the costal cartilages of ribs 7–12, iliac crest, thoracolumbar fascia, and inguinal ligament to the linea alba and via the conjoint tendon to the pecten pubis.

The *rectus abdominus* is the bilateral midline muscle with fibers running superior to inferior. The fibers are attached superiorly to the xiphoid process and the costal cartilages of ribs 5–7. Inferiorly the fibers are attached to the pubic symphysis and pubic crest. The muscle is interrupted by three to four tendinous intersections running laterally across the muscle. Theses tendinous intersections divide the muscle up into smaller sections, giving rise to the term in body builders of 4-pack or 6-pack. The lateral edge of the muscle is referred to as the *linea semilunaris*. The linea semilunaris is not a straight line but has a slight curve to it. Between the two halves of the rectus abdominus is the centrally located *linea alba*.

## Arcuate Line

The fibers from the three circular muscles all have an interesting organization as they approach the linea semilunaris and rectus abdominus. The *arcuate line* is found inferior to the umbilicus and is a landmark for the organization of these muscles. There are differences above versus below the arcuate line in how the muscles surround the rectus abdominus.

Above the arcuate line the external abdominal oblique passes anterior to the rectus abdominus. The internal abdominal oblique splits to go around the rectus abdominus, and the transversus abdominus runs posterior (behind) the rectus abdominus. Above the arcuate line, these circumferential muscles form a strong tough membrane on both sides of the rectus abdominus, referred to, respectively, as either the *anterior layer of the rectus sheath*, or the *posterior layer of the rectus*

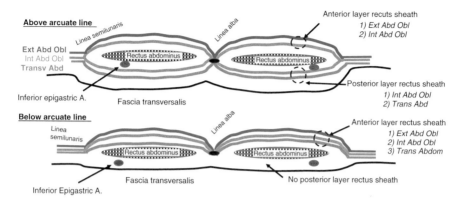

**Fig. 3.2** Rectus sheath. Note the relationship of the three muscles of the anterior abdominal wall and their relationship to the rectus abdominus above versus below the arcuate line. Note the location of inferior epigastric artery above and below the line. (Leo 2022)

*sheath*. Deep (or posterior) to the posterior layer of the rectus sheath is the *transversalis fascia* (Fig. 3.2).

Below the arcuate line there is a somewhat subtle difference in the organization of the layers. The fascia of all three muscles – the external oblique, internal oblique, and transversus abdominus – all pass in front of rectus abdominus. Thus, below the arcuate line, there is an anterior layer of the rectus sheath, but no corresponding posterior layer of rectus sheath. Below the arcuate line, the layer behind the rectus abdominus, is the fascia transversalis.

## Anterior Abdominal Wall Hernias

Because of the potential weak spots in the abdominal wall, abdominal contents can herniate through these weaknesses. *Epigastric* hernias are rare but will be found in the epigastric space. *Umbilical* hernias, also known as paraumbilical hernias, herniate through the umbilicus. *Hypogastric* hernias occur in the midline between umbilicus and pubic symphysis. *Spigelian* hernias are found lateral to the recuts abdominus at the linea alba, typically below the arcuate line. *Incisional* hernias occur along the scars from prior surgeries where two pieces of the abdominal wall were sutured together.

## Blood Supply to Anterior Abdominal Wall

The blood supply to the anterior abdominal wall comes from ascending branches that start in the thoracic, and other branches that start down in the pelvic area. Where these descending and ascending branches meet on the abdominal wall are important sites of anastomoses, all with significant clinical importance. There are essentially two parallel tracts for the vessels, one is superficial to the fascia, and one is deeper.

1. Deep to the fascia, *the superior epigastric artery* comes off the internal thoracic artery near the xiphoid process and descends along the anterior abdominal wall towards the umbilicus. Meanwhile, the *inferior epigastric artery* is a branch of the external iliac artery right before it goes under the inguinal ligament, and it ascends towards the umbilicus. It passes upward along the anterior abdominal wall forming a fold of tissue called the *lateral umbilical ligament*. As the inferior epigastric travels up the anterior wall, initially it is found between the rectus abdominus and the fascia transversalis, but more superiorly it is found between the rectus abdominus and the posterior layer of the rectus sheath. The superior and inferior epigastric arteries form an anastomosis on the anterior abdominal wall. This is an anastomosis between branches of the subclavian artery and branches of the external iliac artery.

2. Superficial to the fascia *the thoracoepigastric veins* meet with the *superficial epigastric veins*. The thoracoepigastric veins, found on the anterolateral abdominal wall in the mid-clavicular line, drain into the lateral thoracic vein (which ultimately drains into the superior vena cava). Meanwhile the superficial epigastric veins drain into the great saphenous vein which in turn drains into the femoral vein located in the femoral triangle. These two veins meet on the lateral abdominal wall and represent an anastomosis between the superior vena cava and inferior vena cava. Thus, swollen veins in the lateral anterior wall could be due to a blockage of the inferior vena cava. Because these veins are superficial, when they become dilated it will be readily apparent on a physical exam (Fig. 3.3).

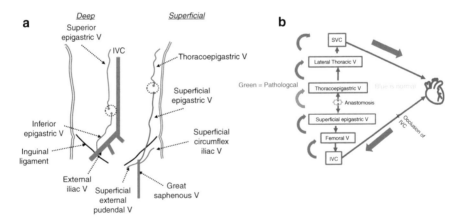

**Fig. 3.3** Anterior Abdominal Wall Venous Drainage. Panel (**a**) On the patient's right side. The deep drainage is shown with the anastomosis between the inferior epigastric vein and the superior epigastric vein. On the patient's left side, the superficial drainage is shown between the superficial epigastric vein and the thoracoepigastric vein. Panel (**b**) shows how a blockage of the IVC could lead to dilated vessels of the anterior abdominal wall. (Leo 2022)

## Paraumbilical Veins with Superficial Epigastric Veins

The *paraumbilical veins* are small veins around the umbilicus which ascend along the anterior wall to drain into the portal vein. The paraumbilical veins anastomose with the *superficial epigastric veins*. This is an anastomosis between portal vein and inferior vena cava. *Portal hypertension* will lead to these veins being dilated.

## Inguinal Canal

During fetal development the testes and ovaries start off in the abdominal region, and then migrate down towards their final adult locations. The ovaries remain in the pelvic cavity, but the testes will push through the anterior abdominal wall to migrate to the scrotum dragging with them all the structures they contact during their migration.

At the fifth month of development the testes are sitting in the abdominal cavity right above the inguinal ligament behind the *fascia transversalis*. They eventually push through this fascia forming an opening called the *deep inguinal ring* which is just lateral to the inferior epigastric artery. Now that they have pushed through the fascia, they continue their migration anterior to the fascia transversalis (Fig. 3.4).

Moving anterior, the next layer is a muscle, *transversus abdominus* which runs from the AISIS, arches over the deep inguinal ring, runs behind the spermatic cord, and attaches to the pubic tubercle (Fig. 3.4).

In front of the transversus abdominus is the *internal abdominal oblique*, which runs from the ASIS and the lateral one-third of the inguinal ligament, passes

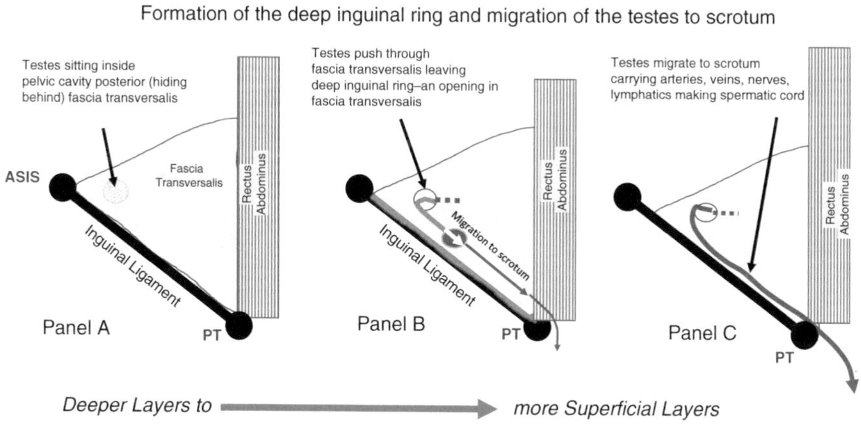

Formation of the deep inguinal ring and migration of the testes to scrotum

**Fig. 3.4** In panel (**a**), at the fifth-month of fetal development, the testes are sitting behind (posterior) to the fascia transversalis. In panel (**b**) the testes have pushed through the fascia transversalis and formed the deep inguinal ring. The testes now descend parallel to the inguinal ligament, and anterior to the fascia transversalis forming the inguinal canal. In panel (**c**), the testes have migrated all the way to the scrotum. (Leo 2022)

anterior to the spermatic cord, and then runs medially behind the spermatic cord, with the transversus abdominus to attach to the pubic tubercle. The combination of the two small pieces of transversus abdominus and internal abdominal oblique that meet behind the spermatic cord near the pubic tubercle is referred to as the *conjoint tendon*, or "falx inguinalis".

The next layer is the external abdominal oblique with is fiber orientation of "hands in the pocket." Medial and superior to the pubic tubercle the spermatic cord pierces the external abdominal oblique at the *superficial inguinal ring* (Fig. 3.5).

As the test migrate through the anterior wall down towards the scrotum, they form the inguinal canal running from deep ring (an opening in fascia transversalis) to the superficial ring (an opening in the external abdominal oblique). In the male running in the inguinal canal is the spermatic cord, the ilioinguinal nerve and the genitofemoral nerve. In the female, is the round ligament and ilioinguinal nerve. Think of the canal as a hallway with a floor, a ceiling, an anterior wall, and a posterior wall. To visualize this, let's take a parasagittal cut through the inguinal canal between the superficial and deep rings.

1. The *floor* is the easiest layer to visualize as it is the inguinal ligament.
2. The *anterior wall* is the internal abdominal oblique, and the external abdominal oblique.
3. Clinically, the *posterior wall* is the most important, and it is subdivided into medial and lateral divisions. The *lateral* posterior wall is the relatively weak area

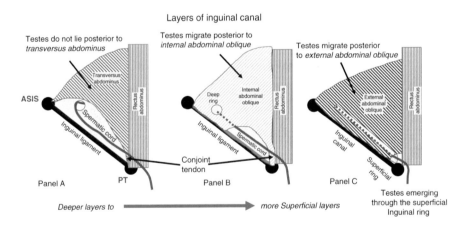

**Fig. 3.5** In panel (**a**), the testes have moved through the deep inguinal ring and migrated to scrotum. The internal abdominal oblique arises from the ASIS and arches over the inguinal canal to insert at the pubic tubercle as part of the conjoint tendon. In panel (**b**) the internal abdominal oblique arises from ASIS and portion of the inguinal ligament to arch over and anterior to the spermatic cord, forming part of the anterior wall of the inguinal canal. The **conjoint tendon** is made up of the combination of the medial corners of the transversus abdominus and internal abdominal oblique. In panel (**c**) the external abdominal oblique arises from ASIS and inguinal ligament to contribute to the anterior wall of the inguinal canal. The spermatic cord emerges through the external abdominal oblique forming the superficial inguinal ring. (Leo 2022)

consisting of the fascia transversalis, while the *medial* posterior wall is relatively strong conjoint tendon – composed of internal abdominal oblique and transversus abdominus.

4. The *roof* is composed of all three muscles (Fig. 3.6).

## Inguinal Ligament

The inguinal ligament is the turned under edge of the external abdominal oblique running from the ASIS to the pubic tubercle. It is an important landmark for various clinical scenarios. The external iliac artery passes from the abdominopelvic cavity underneath the inguinal ligament to enter the thigh in the femoral triangle. Just before it enters the thigh it gives off the inferior epigastric artery which runs in a superomedial direction. The femoral artery runs with the femoral nerve and femoral vein. This is discussed in detail with the lower limb chapter (Fig. 3.7).

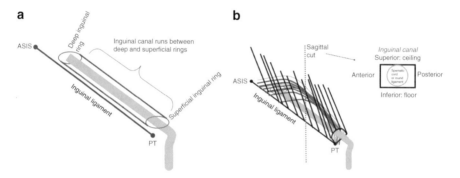

**Fig. 3.6** Panel (**a**) shows the path of the spermatic cord through the inguinal canal from deep to superficial ring. Panel (**b**) shows the inguinal canal covered by the external abdominal oblique and the internal abdominal oblique. The sagittal cut through the canal shows the four sides of the canal. (Leo 2022)

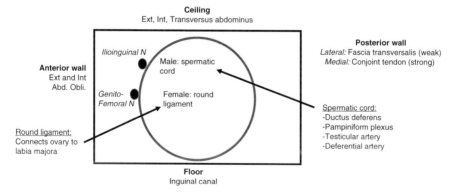

**Fig. 3.7** Boundaries of the inguinal canal. (Leo 2022)

## Indirect Inguinal Hernia

Indirect inguinal hernias start off at the deep inguinal ring. They are more common in males than females. In an elderly male, for instance, because of the defect in the anterior abdominal wall, increased pressure on the anterior wall can lead to abdominal contents herniating through the deep inguinal ring. Thus, the initial outpocketing of the hernia will be lateral to the pulse of the inferior epigastric artery. Once the hernia is in the deep ring it can then travel down through the canal to eventually exit at the superficial ring to continue to the scrotum. If the hernia travels as far as the superficial ring it will be found superior to the pubic tubercle. The indirect inguinal hernia will typically be medial to the pubic tubercle, but it can vary, and it will sometimes be found lateral to it. This is most likely a function of the individual's body weight.

## Direct Inguinal Hernias

In contrast to the pathway of indirect inguinal hernias, a *direct inguinal hernia* will come through the wall at *Hesselbach's triangle*, which is bounded by the inferior epigastric artery, the lateral border of rectus abdominus, and the inguinal ligament. Direct inguinal hernias will be medial to the pulse of the inferior epigastric artery. *Femoral hernias* which are discussed in more detail with the lower limb will push through a weakness in the femoral sheath just medial to the femoral vein. The hernia will enter through the femoral ring and enter the femoral canal, which is the medial compartment of the femoral sheath. On examination, femoral hernias will be inferior to the inguinal ligament and, typically, lateral to the pubic tubercle (Fig. 3.8).

## Process Vaginalis

As the testes descend towards the scrotum, they drag a piece of the peritoneal cavity with them. This *tunica vaginalis* is continuous with the peritoneal cavity via the *processes vaginalis*. This processes vaginalis will eventually degenerate so that the tunica vaginalis is completely separated from the peritoneal cavity. If the communication remains, it is referred to as a *persistent process vaginalis* and is a predisposing factor for a congenital indirect inguinal hernia. A *hydrocele* is a collection of fluid in the tunica vaginalis. A light shown behind it can lead to a red glow.

## Trapezoid of Disaster

If you are inside the pelvic cavity, looking at the posterior surface of the anterior abdominal wall in the region of the inguinal canal there are a significant number of structures that must be considered during surgery in this region. Surgeons

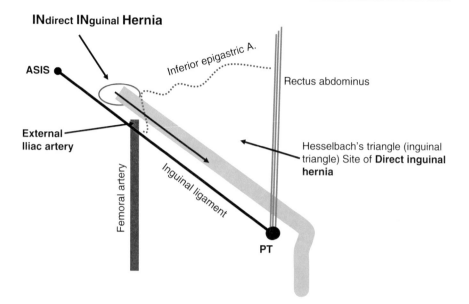

**Fig. 3.8** Inguinal hernias. Indirect hernias start lateral to the inferior epigastric artery. Direct inguinal hernias start medial to the inferior epigastric artery. (Leo 2022)

sometimes refer to this region as the *trapezoid of doom*, which is a combination of two triangles:

1. The *triangle of pain* is made up of iliopubic tract, testicular vessels, and perito-neal fold. It gets its name because there are several nerves in this triangle: femo-ral, lateral femoral cutaneous, genitofemoral, and ilioinguinal.
2. The *triangle of doom* is bounded by the vas deferens, testicular vessels, and peritoneal fold and contains the external iliac artery and vein (Fig. 3.9).

## Layers of Spermatic Cord

As the testes migrate down to scrotum, they will carry with them the layers that they touch on their journey. The fascia transversalis will become the internal spermatic fascia. Because the testes never touch the transversus abdominus on their way, the transversus abdominus does not get dragged down into the scrotum. The internal abdominal oblique becomes the cremaster muscle and fascia. The external abdomi-nal oblique becomes the external spermatic fascia.

There are three important nerves in the region of the inguinal canal.

1. The *genitofemoral nerve* comes from L1 and as it approaches the inguinal canal it splits into two branches: the femoral branch goes deep to the inguinal ligament and is responsible for cutaneous sensation to the anteromedial thigh. The genital

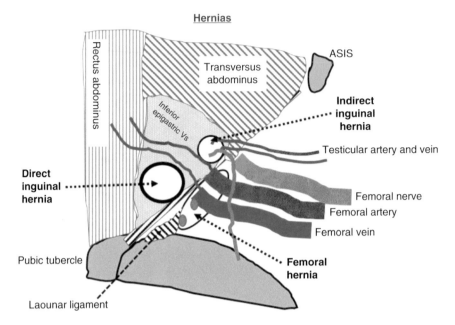

**Fig. 3.9** Hernias. This is an internal view. You are in the abdominal pelvic cavity looking at the structures passing from pelvic cavity to the thigh. Indirect inguinal hernias are located lateral to the inferior epigastric artery. Direct Inguinal hernias are medial to the artery. Femoral hernias are inferior to the inguinal ligament. (Leo 2022)

branch innervates the cremaster muscle and joins the inguinal canal at about the halfway point. It does not travel through the deep ring, but it does travel through the superficial ring. A test for L1 is the cremaster reflex which is tested by scratching the anteromedial thigh which is sensed up by the femoral branch of genitofemoral (or in some cases by ilioinguinal nerve since there is considerable overlap), and then the cremaster muscle contracts via efferent signals in the genital branch of genitofemoral.

2. The *ilioinguinal nerve* comes from L1 and enters the spermatic cord. Along with the genitofemoral nerve, it can be damaged during inguinal surgery.
3. The *iliohypogastric nerve* also comes from L1. It runs parallel but superior to the ilioinguinal nerve. The iliohypogastric can be injured during an appendectomy. Both the ilioinguinal and iliohypogastric nerves go to the anterior abdominal wall muscles.

Within the spermatic cord are several important structures: (1) the *ductus deferens* which is carrying sperm towards the urethra, (2) the *deferential artery* which supplies blood to the vas deferens, (3) the *testicular artery* carrying blood to the testes, and (4) the *pampiniform plexus* which is the beginning of the testicular vein. On the left, the testicular vein drains into the left renal vein; on the right, it drains into the inferior vena cava. A *varicocele* is a collection of blood pooling in the pampiniform plexus due to a blockage of the testicular vein. When the patient goes from standing to lying down, the varicocele will become smaller, as the blood has an easier time draining.

In the females inguinal canal there is the *round ligament* which connects the labia majora to the uterus. Both the *round ligament* and the *ovarian ligament* are remnants of the *gubernaculum.*

Also in this region is *circle of death*, sometimes referred to as the *corona mortis.* This name comes from a common variation formed by an arterial anastomosis in some individuals. Normally the obturator artery comes off the anterior division of the internal iliac artery and perforates the obturator foramen to enter the medial thigh. In addition, the external iliac usually gives off the inferior epigastric artery to ascend along the anterior abdominal wall. In some individuals, there is a small artery that comes off the inferior epigastric artery and connects to the obturator artery. This small communication is in the vicinity of the lacunar ligament and femoral ring. A surgeon making an anterior approach from the medial thigh to the femoral ring needs to be cognizant of this potential variation. If this artery is nicked during this procedure a significant amount of blood will fill the surgical field. In addition, the blood will collect in the abdominopelvic cavity, thus the name *"circle of death."*

## Abdominal Cavity

### The Diaphragm

The abdominal cavity is bounded superiorly by the diaphragm, which is the most important muscle for inspiration. It is a sheet of muscle originating anteriorly from the xiphoid process and ribs 7–12. It runs laterally along rib 12 to insert along the posterior abdominal wall by the crura. The muscle fibers run from the perimeter towards the center, converging to form the *central tendon.* Along the posterior wall the attachment of the diaphragm forms the *medial and lateral arcuate ligaments* around the anterior portions of the psoas major and quadratus lumborum muscles. When the diaphragm contracts, it expands the thoracic space and creates a negative pressure so that air moves into the lungs. There are three major openings in the diaphragm:

1. the *caval hiatus* at the level of T8 with the inferior vena cava, and the right phrenic nerve.
2. the *esophageal hiatus* at the level of T10 with the esophagus and the anterior and posterior vagal trunks, and esophageal branches of the left gastric artery.
3. the *aortic hiatus* at the level of T12 with the aorta, azygous vein, and thoracic duct. The thoracic duct lies just posterior to the esophagus.

A useful saying for the levels and hiatuses is **I E**at **A**pples, 8, 10, 12. **I**nferior vena cava, **E**sophagus, and **A**orta at T8, T10, and T12 respectively.

Another saying for the hiatus is ***Three gooses And A Duck***, standing for the Esophagoose, right vagoose, and left vagoose which travel through the esophageal hiatus, and **A**orta, **A**zygous vein, and thoracic **Duck** traveling together through the aortic hiatus.

The diaphragm develops from four different regions, all of which eventually fuse together to from the mature diaphragm.

1. The central portion of the diaphragm starts in the cervical region. This *septum transversum* will eventually migrate inferiorly to form the *central tendon* of the diaphragm. By the end of week 8 it lies near the lumbar vertebrae.
2. Before all the various regions of the diaphragm fuse, the spaces on either side of the septum transversum are referred to as the *pericardioperitoneal canals*. These canals will eventually be closed by the *pleuroperitoneal membranes* which is the original separation between the pleural and peritoneal cavities.
3. The *dorsal esophageal mesentery* surrounds the esophagus and fuses with the pleuroperitoneal membrane. It will eventually become the *crura* of the diaphragm.
4. All these above-named pieces will eventually fuse with outgrowths of the *lateral body wall* that become the edges or peripheral portions of the diaphragm.

The right and left crura arise from the vertebral bodies of L1-L3 and run anterior to encircle the esophageal hiatus. Some of the fibers of the right crus pass to the left between the aortic and esophageal hiatuses to contribute to the *lower esophageal sphincter. Achalasia* refers to the failure of the sphincter to relax which leads to the bolus backing up in the esophagus. The contracted sphincter leaves a very small opening for the bolus to trickle through. On a radiograph it resembles a bird's beak. The thickening of the crura anterior to the aortic hiatus is the *median arcuate ligament.*

The efferent nerve supply to the diaphragm comes from the *phrenic nerve* which comes from C3, 4, and 5. The afferents from the central tendon of the diaphragm travel on the phrenic nerve so pathology of either the superior or inferior surface of the central diaphragm will refer to the neck, or shoulder region, because of the phrenic nerve. However, pathology out on the lateral side of the diaphragm will refer to the body wall because of the intercostal nerves. As mentioned earlier, when the diaphragm contracts the dome of the diaphragm lowers. And when the diaphragm relaxes the dome elevates. So, damage to a phrenic nerve will lead to the dome moving superiorly. Damage to one phrenic nerve is typically asymptomatic, while bilateral damage can lead to more severe deficits.

The major arteries to the diaphragm come are the *superior phrenic arteries*, which come from the thoracic aorta, and the inferior phrenic arteries, which are branches of the abdominal aorta. As the internal thoracic artery descends on the anterior wall near the sternum it eventually divides into two branches: (1) *the musculophrenic*, and (2) *the superior epigastric.* The musculophrenic branch contributes to the diaphragm. In the neck, the internal thoracic artery gives off a small *pericardiacophrenic* artery which runs with the phrenic nerve to the diaphragm.

A *congenital diaphragmatic hernia* is a malformation that arises because of a failure of the pleuroperitoneal membranes to fuse. This can lead to a defect in the posterolateral portion of the diaphragm, usually found on the left side. In many cases the intestines will be found in the thorax. If the herniation is large enough it can prevent proper lung development and the lung will be smaller than normal *(pulmonary hypoplasia),* which in turn can lead to pulmonary hypertension. Thus, in an infant born with congenital diaphragmatic hernia the pertinent question for viability concerns the state of lung development.

## Abdominal Aorta and Inferior Vena Cava

The abdominal aorta enters the abdomen at the T12 vertebra through the aortic hiatus. Accompanying the aorta are the azygous vein and the thoracic duct. There are unpaired and paired branches coming off the aorta. The three unpaired branches supply the GI tract (Fig. 3.10).

Right as the aorta enters the abdomen it gives two paired branches, *the right and left inferior phrenic arteries* which head towards the diaphragm. Coming off at T12 is the *celiac trunk* supplying the foregut and related structures. Coming off at the superior border of L1 is the *superior mesenteric artery* (SMA) supplying the midgut. Also located at the L1 level, are the paired renal arteries. Moving down the aorta are the *right and left gonadal arteries* to either the testes or ovaries. And coming off at L3 is the *inferior mesenteric artery* (IMA) to the hindgut. Coming off the aorta, between the SMA and IMA, in the lumber region are the four to five lumbar arteries. The aorta ends at the L4 level by bifurcating into the *two common iliac arteries*, which in turn splits into *internal and external iliac arteries.*

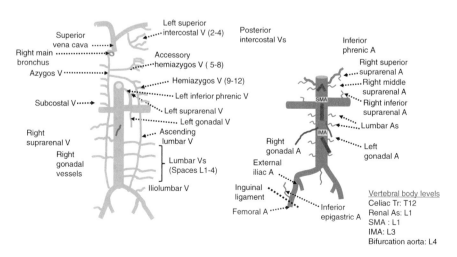

**Fig. 3.10** Panel (**a**) shows the inferior vena cava and its branches. Panel (**b**) shows the abdominal aorta and its branches. (Leo 2022)

## Inferior Vena Cava

The inferior vena cava (IVC) starts at the L5 vertebra where the two common iliac veins merge together. Moving up the IVC there are 4–5 *lumbar veins* draining into the IVC and related structures. There is significant variation here. For instance, in some cases the fifth lumbar vein will drain into the common iliac, and in some cases, the second lumbar vein enters the left renal vein. Because of this variation, various books will show slightly different patterns for the lumbar veins. However, regardless of the variations, an important anastomotic channel is formed by the *ascending lumbar veins* which run parallel to the IVC and connect the common iliac and iliolumbar veins in the pelvic region with the azygous, and hemi-azygos veins in the thorax. If the IVC is blocked these ascending channels provide an alternate path for the return of blood to the heart (Fig. 3.10).

The *right gonadal vein* drains directly into the IVC, while the *left gonadal vein* drains into the left renal vein, which in turn drains into the IVC. Because of this relationship, a mass on the kidney that blocks the left gonadal vein will lead to a varicocele which arises from blood backing up in the gonads. Thus, a swollen left testicle could be indicative of a mass on the left renal vein. Each adrenal gland also has typically one vein. A *varicocele* will tend to enlarge when the patient is standing, and then shrink when they are lying down. On the right side, the adrenal vein drains into the IVC, and on the left it drains into the left renal vein.

Draining into the IVC near the diaphragm are the right and *left inferior phrenic veins*. On the right side this vein has a descending branch that connects with the left renal vein in the vicinity of the left suprarenal vein.

As the IVC it approaches the liver it forms the posterior wall of the epiploic foramen and then continues posterior to the liver making a groove or tunnel that separates the right and caudate lobes of the liver. As the IVC ascends it pushed slightly anteriorly by the diaphragm.

## Abdominal Contents

Let's start with the GI tract as a simple tube with the mouth at one end, and the anal canal at the other end. The entire tract is surrounded by muscle, either smooth or skeletal. At the ends of the tract, the muscles are sphincters formed by a combination of smooth muscle and skeletal muscle. Other than the ends, the rest of the tract is surrounded by smooth muscle. The skeletal muscle at the ends is controlled by somatic nervous system, while the smooth muscle sections are controlled by autonomic nerves, mostly parasympathetic. The organization of the abdomen is all based on the divisions of foregut, midgut, and hindgut. Starting at the beginning of the stomach, the foregut includes the: stomach, the first part of the duodenum, and the top half of the second part of the duodenum. Halfway down the second part of the duodenum, at the greater duodenal papilla, the foregut turns into midgut. The midgut includes the second half of the second part of the duodenum, the third and fourth part of the duodenum, the jejunum, ileum, cecum, ascending colon, and two-thirds of the transverse colon. Close to the splenic flexure, the midgut turns into hindgut. The hindgut then includes the distal one-third of the transverse colon, the descending colon, the sigmoid colon, the rectum, and anal canal. The hindgut ends at the pectinate line. Below the pectinate line we are back to skeletal muscle and somatic nervous system.

There are three main arteries to the GI tract, *the celiac trunk, the superior mesenteric,* and *inferior mesenteric arteries.* All three of these arteries are unpaired arteries arising from the abdominal aorta. The celiac artery goes to the foregut, the superior mesenteric to the midgut, and inferior mesenteric to the hindgut. We will see that the organization of the lymphatics and the nerve supply is all based on these three arteries. For instance, the celiac nodes are responsible for lymphatic drainage from the foregut, superior mesenteric nodes from the midgut, and inferior mesenteric nodes from the hindgut (Fig. 3.11).

## Peritoneum

The peritoneum is a closed empty cavity within the abdominopelvic cavity. There is nothing in the peritoneal cavity. The only thing that normally opens into it is the uterine tube. Imagine you have a balloon filled with air, and you make an incision in

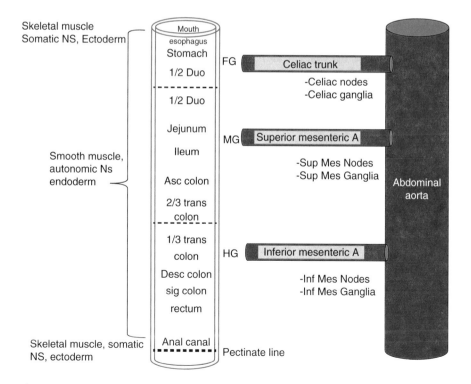

**Fig. 3.11** Foregut, midgut, and hindgut. (Leo 2022)

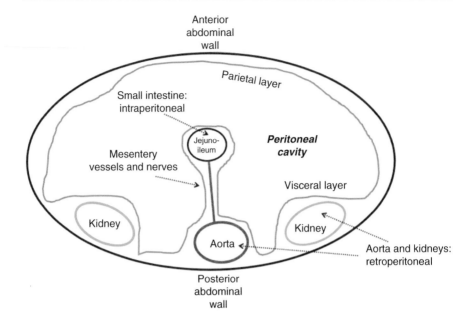

**Fig. 3.12** Peritoneal cavity. The aorta and kidneys are retroperitoneal structures, while the jejunoileum is intraperitoneal. The jejenoileum is connected to the posterior abdominal wall by the
dorsal mesentery. (Leo 2022)

the anterior abdominal wall and stuff the balloon into the abdomen and then suture
the incision closed. The balloon is going to wrap around the abdominal contents.
The cavity of the balloon represents the closed peritoneal cavity. You can see in
Fig. 3.12 that some structures are completely enclosed by the balloon, while other
structures lie behind the balloon. In the diagram, structures like the aorta and kidneys are behind the balloon and are referred to as *retroperitoneal*. Structures like the
jejunoileum are surrounded by peritoneum and are referred to as *intraperitoneal*
(Fig. 3.12).

The portion of the peritoneum that abuts the anterior wall is referred to as *parietal peritoneum*, while the layer surrounding organs is referred to as the *visceral
peritoneum*. Between these two layers – visceral and parietal – is the peritoneal cavity.

The peritoneum is further divided into several compartments. The first major
division is into the *greater sac* and *lesser sac (omental bursa)*. If you make an incision into the anterior abdominal wall, you are entering the greater sac, which makes
up the majority of the peritoneal cavity. However, behind the stomach is another
space – *the lesser sac*. The doorway between the greater and lesser sacs is the *epiploic foramen.* If you are standing at the right side of a donor and you put your finger in the opening behind the *hepatoduodenal ligament*, part of the lesser omentum,
you are moving from the greater sac into the lesser sac. The ceiling of the epiploic
foramen is the caudate lobe of the liver (Fig. 3.13).

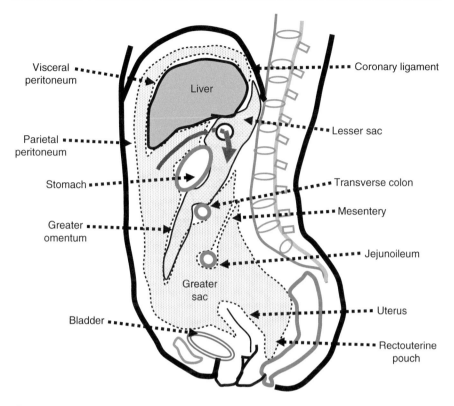

**Fig. 3.13** Greater and lesser sacs. The red arrow is moving from the greater sac (in red) through the epiploic foramen into the lesser sac (in green) behind the lesser omentum. (Leo 2022)

The *hepatoduodenal* and *hepatogastric ligaments* make up the lesser omentum. Running in the hepatoduodenal ligament are three structures: (1) *the portal vein*, (2) *bile duct,* and (3) *common hepatic artery*. However, we also need to pay attention to the organization of these three structures in the ligament. The portal vein is the most posterior structure, with the bile duct being anterolateral, and the hepatic artery being anteromedial. During surgery if you clamp off the hepatoduodenal ligament then you have blocked everything going into and out of the liver. This is called a "pringle maneuver." In Fig. 3.14 the pad of the finger is against the portal vein, and the fingernail is against the inferior vena cava.

Keep in mind that this hepatoduodenal ligament is the anterior wall of the epiploic foramen. If you keep moving your finger towards the midline your finger is now further into the lesser sac, with the lesser omentum and stomach in front of your finger, and the pancreas and posterior abdominal wall behind it. The inferior border of the lesser omentum is the transverse mesocolon. An ulcer of the stomach that burrows through the posterior stomach wall will lead to contents collecting in the lesser sac with subsequent back pain because of aggravation of the pancreas (Fig. 3.14).

The greater sac is further subdivided into the *supracolic* and *infracolic* compartments which are separated by the transverse mesocolon and greater omentum. The supracolic compartment contains the stomach, liver, and spleen. The infra colic compartment contains the small intestine, ascending colon, and descending colon (Fig. 3.15).

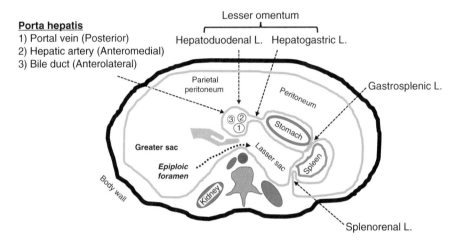

**Fig. 3.14** Porta hepatis. The epiploic foramen is the doorway between the greater sac and the lesser sac of the peritoneal cavity. The finger in the picture is going through the epiploic foramen, posterior to hepatoduodenal ligament. The finger-nail is against the inferior vena cava, and the pad of the finger is against the portal vein. Note the specific location of location of the three structures in the hepatoduodenal ligament making up the porta hepatis. (Leo 2022)

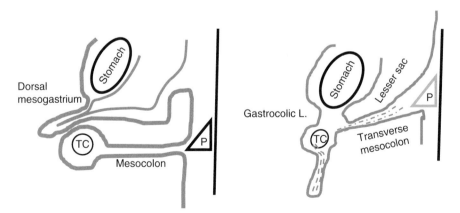

**Fig. 3.15** Panel (**a**) The pancreas becomes a retroperitoneal organ during developmental and is considered a secondary retroperitoneal organ. Panel (**b**) The transverse mesocolon is a derivative of dorsal mesentery formed by the fusion of the posterior leaf of the dorsal mesogastrium with the mesentery of the midgut. Posterior to the stomach is the lesser sac. An ulcer in the posterior wall of the stomach that perforates the wall can drain into the lesser sac. (Leo 2022)

The supracolic and infracolic compartments are connected by two gutters, (1) the *right paracolic gutter* which is to the right of ascending colon, and (2) *left paracolic gutter*, which is to the left of the descending colon. The paracolic gutter on each side connects with the respective right and left anterior subphrenic spaces found on each side between the diaphragm and the liver. Think of the paracolic gutters like hallways connecting one room to another (Fig. 3.16).

The infracolic compartment is in turn divided into the *right and left infracolic spaces* which are separated by the dorsal mesentery.

On the right side, between the liver and the kidney is the *hepatorenal recess* (Morrison's pouch) which is a subdivision of the peritoneal cavity. The posterosuperior edge of this recess is the posterior layer of the coronary ligament. When a patient is lying down, excess fluid in the peritoneal cavity will typically collect here. As the patient sits up, the fluid will tend to drain into *the rectouterine pouch* in the female or the *rectovesical pouch* in the male (Fig. 3.17).

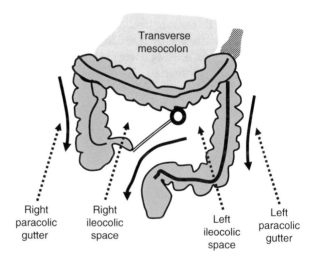

**Fig. 3.16** Ileocolic spaces. (Leo 2022)

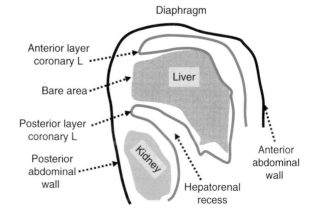

**Fig. 3.17** Peritoneum and the liver. The visceral peritoneum comes up on the diaphragmatic surface of the liver and is reflected onto the undersurface of the diaphragm as the anterior layer of the coronary ligament. On the visceral surface of the liver the reflection creates the hepatorenal recess between the liver and the kidney. (Leo 2022)

Two subdivisions of the peritoneal cavity also surround the liver. On the superior surface of the liver, between the liver and the diaphragm are the right and left *subphrenic spaces* (or suprahepatic spaces) bounded by the coronary ligaments, triangular ligaments, and falciform ligaments. Fluid collecting in the subphrenic space can aggravate the diaphragm leading to pain sensations felt in the neck and shoulder region.

Below the liver the *subhepatic space* (AKA: hepatorenal space or Morrison's Pouch) is a potential space that is normally closed but can open up in the presence of excess fluid. The subhepatic space is between the liver and the right kidney.

## Retroperitoneal Versus Intraperitoneal

The details will follow but it is useful to look at the big picture first when talking about intraperitoneal versus retroperitoneal. If you go down the GI tract from top to bottom, you will see that we alternate between intra and retro. Starting with the stomach and the first part of the duodenum, they are intraperitoneal structures. And intraperitoneal structures by definition have a mesentery. In this case, the greater and lesser omentum. Moving down the tract, the second, third, and fourth part of the duodenum are retroperitoneal. Then the jejunoileum is intraperitoneal (dorsal mesentery). Then the ascending colon is retro; the transverse colon is intraperitoneal (transverse mesocolon); the descending colon is retroperitoneal; and the sigmoid colon is intraperitoneal (sigmoid mesocolon); and finally, the rectum and anal canal are retroperitoneal (or sub peritoneal) (Table 3.1).

**Table 3.1** Intra versus retro peritoneal

### Intra or Retro Peritoneal

|  | Intra or Retro | Peritoneal Folds |
|---|---|---|
| Stomach, 1<sup>st</sup> part Duodenum | Intra | Greater and Lesser Omentum |
| 2, 3, 4<sup>th</sup> parts Duodenum | Retro | |
| Jenuno-illeum | Intra | Dorsal Mesentery "The Mesentery" |
| Ascending Colon | Retro | |
| Transverse Colon | Intra | Transverse Mesocolon |
| Descending Colon | Retro | |
| Sigmoid Colon | Intra | Sigmoid Mesocolon |
| Rectum | Sub | |

## Peritoneal Dialysis

Waste products can be removed from the blood via peritoneal dialysis by using the peritoneum as a filter. A tube is inserted into the peritoneal cavity and fluid (the dialysate) is then passed into the peritoneal cavity. There are several types of peritoneal dialysis, but they are all based on the idea that the dialysate will remain in the peritoneum for a set amount of time (the dwell) to pull the waste products from the blood stream. The dialysate with the waste products is then removed and discarded. Care must be taken so that the catheter site does not become infected as it could lead to peritonitis.

## Foregut

### Stomach

The esophagus turns into the stomach at the diaphragm. This region of the stomach is referred to as the *cardia*. The lower esophageal sphincter, which is a physiological sphincter is present at this junction. Its job is to open when a bolus of food comes down the esophagus to enter the stomach, and to then close after food enters the stomach. The *phrenoesophageal ligament* attaches the diaphragm to the esophagus to help the two structures operate together. The *fundus* is the top of the stomach and is often filed with air on a barium swallow test. As the stomach approaches the duodenum, it looks something like a funnel as it narrows. The large part of the funnel is the antrum, which in turn narrows down to the pyloric region. The *lesser curvature* is towards the right and facing superior. Attached to the lesser curvature is the *lesser omentum,* made up of the hepatoduodenal and hepatogastric ligaments. The *greater curvature* is facing inferior and it is attached to the greater omentum which is made up of the gastro-phrenic, gastro-splenic, and gastro-omental ligaments.

There are several features that help to keep food in the stomach and prevent backflow into the esophagus. The *angle of His* is the angle between the fundus of the stomach and esophagus. In this region, there is also a loose flap of tissue referred to as the *gastroesophageal flap valve* that serves as a flap to prevent contents going back into the esophagus. When contents move into the stomach, air will push up on the fundus which in turn puts pressure on the gastroesophageal flap valve at the angle of His making it harder for stomach contents to move into the esophagus.

There are two related pathologies in the region of the gastroesophageal junction.

1. A *sliding hiatal hernia* occurs when a portion of the stomach herniates into the thorax. The main characteristic of it is that is moves back and forth between stomach and thorax. During swallowing it can move into the thorax but then can move back to stomach – It slides.
2. A *paraesophageal hernia* refers to the stomach herniating into the thorax alongside the esophagus. The herniated stomach becomes lodged in the thorax and

stays there. It does not move back and forth like a sliding hiatal hernia. Thus, the gastroesophageal junction is fixed.

After eating a meal, food will remain in the stomach for several hours. The stomach has three layers of muscle, which are involved in the mechanical aspect of digestion: (1) an outer longitudinal, (2) a circular layer, and (3) and an inner oblique layer. These robust muscles layers allow for strong movements of the stomach to break down food into smaller parts. For the chemical component of digestion, the stomach has two important cell types:

1. *Chief cells* which secrete pepsinogen, which in an acidic environment is converted to pepsin, and gastric lipase.
2. *Parietal cells* secreting HCL, to create an acidic environment, and intrinsic factor which is necessary for the absorption of B12 in the duodenum. Intrinsic factor binds to B12 in the duodenum and is than shuttled across the walls of the ileum to enter the bloodstream. In a patient who has had their stomach removed they need an outside source of intrinsic factor.
3. *G Cells* produced gastrin which increase motility.
4. *D Cells* or somatostatin producing cells produce somatostatin which has inhibitory effects on parietal cells and G cells, thus it reduces the production of HCL and gastrin. D cells are also located in the duodenum and pancreatic islets.
5. *Enterochromaffin cells* produce serotonin which increases peristalsis.
6. *Enterochromaffin-like cells* in the fundus produce histamine which stimulates parietal cells via the H2 receptor to release HCL. Medications such as ranitidine block the H2 receptor.

During this initial phase of digestion, the pyloric sphincter will remain closed. Eventually, typically after 2 or 3 hours, it will open to allow the chyme to move into the duodenum.

Peptic ulcers are found in the stomach and duodenum. Stomach ulcers will typically lead to pain right after eating while duodenal ulcers will cause pain several hours after eating. *Helicobacter pylori* bacteria in the gastrointestinal tract is a predisposing factor for peptic ulcers. Long term use of non-steroidal anti-inflammatory medications (NSAIDs) can cause peptic ulcers.

## Greater and Lesser Omentum

The *lesser omentum* is attached to the lesser curvature. And the greater omentum is attached to the greater curvature. However, there are important subdivisions and details to both of these structures. The lesser omentum is made up of two parts (Fig. 3.18):

1. the *hepatoduodenal ligament* runs from the liver to the first part of the duodenum and forms the anterior wall of the epiploic foramen.

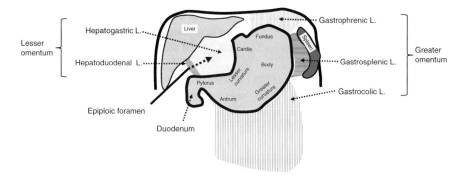

**Fig. 3.18** The stomach is suspended in the abdomen by the lesser and greater omentums. The greater omentum is attached to the greater curvature and is made up of the gastrophrenic, gastrosplenic, and gastrocolic ligaments. The lesser omentum is attached to the lesser curvature and is made up of the hepatogastric and hepatoduodenal ligaments. (Leo 2022)

2. the *hepatogastric ligament* runs from the liver to the stomach and forms the majority of the lesser omentum. It makes up the anterior wall of the lesser sac.

The greater omentum is attached to greater curvature and the fundus of the stomach and is made up of three subdivisions:

1. the *gastrophrenic ligament* runs from the fundus to the diaphragm.
2. The *gastrosplenic ligament* runs from the left side of the greater curvature to the spleen and contains the short gastric arteries.
3. The *gastrocolic ligament* connects the stomach to the transverse colon and contains as the major portion of the greater omentum.

## Duodenum

A prominent characteristic of the duodenum is the presence of circular folds which are easily seen on a barium swallow test. However, the first part of duodenum does not have these folds and its surface is smooth, which is a radiological landmark seen between the stomach and the second part of the duodenum. It is sometimes referred to as the duodenal cap. There are four parts to the duodenum. The first part of the duodenum is intraperitoneal, but the second, third, and fourth parts are retroperitoneal. The first part crosses the L1 vertebra, the second part runs parallel to L2, and the third part crosses L3.

1. The first part of the duodenum starts at the pyloric sphincter. Posterior to the first part is the gastroduodenal artery and the common bile duct. This first part of the duodenum is the most common site for duodenal ulcers. Thus, an ulcer that destroys the posterior wall of the first part of the duodenum will attack the gastroduodenal artery and common bile duct. The hepatoduodenal ligament runs

from the liver to the first part of the duodenum. This ligament forms the anterior wall of the *epiploic foramen* and running in it is the portal vein, and branches of the bile duct, and hepatic artery. The first part of the duodenum is anterior to the hilum of the right kidney.

2. The second part of the duodenum has two prominent landmarks on the medial wall. The superior landmark is the *minor duodenal papilla* which is the opening of the accessory pancreatic duct. Moving inferior, the second landmark is the *greater duodenal papilla* which is the opening of the pancreatic duct. On a laparoscopic view, differentiating one papilla from the other can be difficult. One clue, or aid, is that the greater duodenal papilla has a piece of tissue or fold that descends from its inferior portion called the *longitudinal fold*. Thus, if you see the longitudinal fold then you are looking at the greater duodenal papilla. If you don't see the extra fold, then you are looking at the minor duodenal papilla. The anterior wall of the second part of the duodenum is crossed by the transverse colon. And the body of the gallbladder rests on top of the second part of the duodenum.

3. The third part of the duodenum crosses anterior to the aorta and posterior to the superior mesenteric artery. See below for a more detailed discussion.

4. The fourth and final portion of the duodenum is pulled superior by a ligament which is an extension of the right crus of the diaphragm. This ligament is called the *ligament of Treitz*, or the suspensory muscle of the duodenum, and is the dividing line between the end of the duodenum and the beginning of the jejunum.

At the ligament of Treitz, part of which is an extension of the right crus of the diaphragm, the duodenum turns into the jejunum. The ligament, which is made up of folded peritoneum, pulls up on the duodenum at this point. It is here where the retroperitoneal duodenum turns into the intraperitoneal jejunum. In the vicinity of this ligament, the jejunoileum can become twisted and herniated.

## Gastrinoma Triangle

The *gastrinoma triangle* is bounded by the cystic duct, the lateral side of the second part of the duodenum and part of the head of the pancreas. It is here in this triangle where the majority of gastric tumors are found (Fig. 3.19).

## Celiac Trunk

The celiac trunk is the artery of the foregut. It comes off the abdominal aorta at approximately T12. Right at its origin it has three branches.

1. The *splenic artery* runs behind the pancreas to the spleen where it is found in the *lienorenal ligament*. As it courses along the top of the pancreas it gives off several branches to the pancreas including the *dorsal pancreatic*, and *greater*

**Fig. 3.19** Gastrinoma triangle. The most common site of tumors arising from the gastrin secreting cells in the pancreas. (Leo 2022)

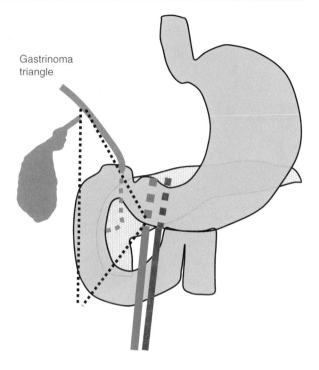

Gastrinoma triangle

*pancreatic* (pancreatica magna). Just before the pancreatic artery enters the spleen, it gives off several branches.

(i) The *short gastric* branches ascend to the fundus of the stomach int the gastrosplenic ligament.

(ii) The *left gastroepiploic* travels along the greater curvature of the stomach to eventually anastomose with the right gastroepiploic coming from the gastroduodenal artery.

2. The left gastric artery gives off *esophageal branches* to the esophagus and *gastric branches* to the lesser curvature of the stomach.

3. The *common hepatic artery* travels towards the right side heading towards the liver. It gives off the gastroduodenal artery. Distal to the branching of the gastroduodenal artery the common hepatic now becomes the proper hepatic.

The gastroduodenal artery terminates into the *anterior and posterior superior pancreaticoduodenal arteries* that perfuse the superior head of the pancreas and the top half of the second part of the duodenum. These two arteries anastomose with their counterparts from the superior mesenteric artery. These anterior and posterior pancreaticoduodenal arteries wrap around the common bile duct.

The *right gastric artery* heads towards the left side of the body run along the lesser curvature of the stomach and anastomoses with the left gastric artery (Fig. 3.20).

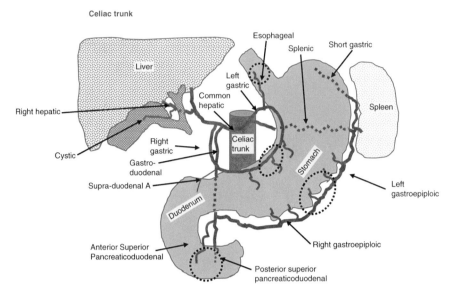

**Fig. 3.20** There are three branches of the celiac trunk: (1) common hepatic, (2) splenic, and (3) the left gastric. Coming off the common hepatic is the gastroduodenal going posterior to the first part of duodenum. Various anastomoses are shown as black circles. (Leo 2022)

## Midgut

The midgut starts halfway down the second part of the duodenum at the major duodenal papilla. The duodenal jejunal flexure is just below the transpyloric plane. The jejunoileum is approximately 20 feet long when uncoiled. Some portion of the jejunoileum is necessary for life because it is responsible for the absorption of nutrients. Its surface area is about the size of a football field when spread out. There is no sharp dividing line between jejunum and ileum, instead there is a transition from one to the other. The walls of the jejunum are thicker and wider than the ileum. Because the jejunum also gets more blood flow it is redder than the ileum.

In the right lower quadrant, the ileum turns into the cecum, which is the beginning of the large intestine. The ileocecal valve is located in the cecum and separates the ileum from the cecum. The valve is normally closed.

The cecum is a bulbous sac like structure which marks the beginning of the ascending colon. Instead of the outer longitudinal layer of muscle wrapping around the entire tube of large intestine, the muscle is consolidated into three longitudinal bands referred to as *tenia coli*. More specifically, the three tenia coli are the: tenia libra, tenia mesocolic, and tenia omental, which all originate or come to a point, at the appendix. The effect of the tenia coli on the large intestine is to cause the intestine to bunch up into a series of sac like structures called *haustra*. Hanging off the tenia coli are *epiploic appendages* which are small fat filled packets.

The *ileocecal valve* is a sphincter that normally stays closed. The *ileocecal reflex* is initiated during eating. As an example, take an individual who was just woken up and is now eating breakfast. During the night, fecal material travelled down the ileum and become lodged in the terminal ileum. At breakfast, when food enters the stomach, gastrin is released by the G-cells in the stomach, duodenum, and pancreas. Gastrin has several effects, one of which is to simulate the ileum to contract. The parasympathetic efferent fibers traveling on the vagus nerve will also stimulate the ileocecal valve to open. The combination of the valve opening, plus the contractions will move material from the ileum to the cecum through the valve.

The cecum is a transition zone for the GI tract to move from peritoneal to retroperitoneal and there is significant variation between individuals of where exactly this transition occurs. There is typically a *superior ileocecal fold* and an *inferior cecal fold* at the junction of where the ileum meets the cecum. These folds form the basis for the *superior* and *inferior ileocecal recesses*. In this region one can also see the appendicular artery, traveling behind the ileum to the appendix. The cecum gives rise to the ascending colon which is a retroperitoneal structure.

At the hepatic flexure, the ascending colon turns into the transverse colon which is an intraperitoneal structure. Its mesentery is the *transverse mesocolon*, whose two layers run towards the pancreas and then split to go either superior or inferior to the pancreas. The attachment of the mesocolon can then be seen anterior to the pancreas which is a retroperitoneal structure. The tail of the pancreas is intraperitoneal and is bounded by the lienorenal ligament. Paralleling the ascending colon, and lateral to the colon, is the right paracolic gutter.

The artery of the midgut is the *superior mesenteric artery,* and its first branch is the *inferior pancreatic duodenal artery*. It heads superior to contribute blood to the inferior portions of the head of the pancreas and the second part of the duodenum. It meets and anastomosis with the superior pancreatic duodenal artery from the gastroduodenal artery. This anastomosis occurs on the head of the pancreas and represents the meeting of the artery of the foregut – celiac trunk- with the artery of the midgut – superior mesenteric artery. Blockage of the aorta just above the celiac trunk would lead to enlarged arteries on the head of the pancreas.

As the superior mesenteric continues, its branches can be divided into those on the left and those on the right. On the left are *10–12 intestinal branches*, some of which are *jejunal branches*, and some of which are *ileal branches*. These *jejunoileal branches* head towards the small intestine with several differences between the two groups. In general, the jejunal branches are straighter, thicker, wider, and more vascular (redder). As each branch approaches its target, it divides in two and meets up with the branches from the neighboring artery which is also branching. Where the branches meet there is an arcade, and there can be several levels of arcades: primary, secondary, or tertiary. And all the arcades are somewhat connected – like a spider web. From the jejunal branches there is typically just one level of arcades, but from the ileal branches it is common to see secondary and tertiary levels. Coming off the arcades are straight branches or vasa recta which eventually pierce the intestinal wall. At the point where the vasa recta pierce the abdominal wall this leads to a weakness in the wall. This weakness predisposes the intestinal wall to *diverticulitis*, which are small outpocketings of the lining. They are typically asymptomatic, but they can lead to a diverticular hemorrhage.

Coming off the right side of the superior mesenteric are branches going to the large intestine. There is significant variation in the pattern of these branches, but regardless of the variation they are named for the portion of the large intestine they are heading for. The *ileocolic artery* heads towards the point where the distal ileum meets the cecum. And coming off the ileocolic artery are the *anterior and posterior cecal arteries*, and the *appendicular artery* which heads posterior to the ileum to travel to the appendix.

The *right colic artery* travels to the ascending colon, while the *middle colic artery* heads towards the transverse colon. Like the intestinal arteries and their arcades, the main arterial branches to the large intestine also branch to meet up with their neighbors, which also branched. This branching forms a continuous channel called the *marginal artery*, which will eventually in turn meet up with the arching branches coming from the inferior mesenteric artery (Figs. 3.20 and 3.21).

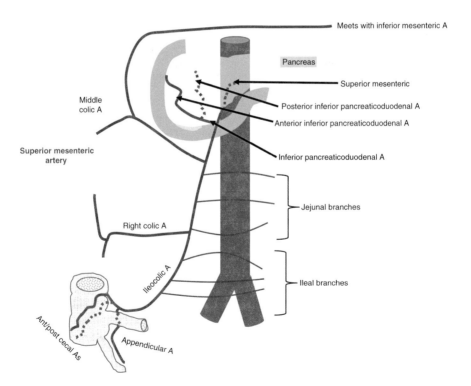

**Fig. 3.21** The superior mesenteric artery arises from the abdominal aorta posterior to the neck of the pancreas. It passes anterior to the duodenum. Its first branch is the inferior pancreaticoduodenal artery which divides into anterior and posterior inferior pancreaticoduodenal arteries. These anastomose with similar branches from the celiac trunk. To the left side, the superior mesenteric artery gives of 10–12 branches to the small intestine, either jejunal or ileal. On the right side it gives off the middle colic, right colic, and ileocolic. The ileocolic gives off cecal branches and an appendicular artery. (Leo 2022)

## Hind Gut

The beginning of the hindgut starts with the last one-third of the transverse colon, close to the splenic flexure, and continues into the descending colon, which then turns into the sigmoid colon, and then the rectum. Paralleling the descending colon is the left paracolic gutter. The sigmoid colon is the S-shaped end of the hindgut and is attached to the sigmoid mesocolon. It has a thick muscular layer and is responsible for the movement of fecal material into the rectum.

The artery of the hindgut is the inferior mesenteric artery. The inferior mesenteric artery comes off the aorta just behind the horizontal third part of the duodenum. The first branch is the *left colic artery* which has two branches, an *ascending branch* heading towards the splenic flexure and a *descending branch* to the descending colon. The ascending branch runs with the inferior mesenteric vein in the *paraduodenal fold*. It is here where *paraduodenal hernias* can migrate behind these two vessels.

The next group of arteries are the 3–5 *sigmoidal arteries* headed towards the sigmoid colon. The terminal branch of the inferior mesenteric artery is the *superior rectal artery,* traveling down along the sacrum towards the rectum.

There are two regions of the descending colon where there are anastomoses between two different arterial systems. These *watershed zones* are susceptible to *ischemic colitis.*

1. *Splenic flexure.* The superior mesenteric artery supplies the proximal two-thirds of the transverse colon. The distal one-third of the transverse colon is supplied by the inferior mesenteric artery. Where these two systems meet is called *Griffith's Point.*
2. *Rectosigmoid junction.* The sigmoidal arteries supply the sigmoid colon. The rectum is supplied by the superior rectal arteries. Where these two systems meet is a potential weak point in the blood supply. This region is referred to as *Sudek's Point*

## Clinical Scenarios

A *volvulus* is a twisting of the small or large intestine and the mesentery that can lead to blockage of the GI tract. It is rare but is more common in children than adults. In the large intestine it can happen at the cecum, transverse colon, and sigmoid colon. Air will often collect in the twisted section and on radiographs will resemble a coffee bean shape. It is considered an emergency situation.

*Intussusception* occurs when one portion of the intestine slips into the neighboring section, like one section of a telescope sliding into the adjacent section. This will lead to blockage of the intestine and often cuts off the blood supply to the affected section. It is considered an emergency situation.

## The Liver

The liver has two surfaces, the *visceral* and *diaphragmatic*, and is divided anatomically into the *right and left lobes* by the *falciform ligament*. The falciform ligament was chosen by early anatomists as the dividing line because of its obvious visual landmark. We will see later that the functional division, based on blood flow, is slightly different. But for now, sticking with the anatomical divisions, the caudate and quadrate lobes are in the anatomical right lobe of the liver. Starting at the inferior border of the liver, the visceral layer of peritoneal membrane is adherent to the diaphragmatic surface, but near the top of the liver it is reflected back onto the inferior surface of the diaphragm. Where the peritoneum is reflected back on itself. This U-turn creates a fold called the *coronary ligament*. As you follow each coronary ligament laterally, each one comes to a point called the triangular ligament - either the *right triangular* or *left triangular ligament*. On the opposite side of each coronary ligament, the surface of the liver does not have a peritoneal covering, which is called the *bare area of the liver*. The peritoneum also travels up the posterior surface creating a space which is a continuation of the lesser sac (Fig. 3.22).

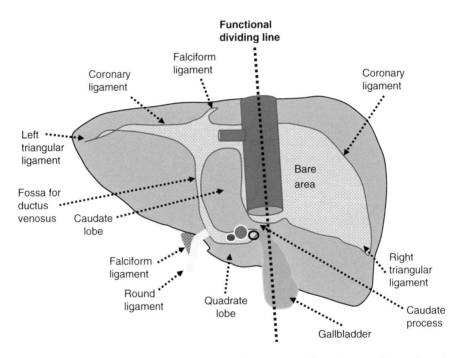

**Fig. 3.22** Visceral surface of liver. The bare area is not covered by peritoneum. The peritoneal folds make up the coronary ligaments. At the corner of the coronary ligaments are the triangular ligaments. The porta hepatis contains branches of the portal vein, bile duct and hepatic arteries. A line running from the Inferior vena cava through the gallbladder divides the liver into the functional right and left lobes. (Leo 2022)

The *porta hepatis* is the doorway to the liver. Several structures pass through the doorway. There are the right and left hepatic arteries and veins going into the liver. And coming out of the liver are the right and left hepatic ducts. Thus, two systems – the artery and vein- are entering the liver at the porta hepatis, and one system is leaving – the biliary system. On the visceral surface of the liver, is the *ligamentum venosum* which is the remanent of the ductus venosus which allowed for blood to bypass the liver during development. During fetal development, it ran from the portal vein to the inferior vena cava.

Based on the blood flow patterns, we now have a more in-depth understanding of the internal architecture of the liver. Using the perfusion territories of the right and left hepatic arteries and veins, the true dividing line between right and left lobes is a line drawn between the gallbladder fossa and the inferior vena cava, which is slightly to the right of the falciform ligament. The *quadrate lobe* and *caudate lobes* are located in the functional left lobe of the liver. However, the caudate lobe receives a dual blood supply from both the right and left hepatic arteries, because it has a small extension called the *caudate process* which is found between the porta hepatis and the inferior vena cava, and it extends over to the right side. Thus, most of the caudate lobe is in the left lobe but the caudate process is in the right lobe.

## Gallbladder and Bile Ducts

The *gallbladder* is divided into *fundus, body, and neck*. The fundus is at the tip of the ninth costal cartilage in the mid-clavicular line and rests on top of the second part of the duodenum and is pointed inferior and anterior. The fundus is encircled by peritoneum. The body is adherent to the visceral surface of the liver and sits in the gallbladder fossa. Its inferior surface is covered by peritoneum. Bile is made in the liver and transported from the liver to gallbladder to be stored until it is needed. Coming out of the liver are the *right* and *left hepatic* ducts which merge to form the *common hepatic duct*, which in turn merges with the *cystic duct* coming out of the gallbladder, to make up the *common bile duct*. The common bile duct heads inferior, going behind (posterior) the first part of duodenum, to enter the second part of the duodenum at the *greater duodenal papilla* along with the main pancreatic duct. The accessory pancreatic duct comes off the pancreatic duct and enters the duodenum at the *minor duodenal papilla.*

At the greater duodenal papilla, the common bile duct is joined by the *pancreatic duct* which sends digestive enzymes into the duodenum. Bile stones that block the great duodenal papilla will block the pancreatic secretions to the duodenum (Fig. 3.23).

The *proper hepatic artery* branches into the *right and left hepatic arteries*, and the right hepatic artery goes behind (posterior) the common hepatic duct and the gives off the *cystic artery* to the gallbladder in the *cystohepatic triangle* (triangle of calot) which is bounded by the liver, cystic duct, and common hepatic duct. The *cystic artery* lies within the triangle. There is significant variation in the origin of the cystic artery, but it is usually from the *right hepatic artery* (Fig. 3.24).

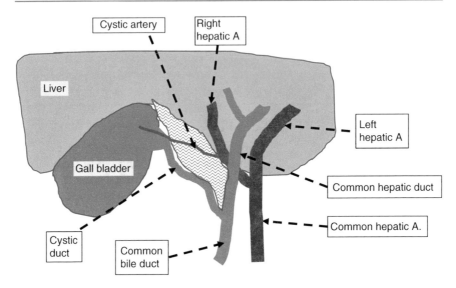

**Fig. 3.23** Cystohepatic triangle (Calot) The triangle is the shaded blue region bounded by visceral surface of liver, cystic duct, and common hepatic duct. Note the cystic artery coming off the right hepatic artery. The right hepatic artery goes behind the bile duct. (Leo 2022)

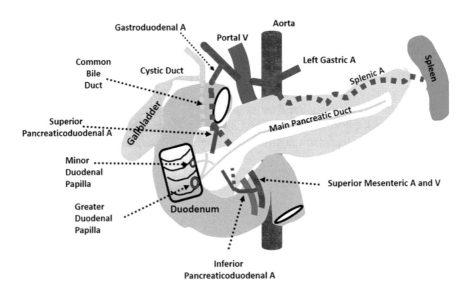

**Fig. 3.24** Pancreas, duodenum, and gallbladder. Note that the gastroduodenal artery and the common bile duct travel posterior to the first part of the duodenum. The common bile duct joins the main pancreatic duct to enter the duodenum at the greater duodenal papilla. The accessory pancreatic duct enters at the minor duodenal papilla. (Leo 2022)

## Liver and Portal System

Blood flow to the limbs involves a single-in-line capillary bed. Oxygen leaves the heart on an artery and travels to the capillary bed where it perfuses across the capillary wall to deliver oxygen to a muscle. The veins then return the oxygen poor blood to the heart. However, a portal system has two capillary beds in-line. There are portal systems in several organs, such as the gastrointestinal tract, the kidney, and the pituitary system. When we talk about the gastrointestinal tract and the hepatic portal system, the first capillary bed is in the wall of the jejunoileum. While the gastrointestinal tract runs from mouth to anus, contents inside the tract are not in the body, per se. Contents that come in through the mouth and leave through the anus have never crossed the body wall. However, within the wall of the jejunoileum are capillary beds so that nutrients such as amino acids, and triglycerides that have been broken down in the gastrointestinal tract are absorbed through the walls of the jejunoileum into veins. These substances along with toxins, such as alcohol and drugs, whether licit or illicit, need to be processed by the liver, thus they travel from that first capillary bed in the jejunoileum to a second capillary bed in the liver via the hepatic portal system.

Pathology in the portal system, such as cirrhosis of the liver, will lead to portal hypertension. This is analogous to putting a dam in the middle of a stream. The water, or in this case the blood, will look for an alternate route around the liver. The blood will now attempt to travel back along the caval system. When blood pressure in the portal veins increases, then pressure in the hepatic veins will typically decrease (Fig. 3.25).

The portal system is made up of three large veins. The *inferior mesenteric vein* ascends and joins the *splenic vein* which in turn meets the *superior mesenteric vein* behind the neck of the pancreas, to form the *portal vein*. The portal vein now ascends

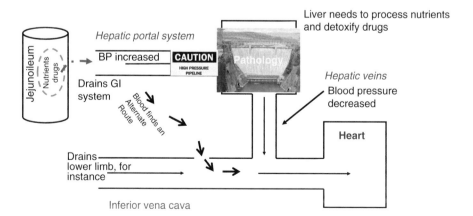

**Fig. 3.25** Hepatic portal versus inferior vena cava. Blood draining the jejunoileum follows the hepatic portal system back to the liver to be processed. Meanwhile, blood from the limbs does not need to go through the liver so it drains via the inferior vena cava back to the heart. (Leo 2022)

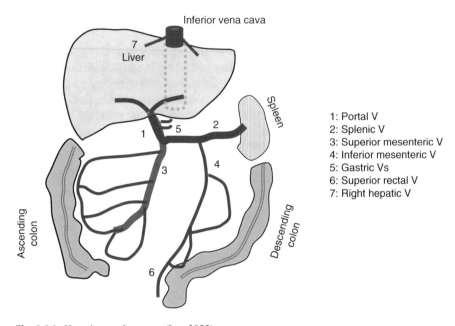

**Fig. 3.26**  Hepatic portal system. (Leo 2022)

to the liver in the *hepatoduodenal ligament* (part of the lesser omentum) to enter at the porta hepatis.

The portal system forms several anastomoses with the caval system, and it is at these sites where pathologies will develop in cases of portal hypertension (Fig. 3.26).

1. *Hemorrhoids.* The dividing line in the rectum is the *pectinate line*. Above the pectinate line, normally blood drains to the superior rectal vein, to the inferior mesenteric vein, to the portal vein. While blood below the pectinate line, drains to the inferior rectal vein, to the internal pudendal vein, and then to the inferior vena cava. In the case of liver pathology, the portal blood pressure rises. At the anastomosis around the pectinate line, blood will now cross the line to drain into the inferior rectal vein, and eventually the inferior vena cava. The veins in this region which are very superficial, can become dilated creating an outpocketing of tissue – referred to as hemorrhoids, which can be classified as internal or external. Internal hemorrhoids are above the pectinate line, while external hemorrhoids are below the pectinate line (Fig. 3.27).
2. *Esophageal Varices.* The terminal esophagus is another site of anastomoses. The esophageal veins in the most distal part of the esophagus drain to the gastric veins and then to the portal vein. Just above this region, the esophagus drains to the caval system. With portal hypertension, the veins in this region become dilated and enlarged. The danger is that they can rupture which is an emergency situation.

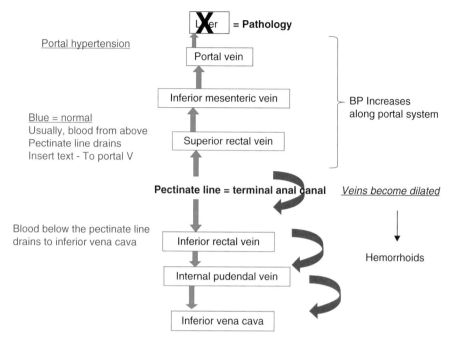

**Fig. 3.27** Portal hypertension. Liver pathology leads to portal hypertension. Venous blood then drains into the inferior rectal vein and back to the Inferior vena cava. (Leo 2022)

3. *Caput Medusa.* In the region of the umbilicus, paraumbilical veins follow the round ligament to drain into the portal vein. Around the umbilicus are also numerous superficial epigastric veins which drain into the femoral vein. With liver pathology, the anastomoses also lead to dilated veins which radiate out from the umbilicus. These dilated veins are thought to resemble the snakes coming out of Medusa's head.
4. *Splenomegaly.* The splenic vein which drains the spleen can also be backed up because of the increased pressure which can lead to an enlarged spleen (Fig. 3.28).

## Liver Subdivisions

There are three ways to divide up the internal architecture of the liver (Fig. 3.29).

1. The most common division is the *classic hepatic lobule* which is a hexagon. As the three structures coming into the liver at the porta hepatis branch they all stay together and are found at the corner of each side of the hexagon. This portal triad thus has a branch of the hepatic artery carrying oxygen into the liver, a branch of the portal vein, carrying nutrients and toxins ready to be metabolized or detoxified, and a branch of the bile duct carrying bile on towards the biliary tract.

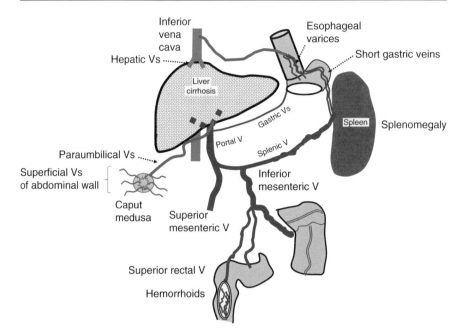

**Fig. 3.28** Portal venous system. Note the inferior mesenteric vein draining into the splenic vein, which then joins the superior mesenteric vein to form the portal vein. Portal hypertension results in esophageal varices, caput medusa and hemorrhoids. (Leo 2022)

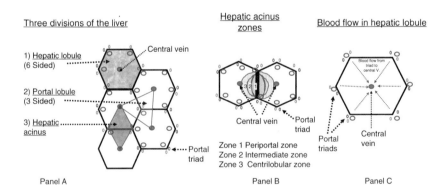

**Fig. 3.29** Panel (**a**) shows the three different ways to divide up the liver into segments. Panel (**b**) shows the organization of the hepatic acinus. Panel (**c**) shows the blood flow in the hepatic lobule from the triads at each corner to the central vein. (Leo 2022)

Blood from the hepatic artery and hepatic portal vein then travels from the corners or periphery of the lobule towards the center to eventually drain into the central vein, which in turn will drain into the hepatic vein and finally the inferior vena cava.

2. The *portal lobule*, a triangle, is simply another way to divide up the liver. Rather than the central vein at the center, the center is one of the portal triads, and the central veins are at the three corners. Thus, the blood is moving from the center, where one finds a branch of hepatic artery and portal vein, to the periphery.

3. The *liver acinus* is a four-sided trapezoid with four points. The center piece is a line drawn between two portal triads. Blood is moving bilaterally from this midline structure to the central veins at the other two points. As the blood moves from the center towards the periphery, pathologists have divided the regions up into three zones. *Zone 1* is closest to the midline structure and will have the highest concentration of oxygen, so it will be the last of the three regions affected by ischemia. *Zone 3* on the other hand is the farthest away from the center, thus it is the least oxygenated and most susceptible to ischemia.

## Pancreas

The pancreas is both an exocrine and endocrine gland. Its exocrine portion involves the production and secretion of pancreatic enzymes. The enzymes travel on the main pancreatic duct to enter the second part of the duodenum at the greater duodenal papilla and minor duodenal papilla. The endocrine portion of the pancreas is handled in physiology textbooks (Fig. 3.30).

## Spleen

The spleen lies against ribs 9, 10, and 11 on the left side in the mid-axillary line. In a patient with trauma to this region the spleen can easily be damaged. There are two

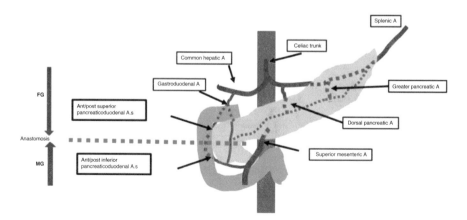

**Fig. 3.30** Blood supply to pancreas. The gastroduodenal comes from celiac trunk and gives off the anterior and posterior pancreaticoduodenal arteries which supply the superior portion of the pancreas and duodenum. The superior mesenteric artery gives of the anterior and posterior pancreaticoduodenal arteries which supply the inferior portion of the pancreas and duodenum. (Leo 2022)

ligaments associated with the spleen. The *lienorenal ligament* connects the spleen to the kidney. The tail of the pancreas and the splenic artery enter the lienorenal ligament. The *gastrosplenic ligament* connects the stomach and spleen and is part of the greater omentum. Just before the splenic artery enters the spleen, it gives off the *short gastric arteries* that head to the fundus of the stomach.

In some cases, the ligaments do not form, and the spleen is able to move within the cavity resulting in a "wandering spleen." Accessory spleens can also be found within the ligaments.

## Referred Pain

The afferent nerve innervation to the GI tract and the visceral peritoneum comes from the autonomic nervous system, which are the thoracic and lumbar splanchnic nerves. The thoracic splanchnic nerves originate in the thorax, descend through the diaphragm, and innervate the GI tract and abdominal organs. These fibers sense pressure and distension from the various portions of the tract. They do not sense pain. Thus, in the initial stages of pathology the patient is unable to precisely localize the source of pain. Instead of pointing to the exact source of the pain, they tend to point to regions. Pain from any foregut structure will refer to the epigastric region. Pain from the midgut will refer to the umbilical region. Pain from the hindgut will refer to the hypogastric region.

Once the pathology has gotten large enough it will aggravate the parietal perineum while will trigger pain sensations along the somatic nervous system, and the patient will now be able to precisely localize the pain (Fig. 3.31).

Take appendicitis as an example. In the initial stages, the patient will complain of pain around the hypogastric region, but as time goes on, say 4–6 hours, and the appendix has gotten larger, it will aggravate the parietal peritoneum and the pain

**Fig. 3.31** Visceral sensation. Pain sensation from foregut travels on greater splanchnic nerves and is referred to epigastric region. From midgut on lesser splanchnic nerves and is referred to umbilical region. From hindgut on least splanchnic nerves and is referred to hypogastric region. (Leo 2022)

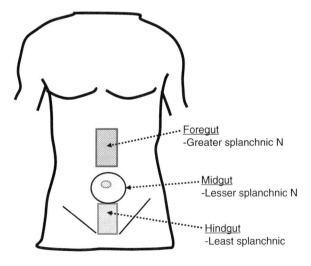

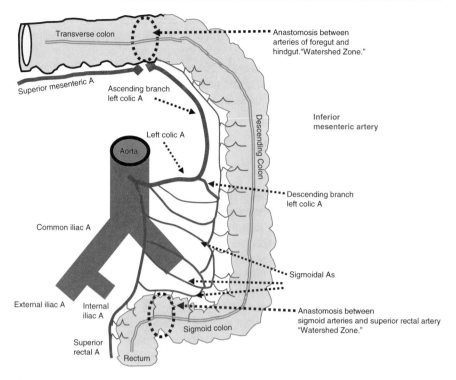

**Fig. 3.32**  Inferior mesenteric artery. (Leo 2022)

will be felt in the right lower quadrant. The appendix lies close to the right iliopsoas and an inflamed appendix can also lead to a positive psoas test, meaning that with the thigh placed against the abdomen, extension of the thigh will lead to pain as the inflamed appendix aggravates the psoas muscle (Fig. 3.32).

## Greater, Lesser, and Least Splanchnic Nerves

In the section above we used the term thoracic splanchnic nerves and pointed out that these are the sympathetic nerves carrying afferent and efferent fibers to and from the viscera. But we can also be more specific. The thoracic splanchnic nerves include the *greater splanchnic nerve* from T5–9, the *lesser splanchnic nerve* from T10–11, and the *least splanchnic nerve* from the T12. These nerves all contain preganglionic sympathetic efferent fibers, and visceral afferent fibers from the GI tract.

The preganglionic sympathetic fibers in the greater splanchnic nerves synapse in the celiac ganglion. The post ganglionic fibers then travel on branches of the celiac trunk to innervate the foregut and related structures. Visceral pain fibers from foregut structures travel on the greater splanchnic nerves back to the spinal cord.

The preganglionic sympathetic fibers in the lesser and least splanchnic nerves travel to the superior mesenteric ganglion and the aorticorenal ganglion, and then travel out on branches of the superior mesenteric artery to reach the midgut structures. Visceral afferents from the midgut structures pass back along these nerves to the spinal cord.

Preganglionic fibers of the lumbar splanchnic nerves travel to the inferior mesenteric ganglion. After synapsing, the fibers pass on branches of the inferior mesenteric artery to the hindgut structures. Visceral afferents also pass on these fibers back to the spinal cord.

## The Rectum and Anal Canal

The rectum is retroperitoneal, or subperitoneal, because it is inferior to the peritoneal cavity. There are three transverse rectal folds resembling three shelves stacked on top of each other. The rectum ends just above the pectinate line. The pectinate line is where the hindgut endoderm meets the skin, or ectoderm. It gets its name from the organization of anal valves, anal sinuses, and anal columns, all of which give the pectinate line the appearance of a comb. The anal columns are outpocketings of tissue housing the terminal branches of the superior rectal artery and veins. On the side of each column is a space called the anal sinus. Running from the terminal end of each anal column is a valve which is a thin piece of tissue connecting each column to its neighboring column. The pectinate line is a line of demarcation for the region. The nerve innervation, the arterial blood supply, the venous drainage pattern, the lymphatic flow, and classification of hemorrhoids are all based on the pectinate line (Table 3.2).

## Venous Drainage of Anal Canal

The venous drainage above the pectinate line is to the *superior rectal vein*, which drains to the inferior mesenteric vein, and then to the portal vein. The drainage below the pectinate line is to the *inferior rectal vein*, then to the *internal pudendal vein*, the internal iliac vein, and finally to the inferior vena cava, so at the pectinate line there is an anastomosis between the portal vein and the inferior vena cava. With liver pathology, for instance, blood pressure in the portal vein will go up which in

**Table 3.2** Differences above and below the pectinate line

| | Tissue | Venous drainage | Arterial supply | Hemorrhoids | Afferent nerve | Efferent nerve | Lymphatic drainage |
|---|---|---|---|---|---|---|---|
| Above pectinate line | Hindgut endoderm | Superior rectal V to portal V | Sup rectal A | Internal | Autonomics | Pelvic splanchnic | Abdominal nodes |
| Below pectinate line | Ectoderm | Inferior rectal V To IVC | Inf rectal A | External | Pudendal | Pudendal | Superficial inguinal nodes |

turn leads to an increase pressure in the superior rectal vein. The blood in the anal canal will now look for an alternate route around the liver and will travel from the superior rectal vein to the inferior rectal vein, which will lead to dilated veins, or hemorrhoids in this area. *Internal hemorrhoids* are outpocketings *above* the pectinate line, while *external hemorrhoids* are outpocketings *below* the pectinate line.

The afferent nerve supply above the pectinate line comes from the autonomic nervous system, mainly the parasympathetic pelvic splanchnic nerves. These nerves are responsible for sensing pressure and have very few pain fibers. The afferent nerve supply below the pectinate line comes from the pudendal nerve which does carry pain sensation. Thus, a patient will typically not feel internal hemorrhoids, however a patient with external hemorrhoids will complain of pain and itching.

The lymphatic drainage above the pectinate line is to internal iliac nodes, while the lymphatic drainage below the line will drain to the superficial inguinal nodes. See the anteromedial thigh section for specifics on the superficial inguinal nodes.

## Superior Mesenteric Artery and Nutcracker Syndrome

The superior mesenteric artery (SMA) comes off the aorta at the L1 vertebra level. The SMA immediately passes anterior to the left renal vein, which is crossing the aorta to enter the inferior vena cava. Because the inferior vena cava lies to the right of the aorta, the left renal vein passes in front of the aorta to enter the inferior vena cava. Just inferior to the left renal vein where it crosses the aorta is the third part of the duodenum. In front of the SMA is the neck of the pancreas. An analogy to these relationships is that the pancreas is like a fist grabbing the superior mesenteric artery. The pancreas is pushing off from the spleen on the left side and pushing into the duodenum on the right side. The fist, or head of the pancreas is now surrounded on all sides by the duodenum. As the hand grabs the SMA, the fingertips extend behind the SMA. The fingertips are analogous to the uncinate process. While most of the hand, or the pancreas, is anterior to the SMA, the tiny uncinate process can slip behind the SMA.

Remember that the pancreas and aorta are retroperitoneal structures, while the superior mesenteric artery is running in the dorsal mesentery. Anterior to the pancreas is the lesser sac, and in front of the lesser sac is the stomach and transverse colon (Fig. 3.33).

Looking anteriorly, as the SMA emerges from the aorta it is surrounded by three veins, like the borders of a window (Fig. 3.34).

1. The *splenic vein* is the top rim of the window, or above the superior mesenteric artery, The splenic vein is coursing from the tail of the pancreas along the pancreas towards the midline. Along the way it is joined by the inferior mesenteric vein, and then behind the neck of the pancreas it meets the superior mesenteric vein to form the portal vein.
2. the *superior mesenteric vein* forms the right side of the window. Keep in mind that the superior mesenteric vein and artery run together. It makes sense the

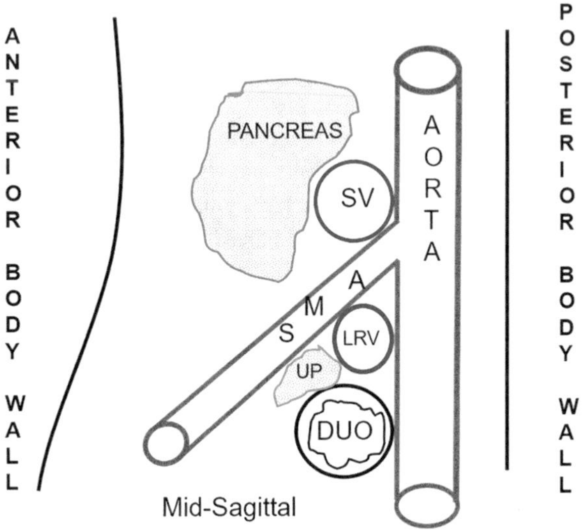

**Fig. 3.33** Superior mesenteric artery. This midsagittal section shows the superior mesenteric artery emerging from the aorta and passing anterior to the left renal vein, uncinate process of pancreas, and the duodenum. (Leo 2022)

SMA is found more to left which is same side as aorta, while the superior mesenteric vein is found on left heading towards the liver, also on left.

3. The *left renal vein* forms the windowsill and lies inferior. As mentioned earlier, it crosses from left kidney, across the aorta, to enter IVC on the right.

## Duodenal Fossae and Folds

In the vicinity of the duodenojejunal flexure where various structures are transitioning from retroperitoneal to intraperitoneal, there is a complicated series of folds and fossae that can lead to weaknesses that in turn can lead to congenital intestinal hernias, classified as either right-sided or left-sided.

Of the two hernias in this region, left-sided are more common. These left-sided hernias are migrations of intestine into the paraduodenal fossa. The ascending branch of the inferior mesenteric artery and the inferior mesenteric vein run parallel and to the left of the fourth part of the duodenum in close proximity to the duodenojejunal flexure. At this point the peritoneum has several folds forming a four-sided window. On the top and bottom of the window are the *superior and inferior duodenal folds* which form the superior and inferior fossae. On the right side of the window is the *paraduodenal fossa* (Landzert's fossa) and on the left side of the window is the *retroduodenal fossa*. The most important fossa in this region is the paraduodenal fossa, or the left side of this window. *Paraduodenal hernias* are herniations of the small intestine into the paraduodenal fossa and are considered left-sided hernias (Fig. 3.34).

Right-sided hernias are associated with the superior mesenteric artery and vein. As the SMA travels over (anterior to) the duodenum, the dorsal mesentery is attached to the superior mesenteric artery. A potential defect at this point can lead to

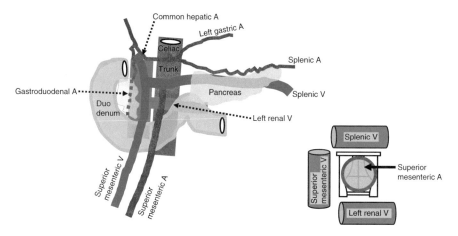

**Fig. 3.34** Superior mesenteric artery. The emergence of the superior mesenteric artery from the aorta is surrounded on three sides by veins. A section of the pancreas has been removed to see the SMA. Think of the SMA as coming through a window. Above the window is the splenic vein. Below the window is the left renal vein. To the right of the window is the superior mesenteric vein. Note the gastroduodenal artery passing behind the first part of the duodenum. The celiac trunk has three branches: (1) left gastric, (2) splenic, and (3) the common hepatic. (Leo 2022)

an opening referred to as Waldayer's fossa which can be a site of intestinal herniation. A hernia's through Waldayer's fossa is a right-sided hernia going behind the superior mesenteric artery (Fig. 3.35).

## Transpyloric Line

The transpyloric plane or line runs across the abdomen through the pyloric region of the stomach at the L1 vertebral body level. It is significant for the structures that it crosses. Rather than just memorize a list, lets first think about what structures we already know intersect the transpyloric plane. We will start with the superior mesenteric artery (SMA). We saw earlier that the SMA emerges from the abdominal aorta at L1. As it emerges, it is crossing the left renal vein. Just inferior to the left renal vein is the ascending portion of the duodenum about to join the jejunum. So, the SMA, the left renal vein, the L1 vertebra, and the conus medullaris all lie in the transpyloric plane. Likewise, the first part of the duodenum also lies in the plane, as does the pyloric region of the stomach.

Anterior to the SMA, is the neck of the pancreas. To the right of the SMA is the superior mesenteric vein, so you can think about the SMA emerging through the window, mentioned earlier, bounded by veins; superior mesenteric to right, splenic vein above, and left renal vein below. All these veins lie in the transpyloric plane.

The pancreas is a retroperitoneal structure. Anterior to the pancreas, the visceral peritoneum both from above and below the pancreas merge to form the transverse mesocolon. So, the transverse mesocolon is also in the transpyloric plane. As the

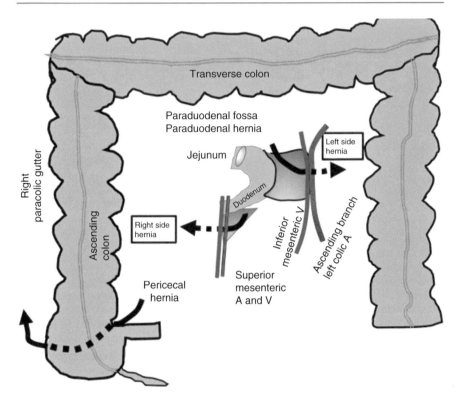

**Fig. 3.35** Three internal Hernias. Just lateral to the duodenum is the paraduodenal fold encasing the inferior mesenteric vein and ascending branch of the middle colic artery. (1) Paraduodenal hernias (left-sided) occur just medial to the fold and move into the paraduodenal fossa. (2) Right-sided hernias move behind the superior mesenteric artery and vein. (3) Pericecal hernias move from right to left behind the cecum and can move into the right paracolic gutter. (Leo 2022)

pancreas pushes off the spleen and into the duodenum it comes to lie on top of the hilum of the right kidney. So, the hilum of the right and left kidneys, pancreas, and the spleen (lower border) all lie in the transpyloric plane.

And as we already discussed the neck of the gallbladder rests on the first part of the duodenum, so the neck of the gallbladder is also on the transpyloric plane.

## Kidneys

The kidneys lie on the posterior abdominal wall running from the T12 to the L3 vertebra. Because of the liver's location on the right side of the body, the right kidney is slightly lower than the left kidney. The posterior surface of the right kidney is crossed by the 12th rib, and the posterior surface of the left kidney by the 11th and 12th ribs. The diaphragm is attached to the 12th rib on each side, so the diaphragm and its accompanying parietal pleura, on the medial side, come down between the

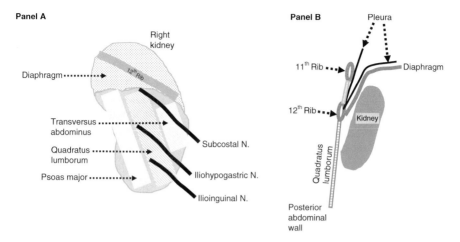

**Fig. 3.36** Panel (**a**) is a posterior view of kidney. Note the top part of the kidney that comes up above rib 12 is covered by the diaphragm. Three nerves of the posterior abdominal wall lie posterior to the kidney. Panel (**b**) shows a view from the side. Note that the pleura adherent to diaphragm comes down between the kidney and posterior abdominal wall. (Leo 2022)

posterior abdominal wall and the kidneys. This relationship needs to be accounted for when performing procedures in this area. For instance, a needle biopsy of the kidney that approached the kidney above the 12th rib could potentially transfer an infection from the liver to the pleural cavity. An approach below the 12th rib would not go through the pleura (Fig. 3.36).

The inferior posterior surface of each kidney abuts three muscles. Moving from medial to lateral:

1. The *iliopsoas* is the chief flexor of the hip. The psoas major originates from the transverse processes of T12-L4 and descends on the posterior wall. Meanwhile, the iliacus arises from the superior pelvic brim. The two muscles come together to make up the iliopsoas to reach the lesser trochanter. Both muscles are innervated by direct branches from L1-L3 (not the femoral nerve). The *genitofemoral nerve* pierces the psoas on its course to the inguinal region. *The Thomas Test* is used to test tightness of the iliopsoas. In brief, with the patient lying on the exam table in the supine position they lift their lower limb off the table and are asked to resist the examiners downward force on the lower limb.
2. The *quadratus lumborum* runs from rib 12 to the iliac crest. When the muscle is active on one side it is a lateral flexor. When both are active it is an extensor. It also assists with stabilizing the 12th rib.
3. The *transversus abdominus* also forms part of the posterior abdominal wall.

The hilum, at the L1 vertebra level, is the opening at the medial border of the kidney. Starting anteriorly and moving posteriorly, the hilum transmits the renal **V**ein, renal **A**rtery, and the renal **P**elvis (VAP). The renal arteries arise at the level of L1, just inferior to the superior mesenteric artery. The origin of the left renal artery is slightly higher than the right renal artery. The right artery is longer because it needs to go posterior to the IVC. On the other hand, the left renal vein is longer because of its longer route to the IVC over (anterior to) the aorta. The left kidney is usually used for transplants because of its longer renal vein. Because the kidneys ascend during development, it is not uncommon to see accessory renal veins.

*Lloyd's test* involves a soft punch, either directly or indirectly, on the posterior abdominal wall just behind the kidney. Pain indicates a kidney stone or infection.

## Renal Fascia

The kidney has a strong fibrous capsule made of dense irregular connective tissue surrounding it. Outside of the capsule is a loose layer of adipose tissue – the perirenal fat, which serves as a shock absorber. And then outside of the perirenal fat is the renal capsule – also known as Gerota's fascia. On the anterior surface, the renal fascia on the right and left sides fuse in front of the aorta and inferior vena cava. Outside of the renal fascia is the pararenal fat. The kidneys are retroperitoneal. The adrenal glands are located in the perirenal space and are also surrounded by perirenal fascia (Fig. 3.37).

## Renal Blood Supply

The blood supply to the kidneys comes from the *right and left renal arteries*, each of which then split into 4–5 *segmental arteries*. The segmental arteries give off *interlobar arteries* which ascend in the renal columns alongside the edges of the renal medulla. The interlobar arteries then make a 90° turn to run along the top of

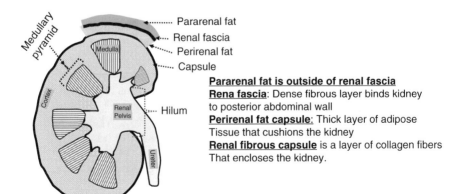

**Fig. 3.37** Internal kidney. Urine formed in the medulla will drain to the renal papilla, which drains into the minor calyx. Several minor calyces will form a major calyx, which in turn will form the renal pelvis. (Leo 2022)

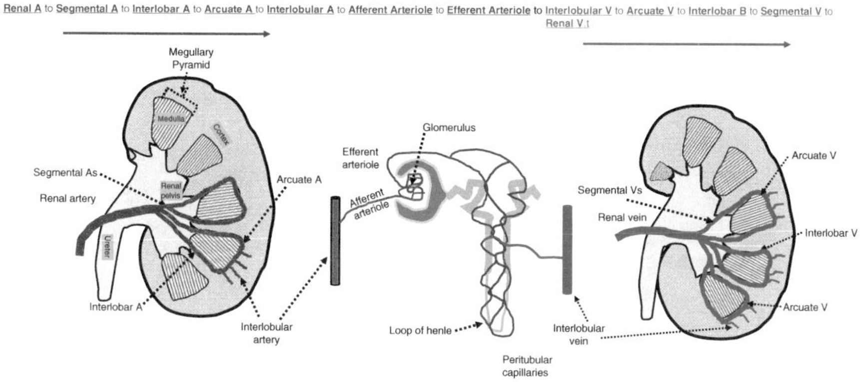

**Fig. 3.38** Panel (**a**) shows the blood coming into the kidney from the renal artery. Panel (**b**) shows the blood leaving the kidney and eventually draining into the renal vein. (Leo 2022)

the medullary pyramids as the *arcuate arteries*. The arcuate arteries then give off the *interlobular arteries* which give off *afferent arterioles* which then enter the glomerulus. Coming out of the glomerulus are the *efferent arterioles* that then wind around the proximal and distal convoluted tubules. Coming out of this network are the *peritubular capillaries* that turn into the *interlobular veins* and then drain back along a similar pattern as the arterial side (Fig. 3.38).

The blood flow of the kidney is a portal system. Remember that portal systems have two capillary beds in line. In the kidneys, the first capillary bed is the glomerulus, and the second capillary bed is the peritubular capillary network. One thing to note, is that in the kidneys the connection between the glomerulus and the peritubular capillary network is the *efferent arteriole*, which is in contrast to the portal vein where the first and second capillary beds are connected by a vein (the portal vein).

## Adrenal Glands

The adrenal glands are triangular in shape and sit on top of the kidneys nestled between the two great vessels. The right adrenal gland abuts the inferior vena cava. The adrenal medulla secretes epinephrine and is functionally equivalent to a post-ganglionic sympathetic neuron. The adrenal medulla has three zones (salt, sugar, and sex):

1. *Zona Glomerulosa* produces aldosterone which causes the distal convoluted tubule and collecting tubule to reabsorb sodium.
2. *Zona Fasciculata* releases cortisol.
3. *Zona Reticulata* produces androgens.

Although there are variations, the arterial pattern is similar on both the right and left sides. Both the *right and left superior suprarenal arteries* come off the *inferior*

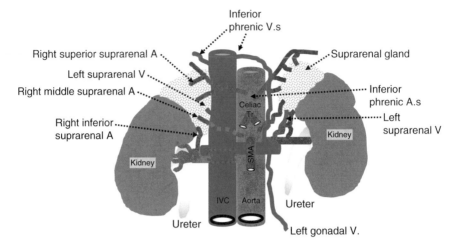

**Fig. 3.39** Blood supply to Suprarenal glands. There are three arteries to the adrenal gland: (1) superior suprarenal from the inferior phrenic artery, (2) middle suprarenal arteries from the abdominal aorta, and (3) the inferior suprarenal arteries from the renal arteries. There is typically only one vein. On the right side the vein drains into the IVC, and on the left it drains into the left renal vein. Note that on the left side, the left inferior phrenic vein sends a branch to the left renal vein. (Leo 2022)

*phrenic arteries*. The *middle suprarenal arteries* come off the abdominal aorta. The *inferior suprarenal arteries* come off the renal arteries. The venous drainage for the adrenals is not symmetrical and is different on the right versus left sides. On the right side, the suprarenal vein drains into inferior vena cava, while on the left the suprarenal vein drains into the left renal vein. At this point an extension of the left inferior phrenic vein sends a branch down to the left renal vein. Given the close proximity of the inferior phrenic vein and the left suprarenal vein to each other where they drain into the left renal vein, it is not uncommon to see a common trunk for these two branches (Fig. 3.39).

## Ureters

The *ureters* descend from the renal pelvis down to the bladder. As they travel down the posterior abdominal wall, they lie on top of the psoas major muscle. They enter the pelvis crossing the pelvic brim Crosses the pelvic brim anterior to the bifurcation of the common iliac artery into internal and external branches. As the ureters descend, they are crossed by either the right or left colic artery traveling to the large intestine, either the ileocolic artery on the left or the sigmoidal arteries on the right, and then the left or right gonadal arteries. And at the pelvic brim, lateral to the ureters are the ovarian vessels entering the pelvis.

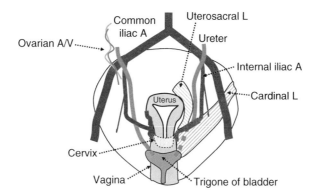

**Fig. 3.40** Uterine artery and pelvic ligaments. The cardinal ligament runs medial to lateral, while the uterosacral runs anterior to posterior. The ureter enters the pelvic cavity just lateral to the origin of the common iliac artery. The ureter then passes under the uterine artery. The uterine artery runs in the cardinal ligament towards the cervix. (Leo 2022)

In females, just lateral to the cervix, the ureter crosses inferior to the uterine artery – "water under the bridge." During a hysterectomy or other pelvic surgeries this relationship is important. In males, just before the ureter enters the bladder it is crossed by the ductus deferens (Fig. 3.40).

Kidney stones can get caught up at either the: (1) the renal pelvis, (2) the pelvic brim, or (3) at the entrance to the bladder. As the stones move down the ureter the patient will complain of pain first in the epigastric region. As the stone descends it will aggravate the psoas major causing the patient to flex at the hip. By assuming the fetal position, the patient is trying to relieve the pressure of the stone on the psoas major. Extension of the patient's lower limb will lead to significant pain because of increased aggravation of the psoas. As the stone enters the bladder the patient will complain of pain in the inguinal canal region – the L1 dermatome (Fig. 3.41).

## Nerves of Posterior Abdominal Wall

Along the posterior abdominal wall are several nerves:

1. The *subcostal nerve* is found just inferior to the 12th rib.
2. The *iliohypogastric nerve* (L1) winds around the abdominal wall running parallel and superior to the inguinal ligament.
3. The *ilioinguinal nerve* also winds around the abdominal wall to travel through the deep ring and enter the inguinal canal.
4. The *lateral femoral cutaneous nerve* travels medial to the ASIS to enter the thigh.
5. The *genitofemoral nerve* splits into a genital and femoral branch. The genital branch innervates the cremaster muscle. The femoral branch carries sensory fibers coming from the anteromedial thigh.

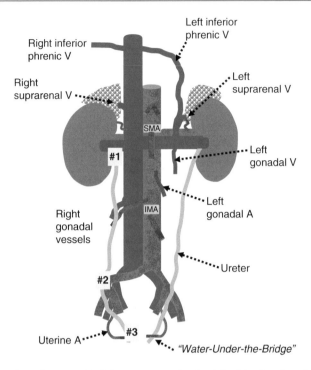

**Fig. 3.41** Branches of aorta and inferior vena cava. On the right side, the adrenal gland and the gonads drain into the IVC. However, on the left side, the gonads and adrenal grand drain into the left renal vein, which then drains into the IVC. The SMA goes anterior to the left renal vein. The ureter enters the pelvis lateral to the common iliac arteries and veins. The ureter then passes under the uterine artery just lateral to the cervix (*Water-under-the-Bridge*). There are three common locations for kidney stone blockage (1) at the renal pelvis, (2) where the ureter crosses the pelvic brim and (3) where the ureter enters the bladder. (Leo 2022)

## Branches of the Abdominal Aorta

As a summary of the abdominal aorta. Consider a stick figure drawing of a person standing up. Their hat is the diaphragm, their eyes are the inferior phrenic arteries, the nose is the celiac trunk, the mouth is the superior mesenteric artery, and the goatee just underneath the mouth is the left renal vein. The upper limbs are the renal arteries with the fingers the segmental arteries of the kidneys. The nipples are the gonadal arteries (either testicular or ovarian), the chest hair represents the lumber arteries, the belly button the inferior mesenteric and the common iliac arteries are the lower limbs (Fig. 3.42).

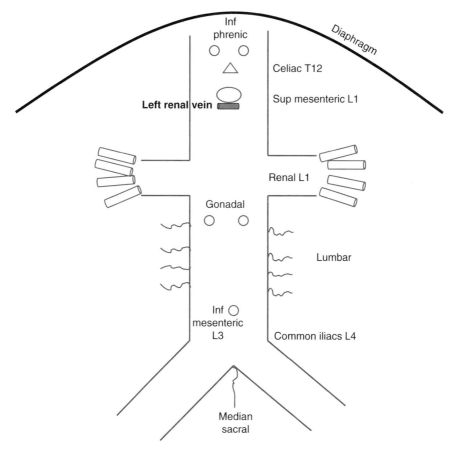

**Fig. 3.42** Abdominal aorta

## Further Reading

Moore K, Dalley AF, Agur A. Clinically oriented anatomy. 7th ed. Baltimore. New York: Lippincott Williams and Wilkin; 2014.

Rosse C, Gaddum-Rosse P. Hollinshead's textbook of anatomy. Philadelphia: Lippincott-Raven; 1997.

Snell R. Clinical anatomy by region. 9th ed. Lippincott Williams and Wilkins; 2012.

# The Pelvis and Perineum

## 4

## Introduction

As an introduction to the pelvic region, imagine the bony pelvis like a bucket, and into this bucket we drop a funnel. And underneath the funnel we are going to add an extra layer of support. The sides of the bucket are the bony pelvis and the obturator internus. The funnel is the muscular pelvic diaphragm. And the extra layer of support is the urogenital diaphragm. The space between the pelvic diaphragm and the urogenital diaphragm is the ischiorectal fossa. And within this fossa, on the medial wall of the obturator internus is the pudendal canal, housing the pudendal nerve and internal pudendal artery and vein (Fig. 4.1). Now for the details.

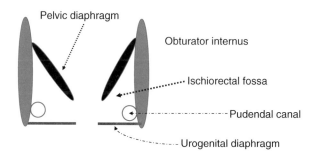

**Fig. 4.1** Pelvic diaphragm. The bony pelvis resembles a bucket, which is obturator internus. Dropped into the bucket is a funnel, the pelvic diaphragm. Inferiorly is the urogenital diaphragm. The pudendal canal is found in the ischiorectal fossa. (Leo 2022)

## Pelvic Diaphragm

The pelvic diaphragm is made up of two muscles: (1) *coccygeus*, and (2) *levator ani,* and the levator ani in turn has three divisions (Fig. 4.2).

1. The fibers of the *pubococcygeus* run from the pubic bone to the coccyx in an anterior to posterior direction.
2. The most medial portion of the pubococcygeus is the *puborectalis.* Starting at the pubic bone, the fibers run posterior towards the rectum, but unlike the pubococcygeus which attaches to the coccyx, the fibers of puborectalis make a 180° turn around the rectum and head towards the contralateral pubic bone. They form a sling around the rectum to keep fecal material inside the rectum.
3. The *iliococcygeus* runs from the ischium to the coccyx with the fibers running in a mediolateral direction, as compared to the anteroposterior running fibers of pubococcygeus. The iliococcygeus also attaches to the tendinous arch of levator ani. In four-legged animals the muscle is attached along the bony rim of the pelvis, but as humans stood up, gravity and the weight of the internal muscles pushed down on the iliococcygeus to push it away from the bone.

The *coccygeus muscle* is fused with the *sacrospinous ligament.*

The pelvic diaphragm muscles – *levator ani* and *coccygeus* – are innervated by direct branches from S3 and 4 (sometimes S2 contributes). During deliveries the pelvic diaphragm is stretched. Kegel exercises help to strengthen the pelvic diaphragm. In some instances, a weak pelvic diaphragm can lead to prolapse of the internal organs. Prolapses are categorized by where in the perineum the organ emerges. Anterior prolapses typically involve the bladder emerging anterior to the

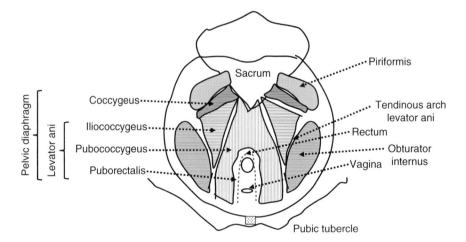

**Fig. 4.2** Pelvic diaphragm. The pelvic diaphragm is made up of levator ani and coccygeus. The levator ani is made up of the iliococcygeus, pubococcygeus and puborectalis. The iliococcygeus arises from the tendinous arch of levator ani. (Leo 2022)

vagina. Posterior prolapses involve the rectum or intestines emerging posterior to the vagina. And apical prolapses involve the uterus emerging thought the vagina.

In the lithotomy position, the perineum can be seen as a diamond shaped pelvic outlet with four points to it. On the sides, the two points are the ischial tuberosities, anterior is the pubic symphysis and posterior is the coccyx. By drawing a line between the two ischial tuberosities, the perineum is further subdivided into two smaller triangles:

1. the *anal triangle* is bounded superiorly by the pelvic diaphragm and contains the internal and external anal sphincters.
2. the *urogenital triangle* has the extra layer of support mentioned earlier. In the lithotomy position the urogenital triangle blocks the view of the pelvic diaphragm.

## Internal Iliac Artery

The internal iliac artery arises from the common iliac artery and enters the pelvic cavity anterior to the sacroiliac joint. There is significant variability in its branching pattern, but it has an anterior and posterior division. The anterior division gives off three branches (Fig. 4.3):

1. The *iliolumbar artery* divides into an *iliac* branch descending towards the ileum and a *lumbar* branch ascending towards the lumbar vertebrae.
2. The *superior gluteal artery* heads inferior and typically runs between the lumbo-sacral trunk and the S1 nerve. It then leaves the pelvis through the greater sciatic foramen and enters the gluteal region superior to piriformis. As it approaches the

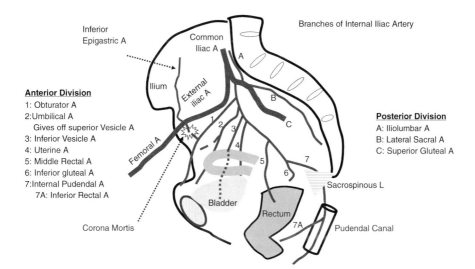

**Fig. 4.3** Branches of the internal iliac artery. (Leo 2022)

gluteal muscles it travels between the gluteus medius and gluteus minimus. In cases of pelvic fractures, the superior gluteal artery is the most often injured vessel.

3. The *lateral sacral artery* heads down along the sacrum lateral to the ventral sacral foramina.

The posterior division of the internal iliac sends branches to the pelvic viscera, the medial thigh, and the gluteal region:

1. The distal portions of the right and left *umbilical arteries*, which transmitted blood to the placenta during development, become obliterated in the adult. Their remnants are found on the posterior surface of the anterior abdominal wall as the medial umbilical ligaments. But the proximal portion remains as the *superior vesicle artery* which goes to the bladder in males. In females this artery is the *vaginal artery,* although in some individuals the vaginal artery will come off the uterine artery.

2. The *obturator artery* leaves the pelvis through the obturator foramen to reach the anterior thigh.

3. The *middle rectal artery* supplies the rectum.

4. The *uterine artery* supplies the uterus. The uterine artery heads towards the cervix in the cardinal ligament traveling over the ureter. As it reaches the uterus it divides into an ascending branch heading towards the uterus, and a descending branch heading towards the vagina. The ascending branch of the uterine artery has a curvy, twisted path so that in a pregnant woman the artery can stretch as the uterus expands.

5. The *inferior gluteal artery* leaves the pelvis through the lesser sciatic foramen inferior to the piriformis to enter the gluteal region.

6. The *internal pudendal artery* leaves the pelvis through the greater sciatic foramen, but then reenters the pelvis through the lesser sciatic foramen. It does a 100° turn around the sacrospinous ligament to enter the pudendal canal which is made up of the fascia of obturator internus.

The visceral peritoneum in the abdominal cavity extends down into the pelvic area and overlays the various organs. The lowest point in the peritoneal cavity is the *rectouterine pouch* in females and *rectovesical pouch* in males. In the supine position, excess fluid in the peritoneal cavity can collect in the rectouterine pouch and also drain via the paracolic gutters to the hepatorenal recess. In the sitting position, the fluid will drain out of the hepatorenal recess and collect in the rectouterine pouch.

## Internal Pudendal Artery

Traveling with the pudendal nerve is the internal pudendal artery. Its branching pattern is very similar to the nerve branches (Fig. 4.4):

**Fig. 4.4** Branches of
internal pudendal artery.
The internal pudendal
artery comes off the
anterior division of the
internal iliac and Leaves
the pelvis through the
greater sciatic foramen. It
then wraps around the
sacrospinous ligament and
renters the pelvis through
the lesser sciatic foramen.
It continues into the
pudendal canal. At the
entrance to the canal, it
gives off an inferior rectal
artery. In the canal it then
gives off a perineal artery.
At the end, the artery
divides into the deep artery
of the penis and the dorsal
artery of the penis or
clitoris. (Leo 2022)

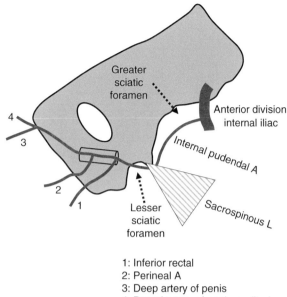

1: Inferior rectal
2: Perineal A
3: Deep artery of penis
4: Dorsal artery of penis or clitoris

1. The *inferior rectal artery* comes off at the beginning of the pudendal canal and crosses the ischiorectal fossa with the inferior rectal nerve.
2. The *perineal artery* supplies the superficial perineum.
3. The *artery to the bulb* supplies the bulb of the vestibule or penis.
4. The *dorsal artery of the penis or clitoris* supplies these two structures.

---

## Pudendal Nerve

The *pudendal nerve* comes from S 2, 3, and 4 and enters the pudendal canal and travels to the perineum. Although there are some autonomic fibers that travel on it, it is primarily a somatic nerve carrying voluntary nerve fibers. On the way it has several branches (Fig. 4.5).

1. The *inferior rectal nerve* has a motor and sensory component. The motor component is to the external anal sphincter. The sensory component is to the skin around the anus. The anal wink is a test for the inferior rectal nerve. In a healthy individual, when the skin around the anus is scratched, the external anal sphincter contracts confirming that the inferior rectal nerve, the pudendal nerve, and S 2, 3, and 4 are all intact.
2. The *perineal nerve* also has motor and sensory branches. The motor nerve supplies all the muscles of the deep and superficial spaces except for the internal urethral sphincter. The sensory branch is the either the posterior scrotal or

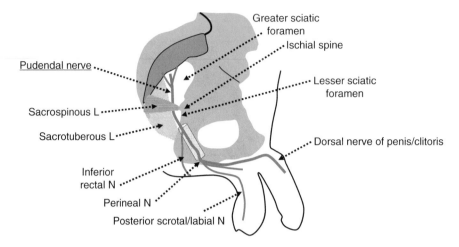

**Fig. 4.5**  Pudendal nerve and its branches. (Leo 2022)

   posterior labial branch. In addition, in females this nerve is responsible for sensation from the terminal one-third of the vagina.
3. The *dorsal nerve of the clitoris or penis* is the terminal branch of the pudendal nerve and is responsible for sensation from the penis or clitoris.

A pudendal nerve block can be used for episiotomies or other surgeries in this region to block pain sensation. The nerve can be anesthetized at the ischial spine.

## The Bladder

The bladder sits just posterior to the pubic bone. The space between the bladder and the pubic bone is the retropubic space which is not part of the peritoneal cavity. Most of the bladder consists of smooth muscle referred to as the *detrusor muscle.* The interior of the bladder has a triangular shaped trigone with three points. Two of the points are made by the ureters entering the bladder. At the center point, the lumen of the bladder turns into the neck of the bladder, which in turn forms the beginning of the urethra. Surrounding the urethra just as it enters the prostate is the *internal urethral sphincter.*

   When the bladder is full it comes up above the pubic bone. Bladder injuries can result in urine draining into the peritoneal cavity (intraperitoneal) or around the peritoneal cavity (extraperitoneal). For instance, in an automobile accident, if the driver has a full bladder, the dome of the bladder can rupture, which in turn tears the visceral peritoneum over the dome. This leads to urine draining into the peritoneal cavity. Pelvic fractures tend to damage the anterior surface of the bladder right behind the pelvic bone. In this case, urine can drain into the retropubic space which is separated from the peritoneal cavity.

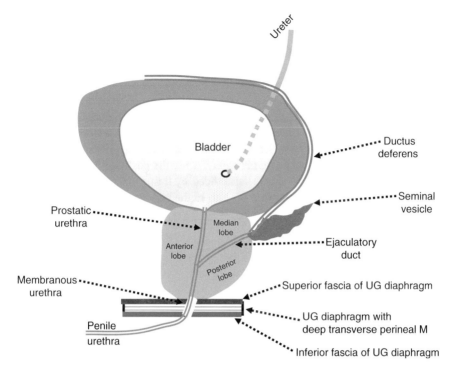

**Fig. 4.6** Urogenital diaphragm. The urogenital diaphragm is located between the superior fascia and inferior fascia of the urogenital diaphragm. Emerging from the bladder is the prostatic urethra, which then travels through the urogenital diaphragm as the membranous urethra, which becomes the penile urethra. (Leo 2022)

At the base of the bladder is the internal urethral sphincter which is also smooth muscle. The detrusor and the internal sphincter work together for voiding and filing of the bladder. When the bladder is filling up, the detrusor relaxes and the internal urethral sphincter contracts. When the bladder is filled and needs to empty, the detrusor will contract, and the internal urethral sphincter will relax. This coordinated activity is under control of the pelvic splanchnic nerves (Fig. 4.6).

The internal urethral is related to the superior surface of the prostate. On the inferior surface of the prostate is the external urethral sphincter which is skeletal muscle under control of the pudendal nerve.

In males, the bladder sits on top of the prostate. The urethra coming out of the bladder passes through the bladder as the prostatic urethrae. Joining the prostatic urethra are the ejaculatory ducts which are the common ducts of the vas deferens and the seminal vesicle.

## Prostate

The prostate sits between the bladder and the urogenital diaphragm. The prostatic urethra leaves the bladder and travels through the prostate. Along the way, the ejaculatory ducts join the prostatic urethra. The prostatic urethra and the ejaculatory ducts divide the prostate up into five lobes. In a mid-sagittal cut one can see the *anterior lobe* in front of the prostatic urethra, the *median lobe* between the prostatic urethra and the ejaculatory duct, and the *posterior lobe*, posterior to the ejaculatory duct. Moving laterally on either side are the *lateral lobes* of the prostate. The median lobe is the site of begin prostatic hypertrophy, while the posterior lobe is the site of prostatic carcinoma. The prostate is surrounded by a fine network of nerve fibers, the prostatic plexus, which in turn gives rise to the cavernous nerves which travel through the urogenital diaphragm to reach the erectile tissue in the superficial perineal space (Fig. 4.6).

The interior of the prostatic urethra is not a simple round tube. On the posterior wall of the prostatic urethra is a protuberance called the *seminal colliculus*. And on the seminal colliculus are three small openings:

1. The *prostatic utricle* is a blind ended sac.
2. On each side of the utricle are the paired *openings of the ejaculatory ducts*.

At the edges of the seminal colliculus are the *prostatic sinuses* where the glands of the prostate open. In the retropubic space is a venous network – the prostatic plexus – which is responsible for the venous drainage of the prostate. This network communicates with the venous networks higher up and can be the cause of prostatic carcinoma spreading to the lungs.

## Uterus

The uterus typically rests on top of the bladder with the cervix pointing posteroinferiorly. It is usually in an anteverted and anteflexed position. There are three layers to the uterus.

1. *Endometrium* is the inner lining with abundant glandular tissue.
2. *Myometrium* is the middle muscular layer.
3. *Perimetrium* is the thin serous layer of peritoneum covering the uterus.

The fundus of the uterus is the superior rounded section. The horns (cornu) are located at each corner Coming into the cornu are the uterine tubes. The cervix is bounded by the superior portion of the vagina. Around the cervix is a continuous space referred to as the fornix which can be divided into anterior, lateral, or posterior fornix.

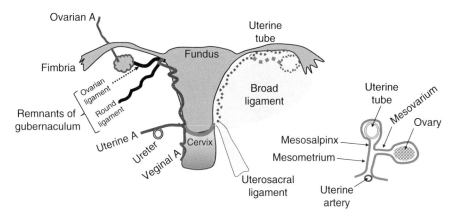

**Fig. 4.7** Broad ligament. The broad ligament is made up of the mesosalpinx, mesometrium, and mesovarium. The ovarian ligament and the round ligament are remnants of the gubernaculum . The ureter runs inferior to the uterine artery. (Leo 2022)

The peritoneum descends along the posterior wall and is reflected onto the superior surface of the bladder at the rectum. This gives rise to the lowest point in the female peritoneal cavity: the rectouterine pouch. Fluid either from an ectopic pregnancy, or an infection in the peritoneal cavity, can be aspirated via the posterior fornix (Fig. 4.7).

## Ovary, Uterine Tube, and Broad Ligament

At ovulation the egg leaves the ovary and crosses the peritoneal cavity and is picked up by the fimbria to enter the uterine tube. From here the ova moves into the ampulla. If sperm are present, fertilization will occur in the ampulla of the uterine tube. It takes approximately 7 days for the developing embryo to move into the uterus. Implantation typically occurs along the posterior surface of the uterus.

The ovary is attached to the cornua of the uterus by the *ovarian ligament*. Also, attached to the cornua is the *round ligament* running from the cornua through the deep inguinal ring, through the inguinal canal to connect to the labia majora. The round ligament and the ovarian ligament are both remnants of the *gubernaculum*. At one point the ligaments are continuous and do not touch the uterus, but during development, the gubernaculum shortens, and as it descends it eventually touches the cornu of the uterus, giving rise to the two different sections: the round ligament and the ovarian ligament (Fig. 4.8).

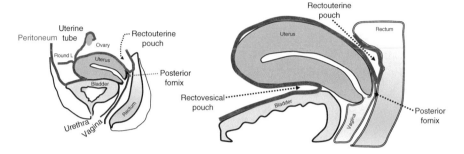

**Fig. 4.8** Peritoneum in the pelvis. Starting on the posterior abdominal wall, the peritoneum, shown in red, descends and is reflected from the rectum to lie on top of the uterus and bladder. Note the proximity of the rectouterine pouch and the posterior fornix. (Leo 2022)

## Broad Ligament

The peritoneum is like a sheet draped over the internal female organs, and as such, it can be divided into three subdivisions:

1. The *mesosalpinx* is the mesentery folded around the uterine tube (salpinx = tube).
2. The *mesovarium* is the mesentery folded around the ovary.
3. The *mesometrium* is the mesentery along the sides of the uterus. Running along the base of the mesometrium is the cardinal ligament.

The blood supply to the uterus comes from the uterine artery which approaches the uterus and divides into an ascending branch which travels up along the edge of the uterus to anastomose with branches of the ovarian artery which came from the descending aorta. The descending branch of the uterine artery descends towards the vagina to anastomose with the vaginal artery. As the uterine artery approaches the uterus if travels superior to the ureter (*water under the bridge*).

## Cardinal and Uterosacral Ligaments

The *cardinal ligament* (Mackenrodt's Ligament) runs transversally from the cervix and vagina to the lateral pelvic wall. It sits at the base of the broad ligament and the uterine artery runs in it on its way to the uterus. The two *uterosacral ligaments* are U-shaped, with each one running from the posterior cervix and vagina towards the sacrum (Fig. 4.4).

## Superficial Space and Deep Perineal Spaces

In the perineal region there are three layers of fascia and two layers of muscle. To talk about these layers, we are going to use a big mac as an analogy. A big mac, remember, has three layers of bun and two hamburger patties. The bottom layer or bun is the *superficial perineal fascia*, the middle layer of bun is the *inferior fascia of the UG diaphragm* (perineal membrane), and the top layer of the bun is the *superior fascia of the UG diaphragm*. Between the bottom bun and middle bun is the *superficial perineal space*. Starting from superficial and moving deep we are going to discuss each layer.

The bottom layer of the bun is the superficial perineal fascia, also known as Colle's fascia. Colle's fascia is continuous with Scarpa's fascia on the anterior abdominal wall, and with the fascia lata on the thigh. At the line between the urogenital and anal triangles, Colle's fascia is attached to the perineal body (Figs. 4.9, 4.10, and 4.11).

In the superficial perineal space, the bottom hamburger layer, are three muscles:

1. The *ischiocavernosus* runs from the inferior pubic rami towards the penis or clitoris.
2. In females the *bulbospongiosus* is found on the sides of the vestibule. In males the bulbospongiosus is fused in the midline on the bulb of the penis.
3. The two *superficial transverse perineal* muscles run from the ischial tuberosities towards the midline and meet at the perineal body. The bulbospongiosus muscle and the external anal sphincter muscle also meet at the perineal body.

These muscles of the superficial space are sitting on top of the erectile tissue which is also in the superficial space:

1. The *crus* of the penis or clitoris are deep to the ischiocavernosus muscle.
2. The *bulb* of the vestibule (females) and the bulb of the penis sit just under the bulbospongiosus.

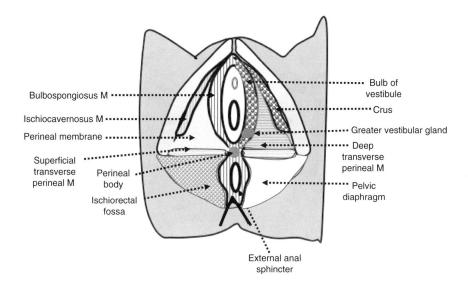

**Fig. 4.9** Perineum. On the patient's right are the muscles of the superficial space and the fat filled ischiorectal fossa. On the patient's left are the structures of the deep perineal space and the pelvic diaphragm. (Leo 2022)

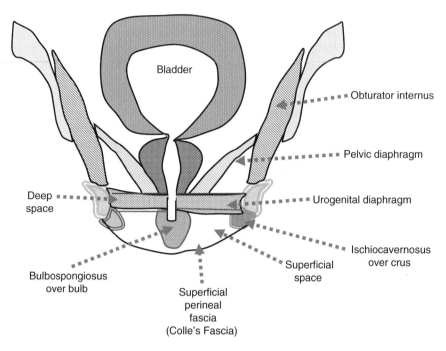

**Fig. 4.10** The urogenital diaphragm is bounded by the superior and inferior fascia of the urogenital diaphragm. In the superficial space are the ischiocavernosus and bulbospongiosus muscles over the crus and bulb, respectively. (Leo 2022)

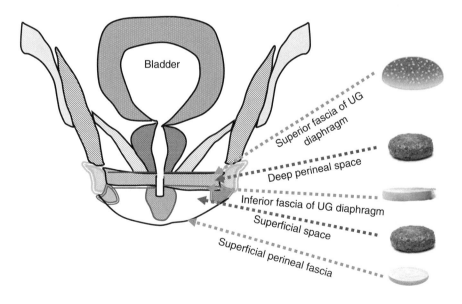

**Fig. 4.11** The perineum. The layers of the perineum are compared to the layers of a big mac. (Leo 2022)

And in females, the *greater vestibular glands* are found in the superficial space located in the posterior one-third of the vestibule.

The middle layer of the bun is the *inferior fascia of the urogenital triangle*, also known as the perineal membrane. This is a thick dense layer that serves as an anchoring point for the erectile tissue (bulbs and crura).

If we peel this layer away, we are now looking at the muscles and structures in the deep space. There are two muscles (Fig. 4.10):

1. The *deep transverse perineal* muscle is a very thin sheet running across the urogenital triangle from one inferior pubic ramus to the other.
2. Within the deep transverse perineal muscle is a small sphincter – the *membranous urethrae*. This sphincter is skeletal muscle which is innervated by the perineal branch of the pudendal nerve.

Also in this deep space, in males are the *bulbourethral glands*. However, while the glands are in the deep space, their ducts drain into the urethra in the superficial space. Of note, remember that in females the greater vestibular glands are in the superficial space.

## Dartos and Cremaster Muscles

The *dartos muscle* (sometimes referred to as the dartos fascia) is smooth muscle that is continuous with Scarpa's fascia. It wrinkles the scrotum to alter the surface area of the scrotum for heat exchange. In cold weather it will contract to pull the testes closer to the body and to decrease the surface area, and in warm weather it relaxes to increase the surface area of the scrotum. It is innervated by sympathetic fibers.

The *cremaster muscle* is an extension of the internal abdominal oblique muscle and travels in the inguinal canal to the testes. It is innervated by the somatic nervous system. Muscle fibers are usually visible running along the spermatic cord. In females there are some rudimentary fibers on the round ligament.

## Episiotomies and Caesarean Sections

During difficult deliveries when the clinician believes that the perineum might tear, episiotomies can be performed. They are typically in either a mediolateral or midline direction. There are advantages and disadvantages to either one. Mediolateral cuts avoid the anal canal, and even if the tear continues it will move laterally and avoid the anal canal region. Midline cuts avoid the nerves and arteries located laterally, but they can continue tearing posterior into the anal canal. And while the tough perineal body can prevent the tear from moving posteriorly, if the tear does go through perineal body, then it will move into the anal canal.

There are two main types of C-sections, a high vertical incision, or a low transverse incision. High incisions used to be more common (thus they are sometimes referred to as a classical incision), but the lower transverse incisions are more common now. The low incision avoids the more vascular superior part of the uterus. In addition, after the delivery the upper portion will contract and retract as it moves back towards its pre-pregnancy state. This contraction and retraction will not happen with the lower portion. The lower incision also gives better access to the actual presenting part of the delivery.

## Pudendal Versus Pelvic Splanchnic Nerves

Both the pudendal nerve and the pelvic splanchnic nerves come from sacral levels 2, 3, 4. However there are important differences between the two. The pelvic splanchnic nerves emerge from the ventral sacral foramina as multiple thread-like fibers to travel down on the walls of the various organs such as the rectum, bladder, and uterus. As they pass over these organs, they also provide the parasympathetic nerve supply to the organs. As the fibers come out of the sacrum they are first referred to as the inferior hypogastric plexus or one of its subsidiary plexuses such as rectal, vesicle, uterine, or prostatic plexus. These nerves are especially susceptible to trauma during pelvic surgery.

The pudendal nerve on the other hand travels through the pudendal canal and approaches the urogenital diaphragm from below. An example of trauma that could injure the pudendal nerve is a bike rider who falls forward off the seat and lands with the cross bar beneath the legs. The pudendal nerve is a somatic or voluntary nerve that carries sensory fibers from the perineal region and provides the motor supply to all the muscles of the deep and superficial spaces. It is not responsible for erection (Fig. 4.12).

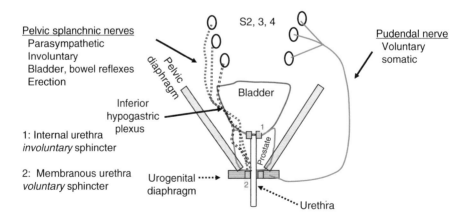

**Fig. 4.12** Both the pelvic splanchnic nerves and the pudendal nerves come from S 2, 3, 4. On one side the figure shows the pelvic splanchnic nerves joining the inferior hypogastric plexus and descending along the pelvic organs to approach the perineal structures from above. On the other side the pudendal nerve is shown leaving the pelvis and approaching the UG diaphragm from below. (Leo 2022)

## Anal Canal

An important division of the anal canal occurs at the pectinate line. This is where the hindgut endoderm meets the ectoderm. Because of this embryological meeting point, there are important structural differences above and below the pectinate line. For instance, the arterial supply above the pectinate line is the superior rectal artery, which comes from the inferior mesenteric artery; and below the pectinate line the blood supply is from the inferior rectal artery via the internal pudendal artery. Likewise, as discussed with the liver, the venous drainage above the line follows the superior rectal vein, to the inferior mesenteric vein, and eventually to the portal vein. The blood below the pectinate line follows the inferior rectal vein, to the internal pudendal vein, and eventually to the inferior vena cava.

The afferent nerve supply to the anal canal above the pectinate line comes from the pelvic splanchnic nerves which are parasympathetic. Because there are no significant pain fibers associated with these nerves, a needle placed in the anal canal above the pectinate line will not cause severe pain. However, the skin below the pectinate line is innervated by the pudendal nerve. Thus, a needle placed below the pectinate line will cause considerable pain (Fig. 4.13).

Above the pectinate line the mucosal layer of the anal canal is thrown into folds called anal folds. Under each fold is a branch of the venous structures. In a patient with portal hypertension, the venous network here can prolapse into the rectum. Hemorrhoids above the pectinate line are referred to as internal hemorrhoids, while those below the pectinate line are referred to as external hemorrhoids. At the distal end of each fold there is a flap of tissue that extends from one fold to another. Thus, the series of anal valves connecting one fold to another end up forming a ring around the terminal rectum. The space above each valve is an anal sinus.

Tears in the anal canal in the region of the anal valves and pectinate line can lead to infections that spread into the ischioanal fossa. Theses can lead to accesses and

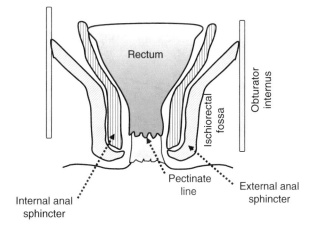

**Fig. 4.13** Anal canal. The pectinate line is the transition from endoderm to ectoderm. Surrounding the terminal anal canal are the internal anal and external anal sphincters. Between the sphincters and the obturator internus is the ischiorectal fossa. (Leo 2022)

fistulas developing in this region. In some cases, these fistulas can run from the anal canal, through the ischioanal fossa, and then open through the skin onto the external environment.

## Bladder and Bowel Control

Bladder and bowel control operate on the same basic mechanisms. The names of the various sphincters change whether you are talking about the bowel or bladder, but the nerve control of the two is similar. We will look at bowel control first. The bowel has internal and external anal sphincters. The internal anal sphincter is smooth muscle under control of the autonomic system via the pelvic splanchnic nerves coming from S 2, 3, and 4. The external anal sphincter is skeletal muscle under control of the somatic nervous system via the inferior rectal nerve, a branch of the pudendal nerve (Fig. 4.14).

The first diagram shows the process of normal voiding – also called the *Urge-to-Purge*. When contents come into the anal canal, the pressure stimulates the afferent nerve fibers that travel into S 2, 3, and 4 of the spinal cord. The information goes onto make a reflex loop with the efferent parasympathetic pathway, but the information also goes up the spinal cord to tell the cerebral cortex that the rectum is full. The efferent fibers of the reflex loop then tell the internal anal sphincter to relax. In an adult, when fecal material moves into the canal and the internal anal sphincter relaxes, however the adult can then voluntarily fire their pudendal nerve and contract the external anal sphincter. The adult will then look for the bathroom, sit down, relax, pick up a magazine or a book, and relax their external anal sphincter to void (Fig. 4.14).

When it comes to the bladder, instead of the internal and external *anal* sphincters, there are the internal and external *urethral* sphincters, plus the detrusor muscle.

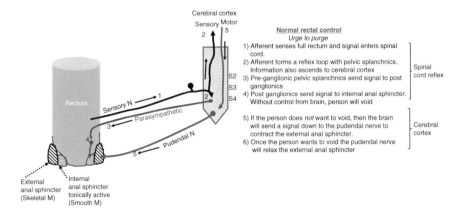

**Fig. 4.14** Autonomic and somatic nerve control of rectum. (Leo 2022)

During the filling stage, the internal urethral sphincter is contracted, and the detrusor is relaxed. During voiding the detrusor contracts, and the internal and external urethral sphincters relax. With this in mind, we have two lesions to discuss.

## Upper Motor Neuron – Spastic Bladder and Bowel

In this first scenario there is a lesion in the cervical or thoracic cord which will lead to blockage of the corticospinal pathway. The sacral regions are still functioning, they are just cut off from cortical control. This person's reflex is still intact, they just have no voluntary control so they will have spontaneous voiding. The bladder fills up, sensory fibers tell the sacral cord that the bladder is full, the reflex loop is active, and the efferent fibers relax the external anal sphincter. The reflex loop is operating on its own and has no cortical involvement (Fig. 4.15).

## Lower Motor Neuron – Flaccid Bladder and Bowel

In this second scenario there is trauma to the sacral region and the lower motor neurons are lost. In this case, the internal anal sphincter remains tonically active, and the individual does not have the ability to relax the muscle, and the patient's anal canal will fill up with material and there will be a slow seepage of contents out of the anal canal and bladder (Fig. 4.16).

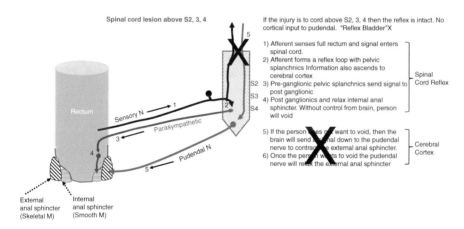

**Fig. 4.15** With a lesion to the cord above S 2, 3, 4 then the reflex arc is still present and internal anal sphincter will relax. Because the patient has no control over pudendal nerve the bowel is only operating at the reflex level. "Upper Motor Neuron Deficit" "Spastic Bowel (Bladder)." (Leo 2022)

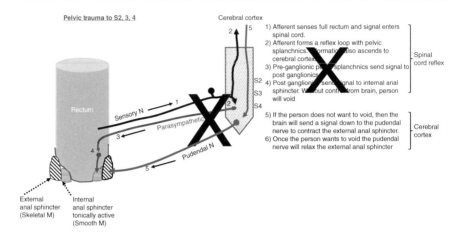

**Fig. 4.16** Bowel Control and LMN Injury. With trauma to the pelvis that damages the conus medullaris (S 2, 3, 4) there is no reflex arc or cortical control. The internal anal sphincter remains tonically active, and person cannot void. Fecal contents will build up until they eventually dribble out. "Lower Motor Neuron Deficit" "Flaccid Bowel (Bladder)". (Leo, 2022)

## Superior Hypogastric Plexus

The superior hypogastric plexus is a collection of fibers resting on top of the sacral promontory. Coming out of it on both sides are the right and left hypogastric nerves, which are sympathetic fibers descending down along the sacrum. Along the way they are joined by the pelvic splanchnic nerves to make up the inferior hypogastric plexus. The most important function of the superior hypogastric plexus is that it receives the pain fibers from the pelvic viscera such as uterus and ovary. A superior hypogastric nerve block is used to block painful sensations from these organs.

## Pelvis

The innominate bone or os coxae is made up of three bones that fuse together. Together these three bones form the lateral sides of the pelvis.

1. the *pubis* has both a superior and an inferior pubic ramus projecting out of its body.
2. the *ischium* has two important landmarks. One is the *ischial spine* where the sacrospinous ligament attaches. The second is the *ischial tuberosity* where the sacrotuberous ligament and hamstring muscles attach. Projecting anteriorly is the ischial ramus which meets the inferior pubic ramus.
3. the *ilium* is the largest of the three bones and has a fan shape look to it. The *iliac crest* runs from the *anterior superior iliac spine* to the *posterior superior iliac spine*. Along the lateral wall, are three lines: the posterior, anterior, and inferior

gluteal lines, for the attachment of the gluteus maximus, gluteus medius, and gluteus minimus respectively.

All three of the bones that comprise the innominate bone: the pubis, ischium, and ilium meet at the *triradiate cartilage* to form the acetabulum of the hip joint. The *obturator foramen is* the large round opening whose boundary is made up of pubis, ischium, and ilium.

The two innominate bones (right and left) meet in the anterior midline at the *pubic symphysis*. Posteriorly, they meet the sacrum. There are important differences between the male and female innominate bones that are based on the fact in females the fetal head moves through the canal during delivery.

The *pelvic inlet* is a line from the superior pubic symphysis to the sacral promontory. It is widest in the transverse section. The pelvic outlet is taken from a line drawn from the lower border of the pubic bone to the coccyx. The widest diameter of the outlet is in the anterior posterior direction. Thus, during delivery, because the fetal head is largest in the anterior to posterior section, as the fetus moves thought the pelvic inlet it will be looking off to the side, but as it moves through the pelvic outlet it will be facing posterior as it passes through the pelvic outlet (Fig. 4.17).

The female innominate bone tends to be lighter and thinner than the male innominate bone. The pelvic inlet in females is oval shaped with the long axis of the oval going from side to side. The pelvic inlet in males, because of the jutting out of the sacral promontory, is shaped like a heart. The pelvic outlet in females is rounder and wider, while in males it is thinner and smaller. The pelvic cavity in females is cylindrical with short parallel sides, while in males it is cone shaped with long sides projecting medially. The pubic arch in females is wide and has a circular shape and is about the size of the angle between your second and third fingers when spread. In females, the ischial tuberosities are everted, while in males they are inverted. The subpubic arch in males is narrow and triangular shaped and can be represented by the angle between your thumb and index finger when spread.

## Sacrum

The sacrum is a wedge-shaped bone made up of the five fused vertebrae of S1-S5. Superiorly it articulates with the L5 vertebra, and inferiorly it articulates with the coccyx. Posterior to the fused vertebrae is the sacral canal with the cauda equina running in it. At the end of the sacral canal is the sacral hiatus where a sacral epidural nerve block can be administered. On the anterior surface are the five anterior sacral foramina, and posterior are the five posterior sacral foramina. On the lateral sides are the two sacral ala (wings) which each form one side of the sacroiliac joint.

The *sacroiliac joint* has a small amount of movement in children, but in adults it is essentially fused. Sacroiliac joint disease is characterized by very small movements at the joint which lead to chronic pain. The *Faber test* is used to evaluate the hip. The patient is in a supine position and places one ankle on the opposite knee – similar to the tailor's position. The lower limb is now abducted, flexed, and

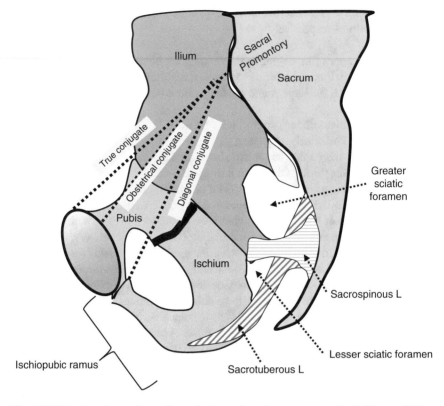

**Fig. 4.17** The three bones that make up the innominate bone are the pubis, ischium and Ilium. Note the pubis and ischium meet to form the ischiopubic ramus. The true conjugate runs from the top of the pubic symphysis to the sacral promontory. The obstetrical conjugate runs from the pubic bone to sacral promontory. The diagonal conjugate runs from the inferior level of the pubic symphysis to the sacral promontory. During a vaginal exam, the diagonal conjugate can be measured. Taking 2 cm off the diagonal conjugate gives a rough estimation of the obstetrical conjugate. (Leo 2022)

externally rotated. The examiner now pushes down on the flexed knee. Pain is thought to be indicative of sacroiliac joint pathology.

On the anterior and posterior surface of the sacrum are the four anterior and posterior sacral foramina through which emerge the ventral and dorsal rami of the sacral nerves. Medial to the anterior sacral foramina are the sympathetic trunks and the lateral sacral arteries. On the posterior surface, one can see the *iliac crest* turning into the *posterior superior iliac spine* which is an important landmark. It marks the middle of the SI joint, the S2 vertebra, and the end of the dural Superficially, the dimple just above the buttocks is directly over the posterior superior iliac spine.

## Further Reading

Boutefnouchet T, Bassett J, Patil S. Anatomy and clinical relevance of the "Corona Mortis": a review of the literature and current aspects of management. J Orthop Rheumatol. 2016;3(2):5.

Moore K, Dalley AF, Agur A. Clinically oriented anatomy. 7th ed. Baltimore: Lippincott Williams and Wilkin; 2014.

Razak L. Pathophysiology of pelvic organ prolapse. In: Rizvi RM, editor. Pelvic floor disorders. IntechOpen; 2018. https://doi.org/10.5772/intechopen.76629. Available from: https://www.intechopen.com/chapters/60935.

Rosse C, Gaddum-Rosse P. Hollinshead's textbook of anatomy. 5th ed. New York: Lippincott-Raven; 1997.

Said H. Endoscopic anatomy of the groin: implications for transabdominal preperitoneal herniorrhaphy. Anat J Africa. 2012;September(1):2–10.

Seif E, Iwanaga J, Oskouian RJ, Loukas M, Tubbs RS. Comprehensive review of the cardinal ligament. Cureus. 2018. https://doi.org/10.7759/cureus.2846.

Simon LV, Sajjad H, Lopez RA, Burns B. Bladder rupture. Stat Pearls. 2020. Available at: https://www.ncbi.nim.nih.gov/books/NBK470226/.

Snell R. Clinical anatomy by region. 9th ed. Lippincott Williams and Wilkins. New York; 2012.

Standring S. Gray's anatomy: the anatomical basis of clinical practice. London: Elsevier; 2005.

Vallabhajosyula R, Mathur M, Kathirvel R, Madan AI, Kang J, Mogali SR. Getting back to the basics: reintroduction of pelvic anatomy concepts for obstetrics and gynecology residents. Proc Singapore Healthc. 2020:1–7. https://doi.org/10.1177/2010105820935913.

# The Lower Limb

5

## Gluteal Region

There are three gluteal muscles (Fig. 5.1):

1. *Gluteus Maximus* is the largest muscle of the buttocks. Its origin is a semi-circular line running from the posterior gluteal line of the ilium, along the sacrum, the sacrospinous ligament, and the coccyx. It inserts into the iliotibial tract, the linea aspera and gluteal tuberosity of the femur. In the standing position, the muscle covers the ischial tuberosity, but in the sitting position, it rises

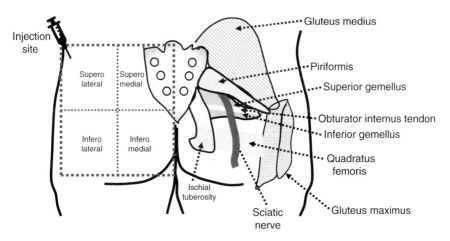

**Fig. 5.1** Gluteal region. The piriformis is a landmark for the gluteal region. Emerging inferior to it is the sciatic nerve which in turn is passing over the superior gemellus, obturator internus and the inferior gemellus. (Leo 2022)

up over the ischial tuberosity so that you sit on your ischial tuberosity and not the gluteus. The gluteus maximus is a strong extensor at the hip joint. Thus, it is important in going from a sitting to a standing position. Running up and down the stairs will strengthen the muscle. It is innervated by the inferior gluteal nerve. Patients with damage to the nerve will have difficulty standing – getting out of a car seat for instance.

2. *Gluteus Medius* is deep to gluteus maximus. It arises from the ilium and inserts into the greater trochanter.
3. *Gluteus Minimus* is deep to gluteus medius. It arises from the ilium and inserts into the greater trochanter. Both gluteus medius and minimus are abductors of the hip.

## Trendelenburg Sign and Trendelenburg Gait

Gluteus medius and minimus work together to stabilize the pelvis when the contra-lateral foot is lifted off the ground. For instance, when you are in a standing posi-tion, and lift your left foot off the ground, the tendency to fall is to the left. As an analogy, imagine kicking out the leg of a dining room table; the table will fall towards the unsupported side. In the healthy human example, lifting the left leg off the ground results in a tendency to fall to the left, but the right gluteus medius and minimus will contract to stabilize the pelvis, and prevent the lean to the left. With damage on the right side, if the person lifts their left leg off the ground they will tend to fall to the left. In the same patient, they will not have a deficit if they lift their right leg off the ground.

If you suspect a patient has a weak gluteus medius and minimus on the right, you ask them to stand and lift the left leg off the ground. If the right muscles are weak, the patient will fall towards the left. This is known as *Trendelenburg's sign*. This patient will also have a "waddling gait" or *Trendelenburg gait*. When they are walk-ing, each time they lift their left leg off the ground they will tend to fall to the left, so they will counteract this tendency by excessively leaning to the right.

Deep to the three gluteal muscles are the six deep lateral rotators. All these mus-cles run from the sacral region laterally to insert along the posterior side of the greater trochanter of the femur (Figs. 5.1 and 5.2).

1. The triangular shaped *piriformis* runs from sacrum to the greater trochanter and is the major landmark in this region. Most of the other muscles and the nerves and arteries in this region are explained based on their relationship to piriformis. They are either superior or inferior to piriformis.
2. Inferior to piriformis are three muscles that form a triangle, sometimes referred to as the triceps coxae (three hip muscles). The middle muscle of the group is the *obturator internus*. If you are dissecting the gluteal region and have removed the three large gluteal muscles, the main muscle belly of obturator internus is out of view, but you can see its tendon sandwiched between two smaller muscle bellies. The tendon is a sharp white line at this point. On either side of the tendon of

**Fig. 5.2** Piriformis relationships. Emerging above piriformis is superior gluteal neurovascular bundle. Emerging below the muscle is the inferior neurovascular bundle. The pudendal nerve also emerges inferior to piriformis, but it does a U-turn and re-enters the pelvis between the sacrotuberous and sacrospinous ligaments. (Leo 2022)

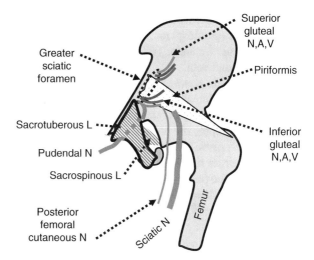

piriformis is the *superior gemellus* and *inferior gemellus*. The two gemelli arise from the ischial spine. The sciatic nerve emerges from the pelvis inferior to piriformis and passes over (posterior to) these three muscles. Obturator internus is discussed in more detail in the pelvis chapter, as its muscle belly forms the lateral wall of the pelvic cavity.

3. *Obturator externus* is not typically visible in the gluteal region with a posterior approach. It also inserts on the greater trochanter. It is discussed in more detail with the medial thigh.
4. *Quadratus femoris* is inferior to the triceps coxae and is also a deep lateral rotator.

## Nerves and Vessels of Gluteal Region

The gluteal region is described as four quadrants. The nerves and arteries of the gluteal region are located in the inferior medial quadrant, thus an injection in this gluteal region is typically given in the superolateral quadrant to avoid these underlying structures.

1. Emerging from the pelvis superior to the piriformis is the *superior gluteal nerve* and *superior gluteal artery* and *vein* which travel between the gluteus medius and minimus. The superior gluteal nerve innervates the gluteus medius and minimus. The superior gluteal vessels are often injured with pelvic fractures.
2. Emerging inferior to the piriformis is the *inferior gluteal nerve and inferior gluteal artery and vein*. The nerve innervates the gluteus maximus.
3. The *pudendal nerve* is the major of the pelvis, but it makes a brief appearance in the gluteal region. It emerges from the pelvis close to the inferior gluteal nerve, but while the inferior gluteal nerve heads posterior to the gluteal region, the

pudendal nerve does a quick 90° turn and heads back into the pelvis by traveling between the sacrospinous and sacrotuberous ligaments, and back through the lesser sciatic foramen. Traveling with the pudendal nerve is the internal pudendal artery and vein.

4. The *posterior femoral cutaneous nerve* also emerges inferior to piriformis through the gluteal region to enter the posterior thigh. It gives a branch to the inferior gluteal region (inferior cluneal nerve) and to the perineum (perineal branch) to supply the posterior regions of the labia majora and the scrotum.

5. The *sciatic nerve* is the largest nerve in the body, even larger than the spinal cord, and it emerges inferior to piriformis to travel medial to the ischial tuberosity on its way to the posterior thigh. The sciatic nerve has two divisions at this point: the *common fibular division*, and the *tibial division*. At this point the two divisions are typically running wrapped together in the same sheath. They will eventually split as they approach the popliteal fossa. However, in some individuals the split occurs in the pelvis with the common fibular division traveling through the piriformis. In this case, the individual may present with sciatica like symptoms and complain of weakness in the muscular compartments innervated by the common fibular nerve.

## Trochanteric Bursitis

As the gluteus medius and minimus pass over the *greater trochanter* there is a bursa between the muscles and the bone. This bursa can become inflamed leading to hip pain. Tendinopathy of the medius and minimus can also lead to pain in this region. In fact, it is hard to tell whether the pain is coming from bursitis or tendinopathy. The tendons of the medius and minimus and the associated bursa can be compressed by the overlying iliotibial band. Exercises to strengthen the medius and minimus are thought to alleviate the pain.

## Cutaneous Sensation in Gluteal Region

Cutaneous sensory information from the superolateral quadrant of the gluteal region travels on the *superior cluneal nerves* which are branches of the dorsal rami of L1, 2, and 3; sensation from the inferolateral quadrant is via the *inferior cluneal nerves* which are branches of the posterior femoral cutaneous nerve; sensation from the superomedial quadrant is via the *medial cluneal nerves* which are branches of the dorsal rami of S 1, 2, and 3; and sensation from the inferomedial quadrant is via the *perforating cutaneous nerve*, from the ventral rami of S, 2 and 3.

# The Thigh

Both the thigh and the leg each have three compartments. In the thigh there are the anterior, posterior, and medial compartments; and in the leg there are the anterior, posterior, and lateral compartments.

## Fascia Lata and Iliotibial Band

The *fascia lata* is a thick tough layer of fascia surrounding the thigh. It is connected to the gluteal fascia which in turn is connected to the thoracolumbar fascia superiorly. The *iliotibial tract* is a thickened layer of the fascia lata on the lateral thigh and runs from the superior iliac crest to *Gerdy's tubercle* on the anterolateral side of the proximal tibia. Within the superior portion of the iliotibial tract is the *tensor fascia lata,* which contracts the iliotibial band, leading to extension and lateral rotation of the leg. It is also involved in adduction and medial rotation of the thigh. It is innervated by the superior gluteal nerve.

*Iliotibial syndrome* occurs when the muscle is overactive which leads to pain on the lateral thigh or knee. It is a common injury in runners. Patients will often complain of pain when standing, getting out of a chair, or getting out of the car for instance. Exercises to develop the gluteus medius, such as running up and down stairs are often recommended.

## Anterior Thigh

The bulk of the anterior thigh is made up of the quadriceps, but it also includes the sartorius and the pectineus. The pectineus is confused as it sits right between the anterior and medial compartments, and some authors will group it with the anterior compartment while other authors will group it with the medial compartment. Since it needs to have a home, I will talk about it as being in the anterior compartment (Fig. 5.2).

The *sartorius,* the longest muscle in the body, is sometimes referred to as the "Tailor's muscle" which alludes to the tailor sitting with the leg crossed with the hip flexed, the knee flexed, and the lower limb laterally rotated at the hip. The tailor would then put a sheet over their thighs to catch anything that they dropped. The sartorius runs from the anterior superior iliac spine (ASIS) to the medial side of the proximal tibia (Fig. 5.3).

Sitting deep to the sartorius is quadriceps group of muscles which include the three vasti and the rectus femoris. The vastus medialis, vastus lateralis, and vastus

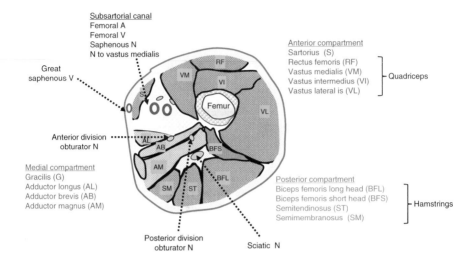

**Fig. 5.3** Cross section of Thigh. In the medial compartment, gracilis is most medial with adductor longus, brevis, and magnus organized in three planes. The adductor brevis is between the anterior and posterior divisions of obturator nerve. In the posterior compartment are the hamstrings: semitendinosus, semimembranosus, and the long head of biceps femoris. In the anterior compartment are the quadriceps and sartorius. The cross section is below pectineus thus it is not in the image. (Leo 2022)

intermedius, all originate from the femur, and come together with the rectus femoris to make up the *quadriceps tendon* which runs over the patella and then continues as the *patellar tendon*. Together with the rectus femoris they are all involved with extension of the knee. In addition, the rectus femoris is a hip flexor.

At first glance one might expect the muscle fibers of vastus medialis to be orientated in a superior to inferior direction. However, if one looks closely at the inferior fibers of vastus medialis, which are easily seen medial to the patella, you will see that they are angled so that they enter the patellar tendon from the side. These fibers then help to counteract the patella's tendency to slip laterally.

Of note is that both the sartorius and the rectus femoris span the hip and the knee joint, and both contribute to hip flexion, however their actions at the knee differ. The rectus femoris arises from the *anterior inferior iliac spine* and runs over the front of the knee and joins the patella tendon to insert into the tibial tuberosity, making it a knee extensor. The sartorius on the other hand runs to the medial side of the knee to insert on the medial surface of the tibia, making is a knee flexor.

*Osgood-Schlatter disease* primarily occurs in adolescents. The patellar tendon attaches to the tibial tuberosity and excessive strain can lead to inflammation of the attachment site.

*Myositis Ossificans* is a somewhat common injury in athletes that arises from repeated trauma or bruising to a muscle that can result in bone forming within the damaged region. It often happens in the quadriceps. Resting after an injury is the best way to prevent bone from forming. With an appropriate amount of rest the bone tissue will typically be reabsorbed.

## Pes Anserinus

The *Pes Anserinus* is a point on the medial tibia where three tendons insert. One mnemonic for remembering this is, Say Grace before Tea standing for the **S**artorius, **G**racilis, and semi**T**endinosus. The three muscles and the Pes Anserinus are like an upside-down tripod, with each muscle, or leg of the tripod coming from a different compartment: sartorius from the anterior compartment, gracilis from the medial compartment, and semitendinosus from the posterior compartment. Deep to the pes anserinus is the *pes anserinus bursa* which can become inflamed (Fig. 5.4).

## Medial Thigh

The bulk of the medial compartment is made up of the three adductors – brevis, longus, and magnus. On the medial edge of the medial compartment is the strap-like *gracilis*. At the superior medial corner, the *pectineus* makes a brief appearance in the medial thigh. The muscles of the medial thigh are organized in three planes. The first plane houses the *adductor longus* and the pectineus. Deep to the adductor longus and pectineus, in the middle layer, is the *adductor brevis.* And then in the deepest layer is the *adductor magnus.* The entire medial thigh is innervated by the obturator nerve. The *obturator nerve* is a branch of the lumbosacral plexus and comes through the obturator foramen and enters the thigh where it splits into *anterior and posterior divisions* proximal to the adductor brevis. The anterior division is

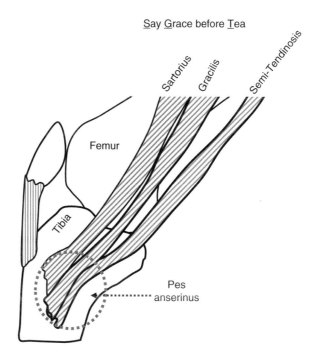

**Fig. 5.4** Pes anserinus. At the medial side of the tibia three muscles come together. From anterior to posterior: the sartorius, gracilis, and semitendinosus – Say Grace Before Tea. (Leo 2022)

easily seen entering the gracilis. Like all the thigh compartments there is one exception. The "hamstring portion" of adductor magnus is innervated by the tibial division of the sciatic nerve. The hamstring portion of adductor magnus is the most medial part of the muscle, it is relatively thin and can be seen attaching to the *adductor tubercle* of the femur. Strain on the adductors is a common injury to horseback riders. The obturator nerve innervates both the hip and knee joint thus a patient can complain of pain in one of these joints when the pathology is in the other joint. In addition, because of the obturator nerve's pathway through the pelvis, a difficult delivery or a pelvic mass can aggravate the obturator nerve (Fig. 5.5).

**Fig. 5.5** Obturator nerve. The obturator nerve comes from L2, 3, and 4. As it enters the medial thigh it splits into and anterior and posterior divisions that are separated by the adductor brevis muscle. (Leo 2022)

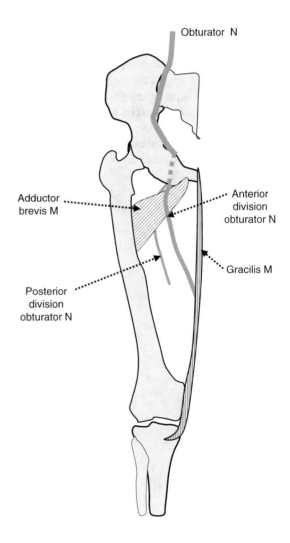

## Posterior Thigh

The posterior thigh is composed of the three hamstrings which all arise as a group from the ischial tuberosity. As the hamstrings travel inferiorly, they separate and go in different directions. The long head of the *biceps femoris* crosses over the sciatic nerve to the lateral side of the tibia, while the *semitendinosus* and *semimembranosus* travel to the medial side. The long head of the biceps femoris is joined by the short head of the biceps femoris at about the midpoint of the posterior thigh. All the hamstrings are innervated by the *tibial division of sciatic*, except for the short head of the biceps which is innervated by the *common fibular nerve*.

The hamstrings extend at the hip and flex at the knee. Hamstring injuries can occur when the muscle is stretched. A good example of this is a "hurdler's injury." When a runner goes over a hurdle, they are putting maximum strain on the hamstrings by flexing at the hip and extending at the knee. If, in the midst of their jump, the hurdler goes down in severe pain and grabs their posterior thigh it is likely that they either tore the hamstrings or avulsed the ischial tuberosity – the origin of the hamstrings.

In the femoral triangle the femoral artery gives off the *profunda femoral artery*. The profunda femoral has several important branches. Close to its origination is the *lateral femoral circumflex artery* which forms a "T."

The profunda also gives off the *medial femoral circumflex*. For the hip joint, the medial is the more important one, but both the medial and lateral femoral circumflex arteries provide blood to the femoral head. To reach the femoral head, the branches of these two arteries travel on the surface of the femoral neck.

It seems counterintuitive at first glance, but the profunda femoral, located in the medial compartment, also supplies blood to the posterior thigh. As the profunda descends in the thigh anterior to the adductor magnus, there are three to four *perforating branches* of profunda that pierce the adductor magnus at various points adjacent to the femur to gain access to the posterior thigh muscles. The second perforating branch supplies blood to the femur.

A slipped capital femoral epiphysis involves the ball of the femoral head slipping off the femoral neck, typically posterior. The femoral head stays in the joint, but the femur moves – the metaphysis shifts relative to the epiphysis. This is most often seen in teenagers.

## Femoral Triangle

The *femoral triangle* is bounded by two muscles and a ligament. The medial border of the triangle is the adductor longus, the lateral border is the sartorius, and the superior border is the inguinal ligament, which runs from the anterior superior iliac spine to the pubic tubercle. The lateral floor is iliopsoas, and the medial floor is pectineus. There are several important structures in the canal. A common mnemonic is NAVL standing for femoral **N**erve, femoral **A**rtery, femoral **V**ein, and **L**ymphatics. Some authors will use the mnemonic NAVEL, where the E stands for empty space, but we will see that both mnemonics mean the same thing. The "L" in the mnemonic stands for Lymphatics and refers to the *deep inguinal nodes.*

Surrounding the femoral artery, femoral vein and lymphatics is the *femoral sheath* which is a continuation of the abdominal sheath. In addition, the sheath can be subdivided into three compartments, appropriately named the: lateral, intermediate, and medial compartments. Furthermore, the medial compartment of the femoral sheath is referred to as the *femoral canal,* and the opening of the femoral canal is the *femoral ring.* Just medial to the femoral ring is the *lacunar ligament* (Fig. 5.6).

When pressure in the abdominal cavity rises, abdominal contents look for a weakness in the anterior wall. The femoral artery and vein act to block contents from herniating through the wall at this point, so the contents will tend to herniate through the femoral ring, which except for some lymph nodes is relatively "empty" and weak.

The NAVL mnemonic will help with numerous scenarios. To start with, the femoral artery sits hallway between the ASIS and the pubic tubercle and lies over the femoral head. If you want to bock the femoral nerve, one way to find it, would be to find the pulse of the femoral artery, and then move laterally. If one wants to find the great saphenous vein, then you could start at the femoral artery, move medially to

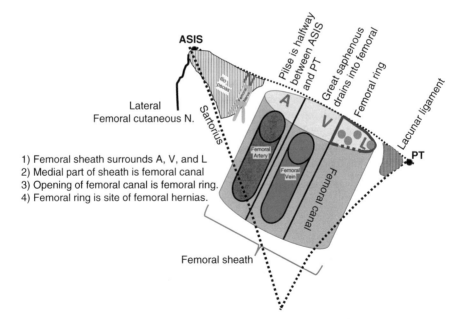

**Fig. 5.6** Femoral triangle. The femoral triangle is bounded by the inguinal ligament, adductor longus, and sartorius. Within the canal, from lateral to medial are the femoral nerve, artery, and vein, and the superficial inguinal nodes. (Leo 2022)

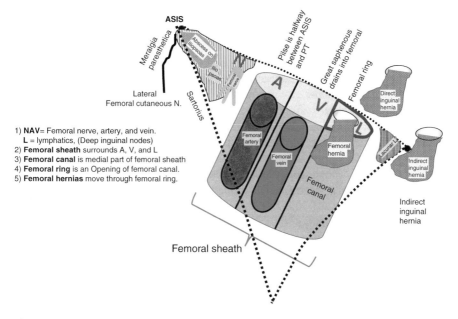

**Fig. 5.7** Hernias. Location of the various hernias and their relationship to the pubic tubercle. (Leo 2022)

the femoral vein, and then find the great saphenous vein opening into the femoral vein. And most importantly, femoral hernias which herniate through the femoral ring will be medial to the femoral vein. And the femoral hernia will be lateral to the lacunar ligament.

The femoral nerve sits on top the medial portion of iliopsoas. An infection inside the abdominal cavity can lie deep to the fascia of psoas major. The infection can then travel down close to the insertion point of iliopsoas to lie mostly lateral to the femoral nerve. Moving even further laterally is the lateral femoral cutaneous nerve which comes under the inguinal ligament just medial to the ASIS (Fig. 5.7).

*Meralgia paresthetica* is a loss of cutaneous sensation to the anterolateral thigh from damage to the lateral femoral cutaneous nerve. Either a belt or jeans that are too tight can aggravate the nerve at this point. Likewise, in the later stages of pregnancy, increased pressure from the abdominopelvic cavity can aggravate the nerve.

## Venous Drainage of the Lower Limb

For all the arteries of the lower limb, there are equivalent veins. For instance, the anterior tibial artery has an equivalent vein. However, there is a separate pattern of drainage for the skin and superficial fascia. The *great saphenous vein* starts as the dorsal venous arch on the dorsum of the foot and runs anterior to the medial malleolus and continues posteromedial to the knee, and then tracks along the medial thigh to drain into the femoral vein by piercing the fascia at the saphenous opening. The vein is sometimes harvested for coronary bypass procedures. To find the vein, one can look anterior to the medial malleolus, or medial to the femoral artery.

The other significant superficial vein of the lower limb is the *popliteal vein* which drains the lateral foot and posterior leg. It pierces the fascia in the popliteal fossa to join the popliteal vein. These superficial veins have a series of valves that assist in moving the blood against gravity. With aging these valves can be compromised which leads to varicose veins.

A deep vein thrombosis (DVT) can develop in the deep veins especially in sedentary individuals. Long airplane flights are a predisposing factor. Symptoms include pain and swelling in the calf. In some patients a deep vein thrombosis can lead to pulmonary embolism (venous thromboembolism). To test for a DVT, the patients lies supine, and the foot is dorsiflexed. A subsequent pain in the posterior leg suggests the presence of a DVT (Homan's sign).

While not as common, a thrombosis can also develop in the superficial veins. These can usually be seen on a physical exam and will typically resolve with time.

## Superficial Inguinal Lymph Nodes

The *superficial inguinal nodes* are found distal to the inguinal ligament and form somewhat of T shape, with the top part of the "T" running parallel to the inguinal ligament, and the descending part of the "T" running down the anterior thigh. The nodes drain the entire superficial lower limb with the exception the lateral leg and the fifth and lateral side of fourth toe, which in turn drain into the popliteal nodes. The superficial nodes also drain the anterior abdominal wall below the umbilicus, the superficial gluteal region, and the superficial perineum. It might seem counterintuitive, but the superficial nodes also drain the cornua of the uterus, because the lymphatics track down the round ligament which is running from the fundus through the inguinal canal to the labia majora. Thus, stepping on a rusty nail with your big toe could lead to swollen superficial inguinal nodes, while stepping on a tack with the little toe could lead to swollen popliteal nodes (Fig. 5.8).

## Femoral Nerve

The *femoral nerve* arises from L 2, 3, and 4 and descends within the abdominal cavity lateral to the *iliopsoas* muscle. In the abdominal cavity the nerve is relatively large. It enters the thigh by passing deep to the inguinal ligament and enters the femoral triangle just lateral to the femoral artery. It is not housed in the femoral sheath. In the femoral triangle the femoral nerve is medial to the iliopsoas muscle. As soon as the nerve passes deep to the inguinal ligament it immediately divides into many small branches that each travel on to innervate the muscles in the anterior thigh. These branches are named for whichever muscle they are innervating.

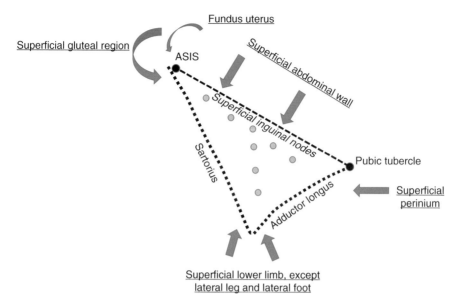

**Fig. 5.8** Superficial inguinal nodes The nodes are shaped like a "T" with one branch running parallel to the inguinal ligament and one branch running down the femoral triangle. The structures draining into the nodes are underlined. (Leo 2022)

## Subsartorial Canal

At the inferomedial corner of the femoral triangle, the femoral artery, femoral vein, and branches of the femoral nerve continue as a group to dive deep to the sartorius in the appropriately named adductor or *subsartorial canal*. At this point, most of the branches of the femoral nerve have terminated in muscles, however there are typically two nerve branches remaining: the *nerve to vastus medialis*, and the *saphenous nerve*. The nerve to vastus medialis will eventually terminate in its muscle but the *saphenous nerve* will continue past the knee by passing just deep to the tendon of sartorius near its insertion point. The saphenous nerve will then continue down to the foot and is responsible for cutaneous sensation to the medial leg and medial foot as far as the ball of the medial foot (Fig. 5.9).

## Adductor Hiatus

As the femoral artery and vein travel down through the adductor canal on top of adductor magnus, they will eventually travel through an opening in adductor magnus called the *adductor hiatus*. They emerge from the hiatus in the popliteal fossa and are now called the popliteal artery and vein.

**Fig. 5.9** The femoral nerve (L2, 3, and 4). As it passes deep to the inguinal ligament it divides into numerous branches that go to the muscles of the anterior thigh. The only branch to go past the knee joint is the saphenous nerve. (Leo 2022)

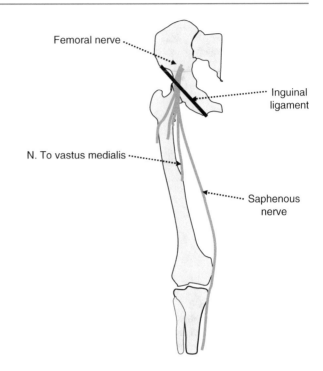

## Femoral Artery

Soon after it comes under the inguinal ligament, the femoral artery gives off the *profunda femoral artery*. Near its origin, there are two important branches. The lateral femoral circumflex artery which proceeds laterally and gives off three appropriately named branches: the *ascending, transverse, and descending*. The descending branch can travel as far as the knee joint and anastomose with the genicular arteries to provide collateral circulation in the event of a blocked femoral artery.

The cruciate anastomosis is a point on the posterior hip where four arteries come together: (1) descending branch of inferior gluteal, (2) an ascending branch of the first perforating artery from the profunda femoral, (3) a transverse branch of lateral femoral circumflex, and (4) an ascending branch of the medial femoral circumflex.

The second important branch of profunda femoral is the *medial femoral circumflex* artery which heads to the hip joint and runs between pectineus and obturator externus. Both the lateral and medial femoral circumflex send retinacular branches to the femoral head.

## Hip Joint

The hip joint, a ball and socket joint, is the strongest joint in the body mainly due to three strong, tough ligaments: the *iliofemoral, ischiofemoral, and pubofemoral*. The

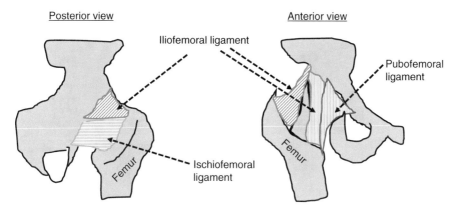

**Fig. 5.10** Hip ligaments. From the anterior view, one can see the two bands of the iliofemoral ligament and the pubofemoral ligament. From the posterior view one can see the top of the iliofemoral plus the whole of the ischiofemoral ligament. (Leo 2022)

iliofemoral ligament (Bigelow Ligament) is the strongest ligament in the body and consists of two bands, resembling a Y and provides support during extension of the hip. The ischiofemoral ligament is located on the posterior surface of the hip joint and prevents excessive internal rotation. The pubofemoral ligament runs inferior to the joint and limits external rotation (Fig. 5.10).

While the hip is the strongest joint in the body, it is at its weakest when an individual is in a seated position. A dashboard injury occurs to a rider in the front-seat of a car when the car's front-end slams into an object and their knees hit the dashboard. The force, combined with the seated position, results in a posterior dislocation of the hip joint such that the femoral head pushes through the acetabulum and ischiofemoral ligament. The femoral head then comes to lie posterior to the ischium. This leads to the lower limb being medially rotated and noticeably shorter (Fig. 5.11).

The *angle of inclination* is determined by drawing one line straight down the femur through the femoral shaft, and another line drawn through the neck of the femur. The normal range is about 105° to 140°. Cox vara is a decreased angle, which predisposes one to femoral neck fracture. Cox valga is an increased angle (Fig. 5.12).

The most important blood supply to the hip and particularly the femoral head comes from the *medial* and *lateral femoral circumflex arteries*, which are typically branches of the profunda femoral artery. They form a continuous ring surrounding the femoral head between the lesser and greater trochanters. Emerging from this ring are several retinacular branches traveling on the outer surface of the femoral neck to reach the femoral head. There is also a tiny artery traveling in the ligament of the head of the femur, the *foveal artery*. In children the foveal artery plays a significant role, but in adults it is virtually non-existent. Fractures to the femoral head will result in the lower limb being laterally rotated and shorter. The lateral rotation occurs because of the attachment of iliopsoas to the lesser trochanter. Fractures here, especially in older individuals, will likely result in avascular necrosis of the femoral head (Fig. 5.13).

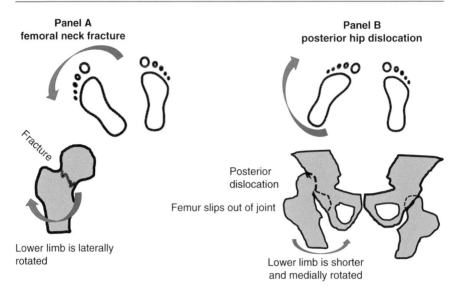

**Panel A**
**femoral neck fracture**

Fracture

Lower limb is laterally
rotated

**Panel B**
**posterior hip dislocation**

Posterior
dislocation

Femur slips out of joint

Lower limb is shorter
and medially rotated

**Fig. 5.11** Panel (**a**) With a fracture of the femoral neck the lower limb will be laterally rotated due to the action of iliopsoas. Panel (**b**) In the case of a posterior dislocation, the lower limb will be medially rotated and shorter. The femur has slipped out of the socket and has come to rest on the posterior ischium. (Leo 2022)

**Fig. 5.12** Angle of inclination. Angle between one line drawn down the femoral neck, and a second line drawn down the femur. Normal is 125°. An increased angle is valgum and a decreased angle is varum. (Leo 2022)

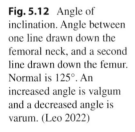
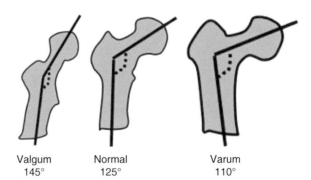

Valgum
145°

Normal
125°

Varum
110°

## Knee Joint

The synovial membrane encases the knee joint to make up the synovial joint. There are several important bursae around the joint. Some of these bursae connect with the knee joint and some are separate compartments. The *suprapatellar bursa* is an out-pocketing of the synovial membrane that extends superior to the patella, which makes it a good location for draining excessive fluid in the knee joint. On the other hand, the *prepatellar bursa* and *infrapatellar bursa* are not continuous with the knee joint. The prepatellar bursa sits directly in front of the patella and patellar tendon, so that excessive friction here can lead to bursitis. The name "housemaid's knee" refers

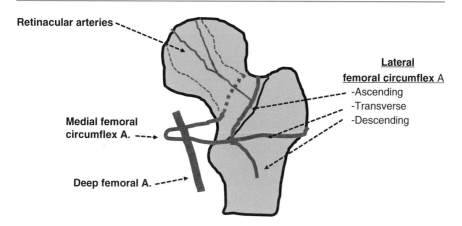

**Fig. 5.13** Femoral head. The blood supply to the head of the femur comes mainly from the medial femoral circumflex artery which sends retinacular branches along the external surface of the femoral neck to reach the head. The lateral femoral circumflex has three branches: ascending, descending, and transverse. (Leo 2022)

to a housemaid who is on her knees putting pressure on the prepatellar bursa. The infrapatellar bursa on the other hand sits anterior to the knee but lower down on the patellar tendon than the prepatellar bursa. The term "clergyman's knee" refers to the praying person who is aggravating this bursa. A *Baker's cyst* refers to an abnormal extension of the synovial membrane in the area of semitendinosus in the posteromedial popliteal fossa. The cyst will typically appear as a small protuberance in this region (Fig. 5.14).

In the center of joint cavity are two important ligaments, the *anterior and posterior cruciate ligaments*. These ligaments are named for their attachment to the tibia. In other words, the anterior cruciate runs from the anteromedial tibia and runs laterally to the femur. The posterior cruciate runs from the posteromedial tibia and runs laterally to the femur. The two ligaments cross each other, making an X, with the anterior cruciate running anterior to the posterior cruciate. The ligaments are surrounded by synovial membrane and are not in the synovial cavity but are extracapsular. The anterior cruciate resists anterior forces. If it is torn then when the patient is sitting on an exam table with the leg free (not touching the floor), the leg can be pulled anterior. This anterior drawer sign is indicative of a torn anterior cruciate ligament. Likewise, a posterior drawer sign is indicative of a torn posterior cruciate ligament. A variant of the anterior drawer test is the *Lachman test*. In brief, with the patient supine on the exam table and the knee flexed 20°, the examiner then checks for stability by pushing on the tibia. The *Reverse Lachman's test* is used to check for PCL stability (Figs. 5.15 and 5.16).

For an easy way to remember the orientation of the ACL and PCL, you can fold your fingers and place your hands on your knee to see the orientation of the ligaments. The ACL is anterior to the PCL. If you are looking at a radiograph of the knee you can take your crossed fingers and hold them up to the radiograph in the anatomical position to help identify which the ligaments on the radiograph.

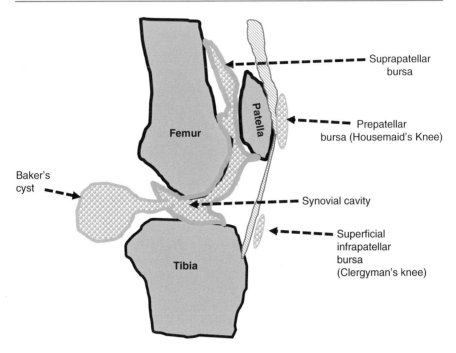

**Fig. 5.14** Knee bursa. The synovial cavity comes between the femur and tibia. It extends superiorly as the suprapatellar bursa. The prepatellar and superficial infrapatellar bursa are separated from the synovial joint. Excess fluid can be drained via the suprapatellar bursa. A Baker's cyst is an extension of the synovial cavity posteriorly. It will usually be found in the region of semimembranosus muscle. (Leo 2022)

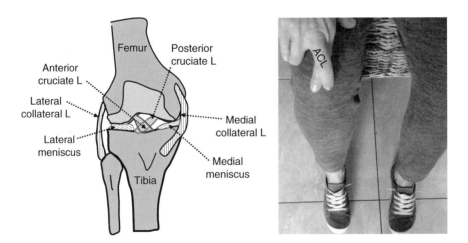

**Fig. 5.15** Cruciate ligaments The cruciate ligaments are named after their attachment to the tibia. The anterior cruciate is attached to the anterior tibia, while the posterior cruciate is attached more posterior to tibia. If you place your crossed fingers on your knee, they are running in the direction of the cruciates. (Leo 2022)

**Fig. 5.16** Orientation of ACL and PCL. The anterior cruciate runs anterior to the posterior cruciate ligament. If you cross your fingers and place your hands on top of your knees, you have the orientation of the ligaments. (Leo 2022)

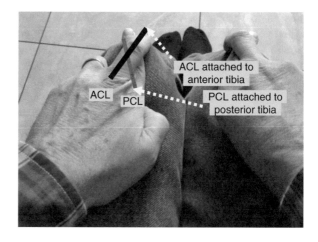

On the sides of the joint are the medial and lateral collateral ligaments. A common injury, often referred to as the *unhappy triad*, involves a blow to the lateral posterior knee that damages the anterior cruciate, the medial collateral ligament and the medial meniscus. Just a word of caution here, this is the traditional definition of the unhappy triad, when in reality, it is not quite so clear cut and the patient does not always present with the textbook scenario (Figs. 5.15 and 5.16).

## The Popliteal Triangle

The *popliteal triangle* is bounded superomedially by the semitendinosus and the semimembranosus; superolaterally by the biceps femoris; and inferomedially and inferolaterally by the medial and lateral heads of the gastrocnemius. Located superficially in the fossa is the sciatic nerve splitting into the common fibular and tibial nerves. Moving deeper is the popliteal vein and then the popliteal artery. The floor of the fossa is made up of the popliteus muscle.

## Popliteus

The *popliteus* is a small triangular shaped muscle deep within the superior portion of the posterior leg. It has a wide attachment on the tibia and runs up laterally to a point on the lateral condyle of the tibia, and the lateral meniscus. Its function is to unlock the knee joint in the initial stages of flexion. It is also involved in rotation. The easiest way to make sense of its function is to start from a sitting position and extend your leg. When you extend your leg fully, you will probably note a slight lateral rotation of your tibia at the very end of extension which is referred to as the "screw home" position. At this point your leg is locked in position. Now start flexing your leg and you will note the tibia medially rotating on the thigh. This action comes from your popliteus unlocking the knee joint. Now, since we are usually not doing this maneuver from a sitting position, we need to think about what is happening when you are standing up. If you are standing, with your knees slightly flexed and you move to a fully upright position by extending at your knee, then your femur is rotating medially on your stationary tibia – remember your foot is on the ground. Now when you flex at your knee, which is unlocking your knee, since your foot is on the ground and your tibia is stationary, you now have the femur laterally rotating on the tibia (instead of the tibia medially rotating in the sitting position) and again this unlocking of the knee is due to popliteus, which although it is a weak flexor of the knee is important. In short: If your leg is straight, with your foot off the ground, the popliteus unscrews the joint with medial rotation of the tibia. With the foot on the ground, it laterally rotates the femur.

## Q Angle

The short version of the *Q angle of the knee* is that it is between the quadriceps tendon above the patella, and the patellar tendon below the patella. The longer version is that the first line is drawn straight down the shaft of the femur from the ASIS to the center of the patella, and the second line is drawn down the tibia from the center of patella to the tibial tubercle. In a standing position the normal angle is about 14° for males and for women about 17° (Fig. 5.17).

## The Leg and Foot

There are three compartments of muscles in the leg, the: anterior, posterior, and lateral. The posterior compartment is further subdivided into a superficial and a deep compartment (Fig. 5.18).

## Posterior Leg

In the superficial compartment there are three muscles, the: *gastrocnemius, soleus*, and *plantaris*. All three come together to form the Achilles tendon which inserts onto the calcaneus. They are all involved with plantar flexion. Deep to these three muscles are *Tom, Dick, and Harry*, standing for **T**ibialis posterior, Flexor **D**igitorum longus, and Flexor **H**allucis longus. Tibialis posterior is a strong inverter, while the names of the other give away their actions. One is a flexor of the big toe, and one is a flexor of the other four toes. All three travel around the medial malleolus deep to the flexor retinaculum in a compartment called the *tarsal tunnel*. Within the tunnel there is also a nerve, artery and vein: the posterior tibial artery, posterior tibial vein, and tibial nerve. Putting the muscles and neurovascular bundle all together gives us the longer mnemonic of **T**om, **D**ick, **A**nd **V**ery **N**ervous **H**arry, with the AVN part standing for the artery, vein and nerve. Note there are variations on the mnemonic. For instance, some authors just refer to the order of the tendons and use Tom, Dick, and Harry (Fig. 5.19).

**Fig. 5.17** Q angle. Angle is taken between two lines. The first line is drawn from ASIS to patella (quadriceps tendon). The second line is drawn from patella down through the tibial tuberosity (patellar tendon). A normal angle for men is 12° and for females is 17°. (Leo 2022)

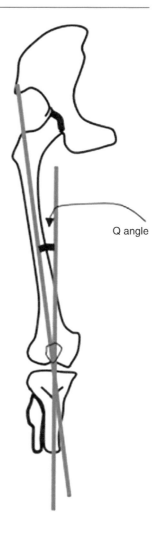

Q angle

The tendons of *tibialis posterior* and the *flexor digitorum longus* pass posterior to the medial malleolus in a groove on the posterior surface of the distal tibia. They then start to curve anterior and diverge to go in different directions. The tibialis posterior passes proximal to the sustentaculum tali and inserts onto the navicular. The flexor digitorum longus passes under the *sustentaculum tali* which is a shelf projecting medially from the talus. Part of the deltoid ligament (tibiocalcaneal L) attaches to it, as does the spring ligament. Just posterior to the flexor digitorum longus is the posterior tibial artery and tibial nerve.

The flexor hallucis longus tendon passes posterior to the tibial nerve and posterior tibial artery. In dancers, this tendon can become overly thick from extended use.

The artery of the posterior leg is the *posterior tibial artery* which is a continuation of the popliteal artery. This posterior tibial artery gives of the *anterior tibial artery* which pierces the interosseus membrane to emerge in the anterior

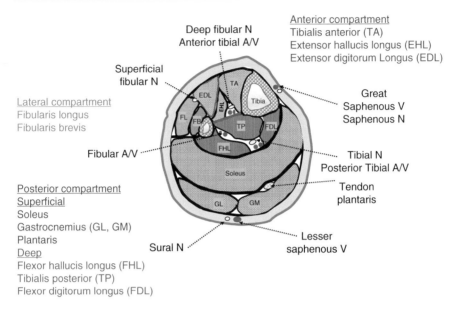

**Fig. 5.18** Cross section through the leg. The anterior compartment includes the tibialis anterior, extensor hallicus longus, and extensor digitorum longus. Also in the anterior compartment, and running together, are the deep fibular nerve and anterior tibial artery. The lateral compartment includes fibularis longus and brevis. The superficial posterior compartment includes the soleus and gastrocnemius. The deep posterior compartment includes tibialis posterior, flexor digitorum longus, and flexor hallicus longus. The nerve and artery of the posterior compartment are the tibial nerve and posterior tibial artery. (Leo 2022)

compartment. The posterior tibial artery also gives off the *fibular artery* which lies in the lateral side of the posterior leg. At the medial malleolus it runs through the *tarsal tunnel* to enter the foot where it divides into the *lateral and medial planter arteries*. The *posterior tibial vein* and its branches run parallel the posterior tibial artery. *Tarsal tunnel syndrome* involves entrapment of the neurovascular bundle in the tarsal tunnel.

The tibial nerve is a branch of the sciatic which runs with the posterior tibial artery through the posterior compartment. It supplies all the muscles of the posterior compartment and then travels through the tarsal tunnel to enter the foot where it divides into the lateral and medial plantar nerves.

It is important to keep in mind that the mnemonic of Tom, Dick and Harry only works at the medial malleolus. If you are looking at the muscles in the calf, the mnemonic does not work. Also keep in mind that in the sole of the foot the tendons of flexor digitorum longus and flexor hallicus longus cross each other (Henry's knot), which means the muscle ending on the medial foot comes from the lateral leg, and the muscle ending on the lateral foot comes from the medial leg – whichever side the muscle inserts on means that it originates from the opposite side. Think of the flexor hallicus longus going to the big toe, which is medial, meaning that it arises from the lateral leg – the fibula. And the flexor digitorum longus ends at the

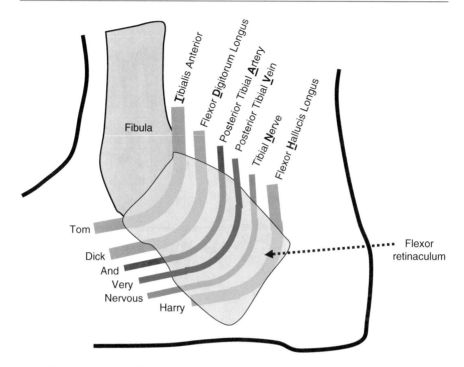

**Fig. 5.19** Tom, Dick, and Harry. At the medial malleolus, the tendons and nerves destined for the sole of the foot pass through the tarsal tunnel. The order of the tendons can be remembered by the saying "Tom, Dick, and Very Nervous Harry." (Leo 2022)

four smaller toes which are lateral, meaning that the muscle originates from the medial side – the tibia. The tibialis posterior sits in the middle of the compartment and arises from both the tibia and fibula (Fig. 5.20).

## Anterior Leg

The anterior leg compartment contains three muscles, all of which are easy to palpate on your own ankle. At the dorsum of the ankle the tendons of these three muscles are held down by the extensor retinaculum. The most medial muscle is the tibialis anterior which is a strong inverter and dorsiflexor. Shin splints are micro tears of the tibialis anterior muscle. Moving laterally, the next muscle is the extensor hallucis longus, and then the extensor digitorum longus. The tendons of extensor digitorum proceed to the distal phalanx of each of the four lateral toes. In addition, there is a slip of this muscle that drops down to the fifth metatarsal that is named the *fibularis tertius*.

The artery of the anterior leg is the *anterior tibial artery* which arises from the popliteal artery in the posterior thigh. Right after it comes of the posterior tibial artery, the anterior tibial artery crosses from the posterior compartment to the

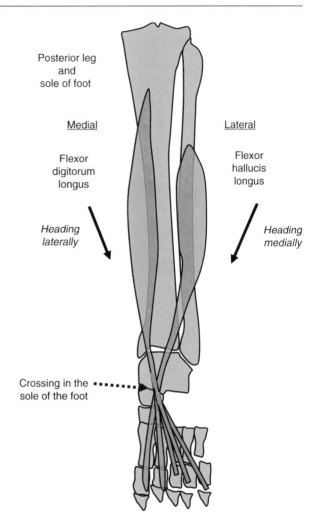

**Fig. 5.20** Two tendons crossing. The FDL starts medial and ends lateral. The tendon of FHL starts lateral and ends medially. The tendon of tibialis posterior is not shown but its insertion is between these two muscles. (Leo 2022)

anterior compartment by passing through the interosseus membrane. It then runs down the anterior leg with the deep fibular nerve between the tibialis anterior and extensor hallucis longus. Just proximal to the ankle joint it dives under the extensor hallucis longus and then enters the dorsum of the foot between extensor hallucis longus and extensor digitorum longus and is now called the *dorsalis pedis artery*. The dorsalis pedis then runs down the dorsum of the foot and gives off the *arcuate artery* which is the arterial arch on the dorsum of the foot. The pulse of the dorsalis pedis can be felt lateral to the extensor hallicus longus tendon. Thus, if you start at the medial malleolus and move laterally, you have two tendons – the tibialis anterior and the extensor hallicus longus – and then the pulse of dorsalis pedis artery (Fig. 5.21).

**Fig. 5.21** Dorsum of foot. The dorsalis pedis pulse can be felt just distal to the navicular between the tendons of the extensor hallicus longus and the extensor digitorum longus. (Leo 2022)

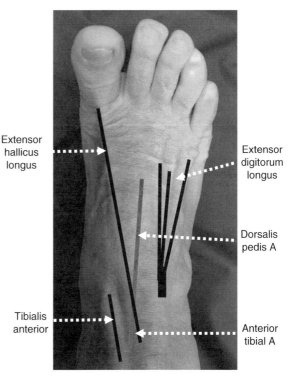

Extensor hallicus longus

Extensor digitorum longus

Dorsalis pedis A

Tibialis anterior

Anterior tibial A

## Lateral Leg

There are two muscles in the lateral leg. The *fibularis longus and brevis*. They both arise from the fibula with the longus slightly higher than the brevis. The fibularis longus enters the sole of the foot posterior to the lateral malleolus and crosses deep to the *long plantar ligament* in a tunnel to insert onto the first metatarsal and the medial cuneiform. The fibularis brevis also arises from the fibula and inserts onto the tuberosity of the fifth metatarsal. Both muscles are evertors of the foot (Fig. 5.22).

## Sciatic Nerve and Branches in the Leg

All of the muscles below the knee are innervated by the sciatic nerve. This is very different than the upper limb. For instance, if you lesion either the radial nerve, the ulnar nerve, or the median nerve in the arm you will lose some but not all motor function below the elbow. However, if you lesion the sciatic nerve in the thigh, you will lose *all* motor function from the knee down (Fig. 5.23).

In the posterior thigh the sciatic nerve splits into the *common fibular* and *tibial nerves.* The common fibular nerve passes around the neck of the fibula between the origins of extensor hallucis longus and fibularis longus. The nerve is very superficial

**Fig. 5.22** The common fibular nerve enters the lateral leg deep to the peroneus longus muscle and splits into the superficial and deep fibular nerves. The superficial fibular innervates the muscles of the lateral leg. The deep fibular innervates the muscles of the anterior leg. (Leo 2022)

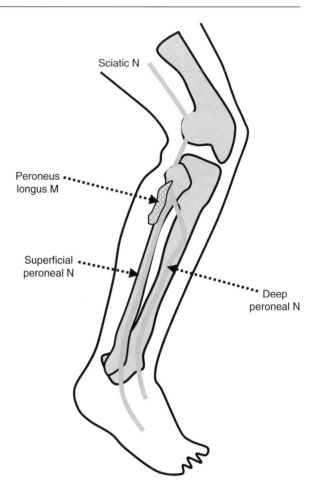

here and easily damaged in injuries to the lateral leg. For instance, in a soccer player who gets kicked on the lateral leg, and fractures the neck of the fibular, the common fibular nerve is at risk. At the fibular head the common fibular splits into the *superficial fibular* and the *deep fibular nerves*. The superficial fibular innervates the lateral compartment of fibularis longus and brevis, while deep fibular nerve goes to the anterior compartment.

Lesions to the deep fibular nerve will result in loss of dorsiflexion. This loss of dorsiflexion can lead to a "foot drop" meaning that when the patient walks, they have difficulty lifting their toes off the ground. They will now counteract this foot drop by lifting their leg higher than normal to keep their toes off the ground. The deep fibular nerve can be compressed by a cast of a ski boot that is too tight.

To think about nerve injuries and motor function to the leg, one should put on an engineer's hat and think of an electrical schematic. As mentioned above, if you lesion the sciatic then all three compartments of the leg are lost, if the common fibular is damaged then both the anterior and lateral compartments are lost, and if the

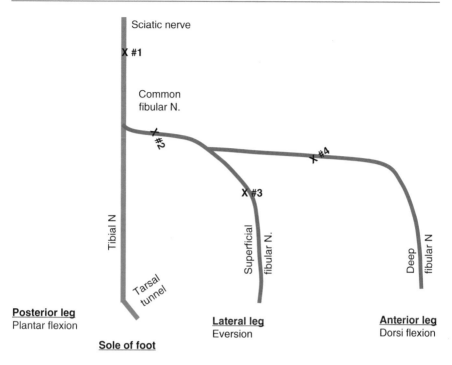

**Fig. 5.23** Leg compartments and nerves. An injury to the sciatic nerve will result in a complete loss of motor function below the knee. Injuries to the common fibular will result in loss of the lateral and anterior leg compartments. (Leo 2022)

deep fibular is damaged the anterior compartment is lost, and with damage to the superficial fibular the lateral compartment is lost. Now we also need to go in reverse here and think about patient scenarios. If a patient has difficulties with eversion, then you would equate this to the lateral compartment which is superficial fibular nerve. If both eversion and dorsiflexion are compromised, then you would conclude that the lateral and anterior compartments are affected which is the common fibular nerve (Fig. 5.23).

## Ankle Joints

The *talocrural joint* or "ankle joint" is a mortis joint with the tibia and fibula each making one side of the joint, and the talus in the middle. Like a hinge, this joint allows the talus to pivot so that the ankle can plantar and dorsiflex. On the medial side of the joint is the strong tough deltoid ligament preventing excessive eversion, On the lateral side is set of ligaments preventing excessive inversion. They are listed here in order of most likely to be involved in an inversion sprain: *anterior talofibular, calcaneofibular*, and *posterior talofibular*. The joint is weakest and thus most susceptible to injury in plantar flexion.

Moving from the leg and the talocrural joint into the foot, as an overview, the foot can be divided into three sections, the forefoot, midfoot, and hindfoot. The forefoot is mainly involved with the toe-off phase of gait. The midfoot is mainly involved with the rotational stability. The hindfoot is involved with absorbing the shock and loads on the foot during walking. The joint between the hindfoot and the ankle is the subtalar joint (Fig. 5.24).

The *subtalar joint* is below the talocrural joint and is formed from the talus sitting on top of the calcaneus. Running from the sustentaculum tali of the calcaneus to the navicular is the all-important "spring" ligament or *plantar calcaneonavicular ligament*. The talus is like the top piece of a medieval arch bounded on either side by navicular and calcaneus. The weight of the body pushing down on the *talus* wants to push the navicular and calcaneus out of the way, but they are held together by the *spring ligament*. The talus is sitting on top of the ligament and is supported by the ligament, but the ligament itself does not attach to the talus (Fig. 5.25).

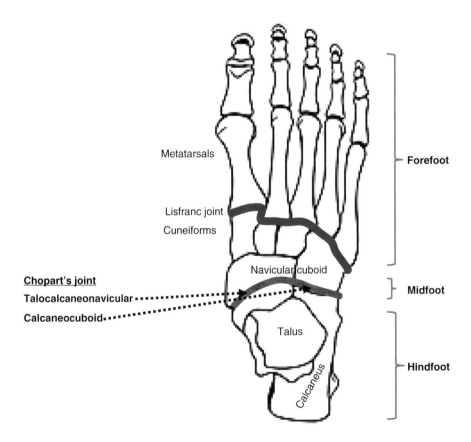

**Fig. 5.24** Foot and ankle joints. Chopart's Joint is made up of the talocalcaneonavicular and calcaneocuboid joints. The Lisfranc joint is between the tarsal bones and the proximal metatarsals. The subtalar joint is between the talus and calcaneus. (Leo 2022)

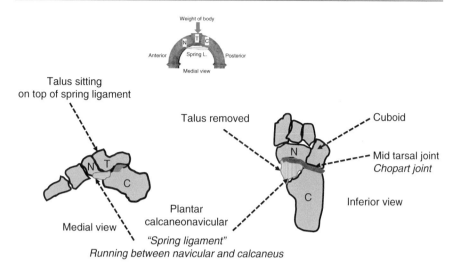

**Fig. 5.25** Spring ligament. The spring ligament runs from the calcaneus to the navicular. The talus is sitting on top of it. The weight of the body is coming down through the talus and onto the spring ligament. The mid tarsal or Chopart's joint is the joint between hindfoot and midfoot. (Leo 2022)

The *Chopart joint* or *midtarsal* or *transverse tarsal joint* is composed of the talonavicular and the calcaneocuboid joints. The Chopart joint separates the hindfoot from the midfoot and is involved in inversion and eversion (Fig. 5.21).

The *Lisfranc joint* is between the proximal metatarsals and the tarsals – the three cuneiforms and the cuboid. The most important ligament here is the shock absorbing Lisfranc ligament running obliquely from the medial cuneiform laterally to the base of the second metatarsal.

## Ankle Fractures

There are two common types of fractures at the ankle that are good to compare and contrast. As mentioned above, inversion sprains, which most of us have had at one point, tend to damage the *anterior talofibular ligament*. However, if the force is severe enough, there can be two ankle fractures with an inversion injury. The inversion force can result in a fracture of the distal one-third of the fibula. Plus, the patient can have an avulsion fracture of the tuberosity of the fifth metatarsal (Jones' Fracture). The fifth metatarsal avulses because the inversion force puts enough strain on the tendon of fibularis brevis to pull off its attachment point which is the tuberosity of the fifth metatarsal.

With excessive eversion, force is exerted on the deltoid ligament which because of its strength does not tear, but rather its attachment to the medial malleolus (distal tibia) is avulsed. In addition, there is often a fracture of the distal fibula. This is referred to as a *Pott's fracture* (Fig. 5.26).

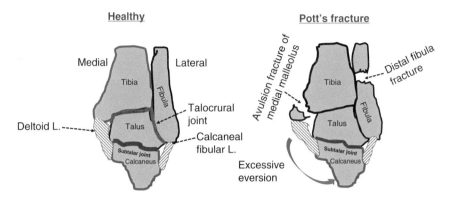

**Fig. 5.26** Talocrural joint. The talocrural joint is the mortise joint with the talus sandwiched between the tibia and fibula. The deltoid ligament is located on the medial side, and the calcaneal fibular ligament is on lateral side. The subtalar joint is between the talus and calcaneus. With excessive eversion, an avulsion fracture of the medial malleolus can occur. In addition, there is often a fracture of the distal fibula. (Leo 2022)

A *trimalleolar fracture* involves the distal tibia and fibula (the medial and lateral malleoli), plus the distal tibia. This is also known as a cotton fracture.

A *maisonneuve fracture* is a fracture of the proximal fibula that results from an inversion injury. The injury can go undetected because often an x-ray of the ankle is taken, and it misses the fracture higher up.

## The Foot

The organization of the foot is somewhat similar to the hand. In the hand we have one compartment of muscles acting on the thumb and another on the little finger, likewise in the foot we have muscles organized into one compartment acting on the big toe and another compartment on the little toe. While the hand muscles are involved in fine motor control, the foot muscles are involved with supporting the weight of the body and gait. The big toe does not have the complicated movements that the thumb has. When dissecting the sole of the foot, the first prominent structure you encounter is the plantar fascia which is a thick tough layer equivalent to the palmar aponeurosis.

The muscles of the foot are conveniently divided into four layers. The number to remember here is "32" – three two; three two. There are three muscles in the first layer, two in the second, three in the third, and two in the fourth.

The *first layer* includes bookends, meaning that the muscles on the lateral and medial sides are similar, while the one in the middle is different. On the lateral side is the *abductor digit minimi brevis*, and on the medial side is the *abductor hallucis,* while the muscle in the middle is the *flexor digitorum brevis*. The abductors are the bookends, and the flexor is in the middle (Fig. 5.24).

In the *second layer*, there are two muscles, the *quadratus plantae* and the *lumbricals*. There are also two tendons in this layer, the tendon of *flexor hallucis longus and flexor digitorum longus*. These two tendons cross each other (Henry's knot) on their way to their insertions. Between the first and second layer, at the medial margin of the foot, we see the posterior tibial artery and tibial nerve emerging from the tarsal tunnel and entering the sole of the foot. And it is here between the first and second layers that both the artery and nerve divide into *lateral* and *medial plantar nerves and arteries*. The medial plantar nerve is equivalent to the median nerve in the hand, and the lateral plantar nerve is equivalent to the ulnar nerve. The lateral plantar artery heads from medial to lateral, crossing the quadratus plantae and it then gives rise to the deep plantar arch which in turn passes deep to the adductor hallucis. Coming off the plantar arch are the plantar metatarsal arteries, which give rise to the common planter digital arteries and then the planter digital arteries going out to the distal toes.

The *quadratus plantae* is a thin muscle running from the calcaneus to the tendon of flexor digitorum longus, and its role is to keep the angle of these long tendons running as straight as possible down the axis of the toes. The lumbricals arise from the tendon of flexor digitorum longus and run towards the toes.

A *bunion* occurs at the metatarsal phalangeal joint. With aging, the action of the flexor hallicus longus tends to pull the distal phalanx of the first toe laterally which results in the metatarsal phalangeal joint moving medially. This is known as a hallux valgus. Think of the distal toe moving Laterally or vaLgus.

In the *third layer*, there are three muscles, and we are back to our bookends. On the medial side is the *flexor hallucis brevis*. And on the lateral side is the *flexor digiti minimi brevis*, and in the middle is *adductor hallucis*. The flexors are on either side while the adductor is in the middle. The adductor hallucis has two heads: a transverse head, and an oblique head. Diving deep to the adductor hallucis is the lateral plantar artery turning into the deep plantar arch.

In the *fourth layer* there are two muscles, the dorsal and plantar interossei. In the hand the axis of rotation for abduction/adduction is the third finger, while in the foot it is the second toe. A major function of most of the muscles in the sole of the foot is to maintain the arch of the foot. They are aided in this function by the ligaments of the foot. In a person who stands all day, the muscles can become tired and strained, which puts more pressure on the ligaments, which leads to the ligaments stretching, the bones moving, and the development of flat feet. As the arch weakens, or falls down, the navicular will be displaced medially.

A *hammer toe* involves abnormal bending of the middle toe joint and usually happens to the second toe, but others can be affected. The toe becomes bent at the middle and assumes a hammer like shape. Instead of pointing forward, the toe will be pointing downward. It often comes from wearing high heels and will result in a callus forming on the dorsum of the toe. Closely related to hammer toe, is *mallet toe* which affects the distal toe joint (Fig. 5.27).

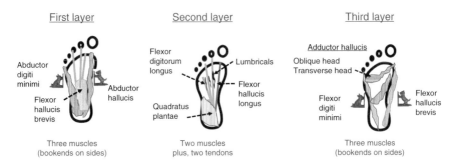

**Fig. 5.27** Foot muscles. The muscles of the foot are arranged in four layers (the image shows the first three layers). In the layers with three muscles there are bookends, meaning the muscles on the sides are similar, with the odd man out in the middle. The first layer is bookended on the sides with the abductor digit minimi and the abductor hallicus, while sandwiched between them is the flexor hallucis brevis. In the second layer are two muscles the quadratus plantae and the lumbricals. Both these muscles are attached to the tendon of flexor digitorum longus. In addition, the tendon of flexor hallucis longus is also in this layer. In the third layer are the bookends of flexor hallucis brevis and flexor digit minimi which are sandwiching the adductor hallicus. In the fourth layer (not shown) are the dorsal and plantar interossei. (Leo 2022)

## Nerves and Arteries in the Sole of the Foot

The tibial nerve passes through the tarsal tunnel and enters the sole of the foot on the medial side where it divides into a lateral and medial plantar nerve. The lateral plantar nerve is equivalent to the ulnar nerve of the hand, while the medial plantar nerve is equivalent to the median nerve. Whereas the median nerve innervates three and half muscles in the hand and the ulnar nerve innervates all the others, in the foot the medial plantar nerve innervates three and quarter muscles and the lateral plantar innervates all the others.

The *medial plantar nerve* passes between the flexor digitorum brevis and abductor hallicus. It innervates both those muscles plus the flexor hallicus brevis, and the first lumbrical. It gives off *common plantar digital nerves* which divide into proper planter digital nerves which carry sensation from the palmar surface of the big toe, and the second, third, and medial half of the fourth toe.

The *lateral planter nerve* passes between the flexor digitorum brevis and the quadratus plantae, and then continues towards the lateral side where it curves back medially to pass deep to the adductor hallicus. It innervates the abductor digiti minimi, flexor digiti minimi brevis, quadratus plantae, the lumbricals, the dorsal and plantar interossei and the adductor hallicus. It gives off a *common plantar digital nerve* which then gives off *proper plantar digital nerves* which carry sensation from the fifth toe and the lateral half of the fourth toe.

The *inferior calcaneal nerve* (Baxter's Nerve) is the first branch of the lateral plantar nerve. It arises in the vicinity of the bifurcation of the tibial nerve. It runs between the quadratus plantae and the flexor digitorum brevis where it can become compressed leading to chronic heel pain. The pain is similar to the pain felt from plantar fasciitis, however, with Baxter's nerve entrapment the pain is felt more on the inside of the heel and the pain tends to be more persistent, while plantar fasciitis is usually worse in the morning, or after sitting for extended times.

*Morton's neuroma* occurs from the metatarsals rubbing against each other and pinching the nerves which leads to the nerve becoming swollen and scarred. This most often occurs to the nerves located between the third and fourth toes where the medial and lateral plantar nerves meet.

The *deep plantar arch* gives of plantar metatarsal arteries. It also forms an anastomosis with the dorsalis pedis artery located on the dorsal surface of the foot. The location of the plantar arch deep in the foot makes it difficult to stop the bleeding from lacerations – for instance steeping on a nail.

## Plantar Fasciitis

Just deep to the skin of the sole is the very thick, tough *planter aponeurosis* that runs from the calcaneus to the toes. With age this layer can tighten, leading to pain in the sole of the foot, which is usually worse after extended periods of sitting. For instance, patients will usually say the pain is the worse in the early morning, and that as they move around it will lessen. Over time these patients often develop a calcaneal spur from the fascia pulling at its attachment point. Stretching can help to relieve the pain. For office workers, one suggestion is to roll their foot back and forth during the day on top of a tennis ball.

## Lumbar Disc Herniations

The most common disc herniations in the lower limb region are to either L4, L5, or S1. With a disc injury you want to think of three tests. The first is the reflex test, the second is the muscle test (the myotome), and the third is the sensory loss related to dermatome. Not every level has a good reflex test (Table 5.1).

## Dermatomes and Peripheral Nerve Map of Lower Limb

The dermatome map shows which *spinal cord levels* are responsible for sensation from the lower limb. The peripheral nerve map shows which *peripheral nerves* are responsible for sensation from the lower limb. For a more in-depth discussion of the

**Table 5.1** Lumbar disc herniations

|              | L4                                            | L5                   | S1                             |
| ------------ | --------------------------------------------- | -------------------- | ------------------------------ |
| Reflex test  | Patellar tendon                               | No good reflex       | Achilles reflex                |
| Muscle test  | Quadriceps                                    | Dorsiflexing toes    | Plantarflex ankle              |
| Sensory loss | Lateral thigh, medial leg, and medial foot    | Lateral leg, dorsum of foot | Posterior thigh, lateral leg, and lateral foot |

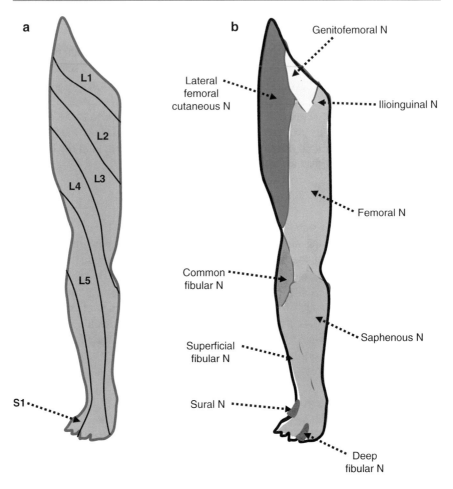

**Fig. 5.28** Roots versus peripheral nerves. Panel (**a**) is the dermatome map of the lower limb. Panel (**b**) is the peripheral nerve map of the lower limb. (Leo 2022)

difference, chapter eight compares root injuries to peripheral nerve injuries. When it comes to the lower limb and dermatomes, the most important roots are: L4 is medial foot; L5 is dorsum of the foot; and S1 is the lateral foot. In addition, L1 is the inguinal region (Fig. 5.28).

For the peripheral nerve map, note that the medial leg and medial foot are saphenous nerve territory. The dorsum of the foot is mostly the superficial fibular nerve, although the first dorsal web space is the deep fibular nerve. The lateral foot is the sural nerve (Fig. 5.28, Table 5.2).

**Table 5.2** Summary of lower limb nerves

| Nerve | Sensory deficit | Motor deficit | Typical causes |
|---|---|---|---|
| Ilioinguinal | Groin | Weak ant wall | Hernia surgery |
| Genitofemoral | Anteromedial thigh | Cremaster | Surgery |
| Lateral femoral cutaneous | Lateral thigh | | ASIS trauma |
| Femoral | Anterior thigh/knee | Quadriceps | Trauma, pelvic mass |
| Saphenous | Medial knee/leg | | Entrapment medial epicondyle |
| Obturator | Medial thigh | Adductors of thigh | Pelvic mass |
| Superior gluteal | Buttock | Gluteus medius and minimus | Trendelenburg gait |
| Inferior gluteal | Buttock | Fall | Trauma |
| Sciatic | Posterior thigh, leg except for medial side | Hamstrings and all muscles below the knee | Trauma |
| Commo peroneal | Dorsum and lateral foot | Anterior, lateral leg | Fracture of fibular head, Baker's cyst |
| Superficial peroneal | Dorsum of foot | Lateral leg | Trauma |
| Deep peroneal | First dorsal web space | Anterior leg | Ski boot syndrome, cast |
| Tibial | Sole of foot | Posterior compartment | Tarsal tunnel Fractures |

# Further Reading

Grimaldi A, Fearon A. Gluteal tendinopathy: integrating pathomechanics and clinical features in its management. J Orthop Sports Phys Ther. 2015;45(11):910–22.

Moore K, Daley AF, Agur A. Moore clinically oriented anatomy. 7th ed. New York: Lippincott Williams and Wilkins; 2014.

Rosse C, Gaddum-Rosse P. Hollinshead's textbook of anatomy. 5th ed. New York: Lippincott-Raven Publishers; 1997.

Standring S. Gray's anatomy: the anatomical basis of clinical practice. London: Elsevier; 2005.

# The Upper Limb

**6**

## Introduction

All the details will follow, but before getting into the specifics it helps to have an overview of the compartments. Just like the lower limb, it is important to organize the upper limb around compartments. When you lose a nerve, you typically lose a compartment, or two, and if you know the function of that compartment then the nerve palsies are easier to understand. Both the arm and forearm each have an anterior and posterior compartment. Both the posterior arm and forearm are radial nerve territory, the anterior forearm is musculocutaneous nerve territory, and the anterior forearm is innervated by the median nerve with the exception of one and a half muscles – the flexor carpi ulnaris, and half of flexor digitorum profundus. And in the hand the median innervates three-and-a-half muscles, and the ulnar innervates everything else (Fig. 6.1). The "three" refers to the three thenar muscles, and the "half" refers to two of the four lumbricals.

## The Shoulder

### There are several muscles that attach the upper limb to the trunk

1. The *trapezius* is a large flat trapezoid shaped muscle that originates from a line running down the midline from the skull along the cervical, and thoracic vertebrae. It inserts along the spine of the scapula. It can be divided into an upper, middle, and lower divisions. The trapezius can move the scapula in several different directions. If we look at the location of its divisions and the orientation of their muscle fibers, the actions should make sense. The superior border elevates the scapula, the middle border, retracts it, and the lower division depresses the lateral corner of the scapula.

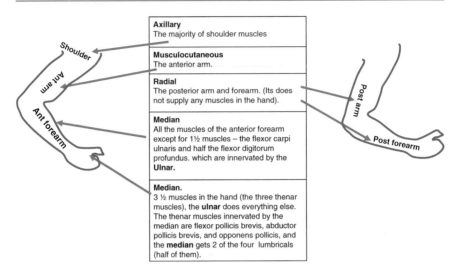

**Fig. 6.1**  Overview of nerve supply to upper limb. (Leo 2022)

2. The *rhomboid major* and *rhomboid minor* together form a thin sheet of muscle originating from the midline from the C7 to T5 spinous processes. They attach along the medial border of the scapula and are involved in retraction. They are innervated by the dorsal scapular nerve.

3. The *levator scapulae* is a strap like muscle originating from the transverse processes of C1-C4 and inserting on superior portion of the medial border of the scapula. When it fires it will pull this medial angle superior, which tilts the glenoid cavity inferiorly. It is innervated by the dorsal scapular nerve.

4. The *pectoralis major* arises from the sternum and ribs, and medial portion of the clavicle. Its muscle fibers head towards the humerus but on the way the fibers rotate such that the inferior fibers end up forming the posterior lamina of the tendon while the upper fibers form the anterior lamina of the tendon. The tendon attaches to the medial lip of the intertubercular groove on the humerus. It is innervated by the medial and lateral pectoral nerves.

5. The *pectoralis minor* arises from ribs 3–5 and inserts onto the coracoid process and is involved in stabilizing the shoulder.

6. The *deltoid muscle* has three heads which overlie the shoulder. The three heads are named for their relative locations: the anterior portion is over the clavicle, the intermediate portion over the acromion, and the posterior portion over the scapula. Each head arises from the structure it covers, and all three heads insert onto the deltoid tuberosity. Its actions are abduction, flexion, and extension. It is innervated by the axillary nerve.

## The Shoulder Joint

The shoulder joint is made up of three joints: the acromioclavicular, the glenohumeral, and sternoclavicular.

The *acromioclavicular ligament* is the attachment between the lateral end of the clavicle and the acromion. Surrounding the joint is a weak capsule which is surrounded by superior and inferior capsular ligaments. In addition, the joint is strengthened by the *coracoclavicular ligament* which in turn is composed of two parts. The medially located *conoid ligament* is shaped like a fan, and the *trapezoid ligament* is the more laterally located portion which is shaped like a quadrangle. The clavicle is essentially suspended from the scapula by the coracoclavicular ligament (Fig. 6.2).

Dislocation of the acromioclavicular joint often follows blows to the shoulder in traffic accidents or sporting injuries. The severity of shoulder separations occur on a spectrum but can involve the acromioclavicular ligament, coracoclavicular ligament, or both.

1. A mild sprain of the acromioclavicular ligament may not show up on an x-ray and will not cause a shoulder deformity.
2. A minor tear of the acromioclavicular ligament can result in a mild misalignment of the collar bone.
3. A complete tear of the acromioclavicular and coracoclavicular ligaments will lead to the shoulder sagging and large bump over the shoulder.

You can test someone else's shoulder mobility, or your own, by asking them to reach over and touch the opposite shoulder with their hand (Apley Scratch Test). It should be symmetrical for each side.

**Fig. 6.2** Shoulder ligaments. The coracoclavicular ligament is composed of two parts: trapezoid and conoid Ls. The coracoacromial ligament connects the coracoid process to the coracoid. (Leo 2022)

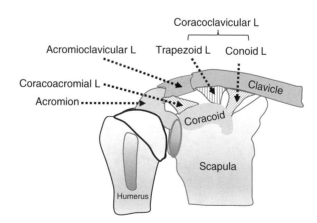

## The Clavicle

The clavicle is a long thin "S" shaped bone that via the sternoclavicular joint attaches the upper limb to the axial skeleton. It is the most often fractured bone in the body. Superomedially it is attached to the sternocleidomastoid, and inferolaterally it is attached to the pectoralis major. Fractures to the clavicle often occur following a fall on the outstretched hand. The patient will typically present with the medial portion of the scapula pulled superiorly by the sternocleidomastoid, and the lateral portion pulled inferiorly by the pectoralis major.

## The Manubrium

The *manubrium* is a quadrangular shaped structure that articulates with the clavicle, first rib, second rib, and the sternum. The *sternoclavicular joint* between the manubrium and the clavicle has an articular disk between the two boney features. On either side of the joint are the anterior and posterior sternoclavicular ligaments. Running across the manubrium from one clavicle to another is the *interclavicular ligament*. Running from the clavicle to the first rib is the *costoclavicular ligament* (Fig. 6.3).

Between the first rib and the manubrium is a strong immobile synchondrosis that allows the clavicle and manubrium to move together. Starting with the second rib and moving down the sternum the remaining joints are synovial joints. Note that anteriorly the second rib articulates with both the manubrium and sternum, while ribs 2–7 articulate just with the sternum. Costochondritis is inflammation of the cartilage between the ribs and the sternum.

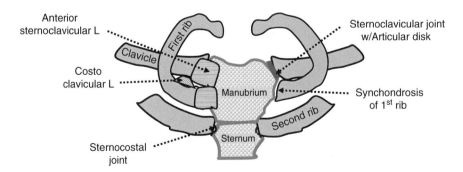

**Fig. 6.3** Manubrium. The manubrium joins the first two ribs and the clavicle. The sternoclavicular joint is between the manubrium and the clavicle. There is an articular disk between the two bones. The first rib joins the manubrium just inferior to the clavicle. The second rib joint the manubrium and the sternum. (Leo 2022)

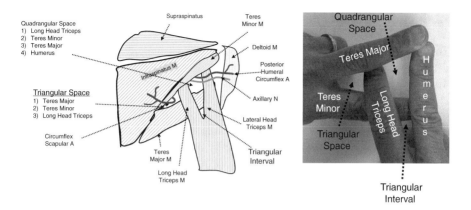

**Fig. 6.4** Triangular and quadrangular spaces. (Leo 2022)

## Rotator Cuff

The four rotator cuff muscles surround and hold the humeral held in place against the glenoid fossa. They are often referred to as the SITS muscles. They all insert on the superior aspect of the humerus in the region of the greater and lesser tuberosities (Fig. 6.4).

1. The *supraspinatus* originates from the supraspinous fossa and inserts on the superior aspect of the greater tuberosity. It is innervated by the suprascapular nerve. It is responsible for the first 15° of shoulder abduction. If it is injured, the patient can initiate abduction by swinging their hip and pushing the upper limb laterally, or they can lean towards the damaged side which will result in the upper limb being abducted 10–15° relative to the trunk. They can use other muscles to keep the abduction going.
2. The *infraspinatus* has a wide origin from the infraspinous fossa of the scapula and comes to a point to insert on the posterior aspect of the greater tuberosity. It is innervated by the suprascapular nerve.
3. The *teres minor* is very closely related to the infraspinatus and at first glance seems to be part of infraspinatus. It inserts on the greater tuberosity. It is a lateral rotator at the shoulder.
4. The *subscapular* muscle is located on the inner surface of the scapula in the subscapular fossa. It inserts on the lesser tuberosity. It is a medial rotator of the shoulder. It is innervated by the upper and lower subscapular nerves.

Note that in the above discussion, three of the SITS muscles, the supraspinatus, infraspinatus, and the teres minor all insert on the greater tuberosity. Fractures of the greater tuberosity would compromise these three muscles. Meanwhile the subscapularis attaches to the lesser tuberosity so fractures here would involve the subscapularis.

## Abduction of the Upper Limb

To discuss abduction of the upper limb, start with an individual standing up with their upper limb by their side. When they go from this position to moving their upper limb straight over their head, several muscles are involved. The supraspinatus is responsible for the first 15° of abduction, from here the deltoid takes over and moves the upper limb to the 90° position. At this point the glenoid cavity is pointing off to the side. To continue moving the upper limb to straight over the head, the serratus anterior and trapezius also contribute by rotating the scapula so that the glenoid cavity now pivots to point more superiorly.

*Painful Arc Syndrome* refers to a patient who complains of pain on attempted abduction of the upper limb. The source of the pain can come from several different structures. The supraspinatus tendon lies in a small tight space between the acromion and the humeral head. Also in this small space is the *subacromial bursa*. Pain in is region can come from impingement of either of these structures. Besides inflammation, impingement can also result from bone spurs forming in the bones around the space (Fig. 6.5).

Supraspinatus is the most commonly injured of the SITS muscles which can lead to pain in the shoulder. The tendon can become frayed or torn away at its origin. In some cases, there will be crackling sensations on shoulder movement.

## Glenohumeral Joint

The humeral head is the ball, and the glenoid fossa is the socket of the ball-and-socket *glenohumeral joint*. The socket is strengthened by the *glenoid labrum*. The joint is strengthened by the *superior, middle, and inferior glenohumeral ligaments*. The humeral head can be dislocated anteriorly, posteriorly, or inferiorly. The most common direction is anteriorly and involves rupture of the inferior glenohumeral ligament. The patient will often present with a lump on the anterior shoulder which represents the head of the humerus coming to lie deep to the pectoralis minor. The glenohumeral joint is the most mobile joint in the body, and also the most common

**Fig. 6.5** Subacromial space. The subacromial space is bounded superiorly by the coracoacromial ligament. The humeral head is inferior. Within the space is the tendon of supraspinatus and the subacromial bursa. (Leo 2022)

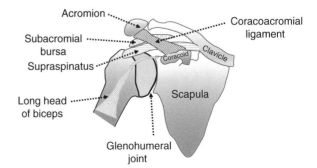

site for dislocations. *Adhesive capsulitis* also known as frozen shoulder refers to the joint becoming tight and stiff usually from immobility.

## SLAP Tear and the Long Head of the Biceps

The long head of the biceps enters the glenohumeral joint and attaches to the *supraglenoid tubercle*. A slap tear refers to a tear of the *superior labrum* on either side – anterior and posterior of the attachment of the long head of the biceps tendon thus the mnemonic **S**uperior **L**abrum **A**nterior **P**osterior. Slap tears can occur as a result of trauma such as car accidents or falling on the outstretched hand, or from repetitive overuse injuries such as weightlifting (Fig. 6.6).

## Bankart Tears

A Bankart tear occurs at the anterior labrum usually following a shoulder dislocation, especially in those under 30 years of age (Fig. 6.6).

## Axilla

The *axilla* is a triangular shaped area bounded by the serratus anterior medially, the pectoralis major anteriorly, and the subscapularis muscle posterior. The axilla contains the axillary artery, axillary vein, cords of the brachial plexus, and the axillary nodes. Some authors refer to the thin layer of fascia encompassing the neurovascular structures as the axillary sheath, but its existence is debated (Fig. 6.7).

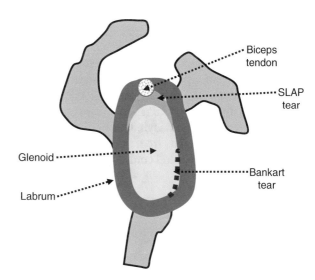

**Fig. 6.6** Labrum tears. Bankart tears occur on the anterior inferior margin of the labrum. SLAP tears occur anterior and posterior of the attachment of the biceps tendon. (Leo 2022)

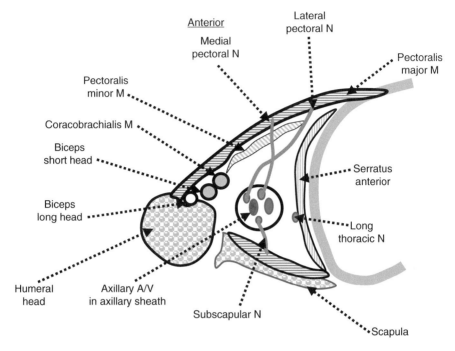

**Fig. 6.7** Axilla. The axilla is bounded by the serratus anterior, the pectoralis major and the subscapularis. The axillary sheath is seen surrounding the axillary artery and vein. (Leo 2022)

## Clavipectoral Fascia

The *clavipectoral fascia* is a strong layer that starts from the clavicle and heads inferiorly to wrap around the pectoralis minor, and then continues inferiorly to blend in with the axillary fascia. Between the pectoralis minor and the clavicle, the lateral thoracic artery and the cephalic vein pierce the fascia. Deep to the fascia is the axillary artery and the medial, lateral, and posterior cords of the brachial plexus. The medial cord gives off the medial pectoral nerve, and the lateral cord gives off the lateral pectoral nerve both of which travel anteriorly. When these two nerves reach the anterior abdominal wall, note that the lateral pectoral nerve is found medial to the medial pectoral nerve. Keep in mind that nerves are named for where they come from, thus, although the medial pectoral nerve is found laterally, it gets its name because it comes from the medial cord, and likewise the lateral pectoral nerve comes from the lateral cord (Fig. 6.8).

## Axillary Artery

The *axillary artery* runs from the first rib to the inferior border of teres minor. There are three parts to the axillary artery based on their relationship to the pectoralis

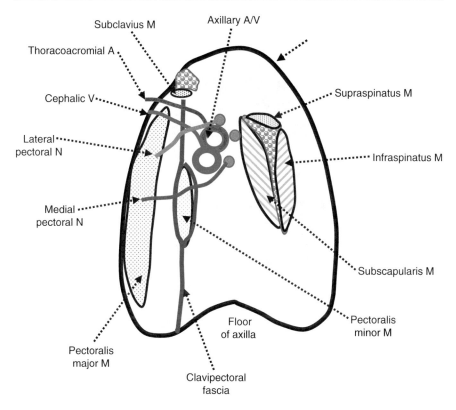

**Fig. 6.8** Clavipectoral fascia. Extension of the investing deep cervical fascia. It is pierced by the thoracoacromial artery, and the cephalic vein. Within the axilla is the axillary artery and axillary vein and the cords of the brachial plexus. (Leo 2022)

minor muscle. The pectoralis muscle runs from the ribs medially to the corocoid process of the scapula and overlies the axillary artery. The first part of the artery is proximal to pectoralis minor, the second part of the artery is posterior to pectoralis minor, and the third part is distal to pectoralis minor. There are six branches of the axillary artery, and it is organized very conveniently. There is one branch off the first part, two branches off the second part, and three branches off the third part (Fig. 6.9).

**First Part of Axillary Artery**

1. The *supreme thoracic artery* goes to the superior thoracic wall.

**Second Part of Axillary Artery**

2. The *thoracoacromial artery* comes off right at the superior border of pectoralis minor and pierces the clavipectoral fascia. It has several branches: pectoral, acromial, clavicular, and humeral.
3. The *lateral thoracic artery* runs to the lateral thoracic wall and supplies the lateral breast. It runs with the long thoracic nerve which innervates the serratus anterior muscle. During breast surgery, the lateral thoracic artery may need to be

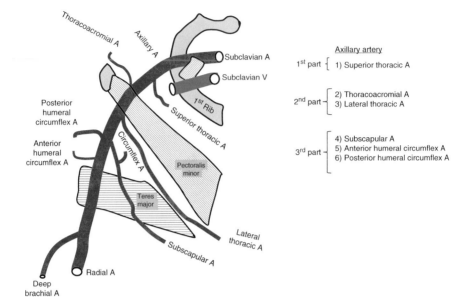

**Fig. 6.9** Axillary artery. There are three parts to the axillary artery based on their relationship to the pectoralis minor muscle. Off the first part is one branch, off the second part are two branches, and off the third part are three branches. (Leo 2022)

ligated. If the surgeon damages the long thoracic nerve the patient will have a winged scapula.

### Third Part of Axillary Artery

4. The *subscapular artery* comes off the medial side of the axillary artery and quickly gives off the circumflex scapular artery which travels through the triangular space. The subscapular artery continues to the medial inferior scapula. It runs with the thoracodorsal nerve which innervates the latissimus dorsi muscle.
5. The *anterior humeral circumflex artery* comes off the lateral side of the axillary artery and heads to the anterior surface of the neck of the humerus.
6. The *posterior humeral circumflex artery* comes off right next to the anterior humeral circumflex artery and these two arteries form an anastomosis. Of the two, the posterior humeral circumflex is usually larger, and it runs through the quadrangular space with the axillary nerve.

## Brachial Plexus

The brachial plexus arises from the ventral roots of C5, C6, C7, C8, and T1. In some individuals, C4 or T2 may contribute (Fig. 6.10).

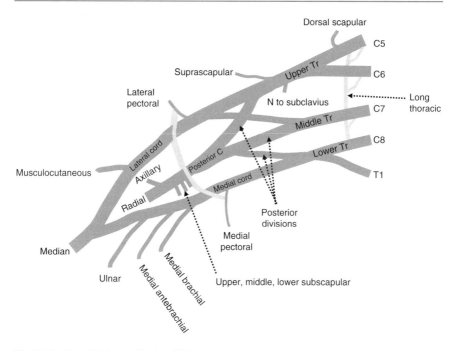

**Fig. 6.10** Brachial plexus. The brachial plexus arises from the roots of C5-T1, which in turn gives rise to the trunks, divisions, cords and branches. (Leo 2022)

1. The *long thoracic nerve* comes from branches of the C5, C6, and 7 roots and supplies the serratus anterior.
2. The *dorsal scapular nerve* come directly from the C5 root and supplies the rhomboid major and minor plus the levator scapulae.
3. The *nerve to subclavius* comes from the roots of C5 and C6 and innervates subclavius.

The roots then form the trunks. The superior trunk comes from C5 and C6, the middle trunk from C7, and the inferior trunk from C8 and T1. The trunks lie in the scalene triangle with the subclavian artery. They are susceptible here to impingement and fractures of the first rib.

1. The *suprascapular nerve* arises from the superior trunk and innervates the supraspinatus and infraspinatus muscles.
2. The *nerve to subclavius* also arises from the upper trunk

All three trunks split into two divisions, an anterior and a posterior division.

The lateral cord is formed by the combination of the anterior divisions of the superior and middle trunks, the posterior cord is formed from all three posterior divisions, and the medial cord comes from the inferior trunk. The cords are named for their relationship to the axillary artery. The cords go on to form the branches to the upper limb muscles. There are five main branches and several smaller branches.

The posterior cord gives rise to two of the five main branches, the axillary and radial nerves. It also gives rise to three smaller branches lined up in a row: the upper, middle, and lower subscapular nerves.

1. The *axillary nerve* innervates several muscles of the shoulder, the deltoid, and the teres minor muscles.
2. The *radial nerve* innervates the muscles of the posterior arm and posterior forearm.
3. Both the *upper and lower subscapular nerves* innervate the subscapularis muscle. The lower subscapular nerve also innervates the teres major muscle.
4. The *middle subscapular nerve* also known as the thoracodorsal nerve innervates the latissimus dorsi muscle.

The lateral cord sends a contribution to the median nerve, and it also forms:

1. the *musculocutaneous nerve* which supplies the anterior forearm muscles. The musculocutaneous nerve then continues past the elbow as the lateral cutaneous nerve of the forearm.
2. The *lateral pectoral nerve* which goes to the pectoralis major.

The medial cord gives off the medial cutaneous nerve of the forearm and the medial cutaneous nerve of the arm and sends a contribution to the median nerve. It also forms:

1. the *ulnar nerve* which supplies one and a half muscles in the anterior forearm and many of the hand muscles.
2. The *medial pectoral nerve* which goes to the pectoralis minor and major.

The *intercostobrachial nerves* carry sensory information from the medial arm. It comes from the T2 level. Patients having a heart attack often complain of pain in the left arm. This is because the heart also travels back to T2 thus the pain is referred to the arm.

## The Compartments of the Upper Limb

### Anterior Arm Compartment

The anterior compartment of the arm contains three muscles all innervated by the musculocutaneous nerve. The muscles have several functions at the shoulder and are the main flexors at the elbow (Fig. 6.11).

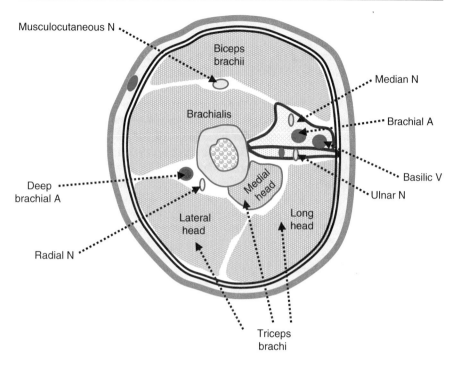

**Fig. 6.11** Cross section of the arm. On the posterior side are the three heads of the triceps. On the anterior side are the biceps and brachialis. On the medial side note the median nerve, brachial artery, and basilic vein. The musculocutaneous nerve is located between the biceps brachii and the brachialis. The radial nerve and the deep brachial artery wrap around the humerus in the radial groove. (Leo 2022)

1. The *biceps brachii muscle* has two heads. The long head arises from the supraglenoid tubercle and runs through the glenohumeral joint cavity to go over the superior surface of the humerus. It then travels through the intertubercular groove covered by the *transverse humeral ligament*. The short head arises from the coracoid process and joins the long head in the upper third of the arm. The biceps continues to the radial tuberosity. The bicipital aponeurosis runs from lateral to medial to insert on the ulnar fascia. The best way to think about the action of the biceps is opening a wine bottle with a corkscrew. The biceps is a flexor at the elbow and a supinator. When you are removing the cork from a wine bottle, you are flexing and supinating. The muscle also acts at the shoulder as an abductor. In some patients, the long head of the biceps can avulse the supraglenoid tubercle of the scapula. The muscle belly will then pull the tendon inferiorly which leads to a large bump in the anterior forearm known as a *Popeye deformity*.

2. The *coracobrachialis muscle* arises at the coracoid process with the short head of the biceps. It inserts on the medial side of the humerus. It is a flexor and adductor at the shoulder.

3. The *brachialis muscle* runs from the humerus to the ulna and is a flexor at the elbow.

## Posterior Arm Compartment

The posterior compartment of the arm is involved with extension at the shoulder and the elbow. All the muscles of the posterior compartment are innervated by the radial nerve.

1. The *triceps muscle* has three heads. The long head arises from the infraglenoid tubercle, the medial head from the humerus, and the lateral head from the humerus. The three heads meet, and the triceps attaches to the olecranon process of the ulna. Just under the skin, over the olecranon process, at the insertion of the triceps is the *olecranon bursa*. Resting on one's elbow while sitting at a desk for prolonged periods can lead to olecranon bursitis – student's elbow. The triceps contributes to extension at the shoulder and is the main extensor at the elbow.

## Arteries of the Upper Limb

The brachial artery gives off the profunda brachial artery which wraps around the humerus between the medial and lateral heads of the triceps in the triangular interval. It runs with the radial nerve. Behind the humerus the artery splits into the middle collateral artery and the radial collateral which follows the radial nerve (Fig. 6.12).

The radial artery also gives off the *superior ulnar collateral artery* which travels posterior to the medial epicondyle with the ulnar nerve. The superior ulnar

**Fig. 6.12** The common interosseus artery splits into anterior and posterior interosseus arteries. The Radial collateral artery arises from the profunda brachii artery and passes anterior to the lateral epicondyle. The superior and inferior ulnar collateral arteries head towards the medial side of the elbow joint. (Leo 2022)

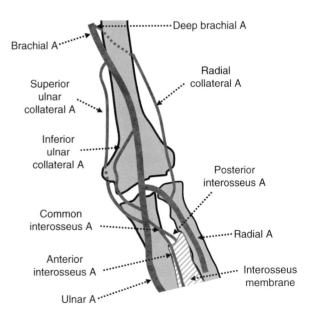

collateral anastomoses with the *posterior ulnar recurrent* artery which is a branch of the ulnar artery. In a similar fashion the *inferior ulnar collateral artery* arises from the radial artery and travels anterior to the elbow joint to meet up with the *anterior ulnar recurrent artery* which is a branch of the ulnar artery.

## Nerves of the Posterior Compartment

The *musculocutaneous nerve* is the continuation of the lateral cord. It enters the superior aspect of the coracobrachialis and continues down the arm between the biceps brachii and the brachialis muscles. It supplies these three muscles: coracobrachialis, biceps brachii, and brachialis.

The radial nerve is a branch of the posterior cord. It travels with the profunda brachii artery in the radial groove deep to the lateral head of the triceps. The median nerve travels with the brachial artery on the medial side. Likewise. the ulnar nerve is located medially. Neither the ulnar nor the median nerve innervate any muscles in the arm (Table 6.1).

## The Elbow Joint

At the elbow, the *capitulum* of the humerus meets with *radial head*, and the *trochlea* of the humerus rests in the *trochlea notch* of the ulna. The anterior prominence of the trochlea is the coronoid process, which on flexion moves into the coronoid fossa of the anterior distal humerus. The posterior process of the superior ulna is the *olecranon*, which on extension moves into the olecranon fossa on the posterior distal humerus.

**Table 6.1** Pathways and landmarks for the three major nerves of the upper limb as they pass through the arm, elbow, forearm, wrist, and hand. (Leo 2022)

|  | Ulnar nerve | Median nerve | Radial nerve |
|---|---|---|---|
| **Arm** | Passes medial to brachial artery, enters the posterior compartment and then joins the superior ulnar collateral artery. | Found lateral to brachial artery in cubital fossa. | Runs with profunda brachial artery in radial groove. |
| **Elbow region** | Passes posterior to the medial epicondyle and then passes through the cubital tunnel | Passes between the two heads of pronator teres | Located anterior to the lateral epicondyle. |
| **Forearm** | Deep to flexor carpi ulnaris. Runs with ulnar artery | In distal forearm it gives off the recurrent branch of median nerve. Runs with anterior interosseus artery. | Splits into superficial and deep branches. Deep branch pierces supinator to reach posterior compartment. The superficial branch runs under brachioradialis. |
| **Wrist** | Lateral to pisiform | Between | Superficial branch enters superficial to the extensor retinaculum and send branches to the thumb and index finger |
| **Hand** | Travels through Guyon's canal and splits into superficial and deep branches | Passes through the carpal tunnel. Gives off recurrent branch to the thenar muscles. | Superficial radial nerve crosses snuff box. Is superficial to radial artery in snuff box. |

With the elbow flexed to 90°, the olecranon process forms an isosceles triangle with the medial and lateral epicondyle. On extension these three points line up in a row. With elbow injuries these relationships are disrupted.

On the lateral side the *radial collateral ligament* and *lateral ulnar collateral ligament* maintain stability. On the medial side, the ulnar collateral ligament is composed of the anterior, lateral bundle, and posterior bundles. *Tommy John Surgery* refers to restoration of the ulnar collateral ligament by using a ligament harvested from somewhere else in the body. Often the palmaris longus tendon is used for the graft. The surgery was first performed on the baseball player Tommy John in 1974. The ulnar nerve enters the elbow around the medial epicondyle and crosses the ulnar collateral ligament. (Note, don't confuse the ulnar collateral ligament and its three sections with the lateral ulnar collateral ligament – they names are very similar, but they are different).

Wrapping around the radial head is the *annular ligament* which allows the radial head to spin within the ligament for supination and pronation. The ligament is attached to the notch of the ulna making up the *proximal radioulnar joint* which is encased by the articular capsule. In adults this ligament is very strong however in infants it is weaker and a strong pull on the arm can subluxate (dislocate) the radial head. Over the years this has unfortunately taken on the pejorative term of *nurse-maid's elbow*.

The *terrible triad of the elbow* refers to an injury of the elbow joint that involves: (1) a radial head fracture, (2) a fracture of the ulnar coracoid process, and (3) a posterior dislocation of the elbow joint. It typically results from trauma where large forces push on the extended and supinated elbow joint; for instance, a car accident where the hand strikes the dashboard or other immoveable object. In addition to the three structures mentioned above, collateral ligaments of the elbow can also be injured.

As the ulnar nerve approaches the medial elbow, it enters the cubital tunnel with the ulnar collateral ligament making up the floor, and the cubital tunnel retinaculum making up the ceiling. Nerve impingement in this area is common (Fig. 6.13).

As the nerve moves emerges from the tunnel, it dives deep to the arcuate ligament (of Osborne) that lies between the two heads of the flexor carpi ulnaris.

In summary, as the three major nerves to the forearm and hand cross the elbow, they all pierce a muscle which can be a source of aggravation: the ulnar nerve travels between the two heads of flexor carpi ulnaris; the median nerve travels between the two heads of the pronator teres; and the deep radial nerve pierces the supinator muscle.

## Cubital Fossa

The *cubital fossa* is found on the anterior surface of the elbow. It is a triangular shaped space transmitting several structures from the arm to the forearm. It is bounded by the medial border of brachioradialis, the lateral border of pronator teres,

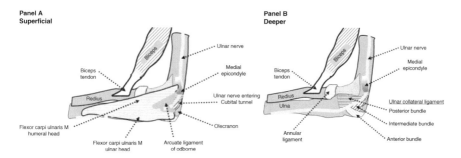

**Fig. 6.13** Medial view of elbow. Panel **a** shows the ulnar nerve entering the cubital tunnel which is deep to the arcuate ligament of Osborne. In Panel **b** the flexor carpi ulnaris has been removed to show the ulnar nerve wrapping around the medial epicondyle. The ulnar collateral ligament has three divisions. (Leo 2022)

and a horizontal line across the elbow. The order of the structures from lateral to medial is the biceps tendon, the brachial artery, and the median nerve. This gives us the mnemonic TAN for tendon, artery, and nerve. However, realize that the radial nerve is also found in the far lateral side of the compartment where it divides into superficial and deep branches (Fig. 6.14).

## Forearm

Many of the muscles responsible for hand movements arise in the forearm. The common flexor origin is located on the medial epicondyle and the many of the extensors are located on the lateral epicondyle. Keep in mind that in most cases when you talk about muscles to the thumb and little finger there are redundant muscles – a longus and a brevis. And in some cases, losing one muscle, say the longus, does not mean the associated movement is lost, because the brevis takes over, or vice versa (Fig. 6.15).

Flexion of the fingers involves moving your fingertips towards your palm, and extension involves moving the fingertips away. Abduction of the fingers involves spreading your fingers apart, while adduction involves moving them closer together.

Because of the thumb's rotation, its movements are in a plane that is 90° to the fingers. Flexion of the thumb involves moving it in towards the little finger and crossing over the palm, while extension involves spreading it out laterally (Fig. 6.16).

Abduction of the thumb involves moving the thumb away from the hand at a right angle to the palm, while adduction brings it back in to the palm (Fig. 6.17).

**Fig. 6.14** The cubital fossa is bounded by the medial border of the pronator teres, the lateral border of the brachioradialis and a line above the elbow. Within the fossa, from lateral to medial is the biceps Tendon, the brachial Artery, and the median Nerve. Remember TAN for the order of the structures. (Leo 2022)

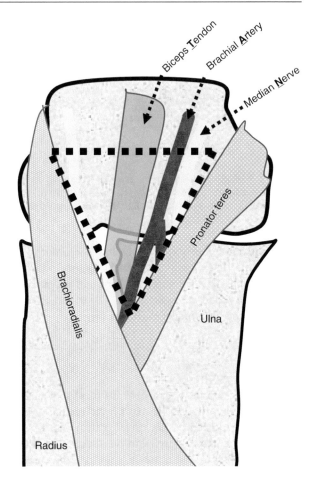

## Anterior Forearm

There are five muscles that arise together from the common flexor origin along the medial epicondyle and travel in the anterior forearm. Starting with the most lateral muscle:

1. The *pronator teres muscle* has two heads. One arises from the humerus, and one from the ulna tuberosity. They merge together to insert onto the radius. It is a flexor and pronator of the elbow. Median nerve.
2. The *flexor carpi radialis muscle* arises from the common flexor tendon and inserts onto the radial tuberosity and the bases of the second and third metacarpals. It is a flexor at the elbow and an abductor at the wrist. Median nerve.
3. The *palmaris longus muscle* also arises from the common flexor origin and inserts into the palmar aponeurosis. Median nerve.

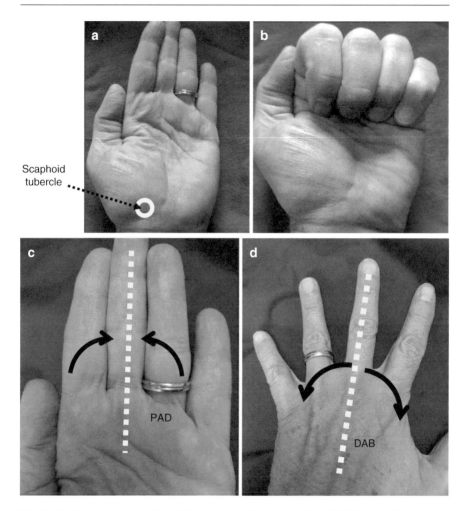

**Fig. 6.15** Finger movements Panel (**a**) extension of the fingers. Panel (**b**) Flexion of the fingers., Panel (**c**) Adduction (Palmar Interossei) Panel (**d**) Abduction (Dorsal Interossei) (Leo 2022)

4. The *flexor carpi ulnaris muscle* also arises from the common flexor origin and inserts onto the fifth metacarpal, the hook of the hamate and the pisiform. It is a flexor at the elbow and an adductor at the wrist. Ulnar nerve

5. The *flexor digitorum superficialis muscle* has two heads. A humeroulnar head which arises in part from the common flexor tendon but in part from the coronoid process of the ulna. It is also has a radial head arising from the radius. The tendons travel down the arm to insert on the middle phalanges of digits 2–5. Its action is flexion of the metacarpal phalangeal and proximal interphalangeal joints. It is innervated by the median nerve. Note that when it comes to organizing these muscles some authors place this muscle in an intermediate compartment. It is really just a matter of how you would like to organize it. When it

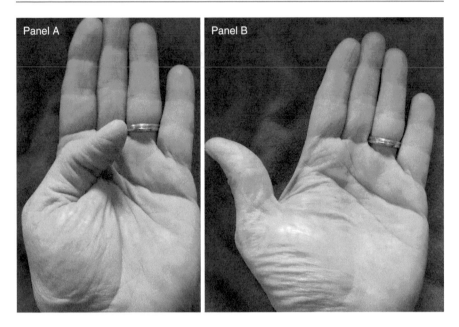

**Fig. 6.16**   Panel (**a**) Flexion of the thumb. Panel (**b**) Extension of the thumb. (Leo 2022)

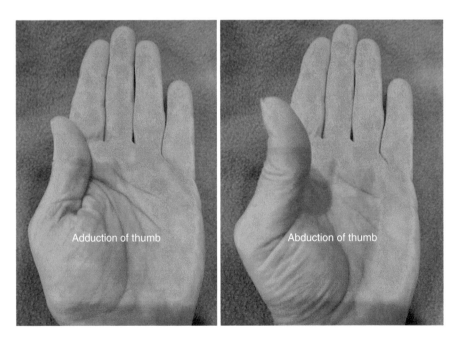

**Fig. 6.17**   Thumb adduction and abduction. (Leo 2022)

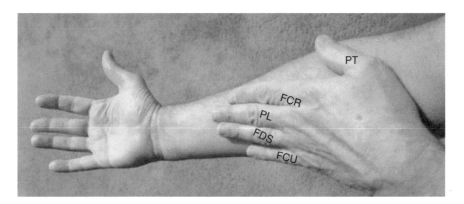

**Fig. 6.18** Common flexor origin. There are five superficial flexors originating from the medial epicondyle. If you lay you hand on the medial elbow, your five fingers represent the five muscles. PT pronator teres, FCR flexor carpi radialis, PL palmaris longus, FDS flexor digitorum superficialis, FCU flexor carpi ulnaris. (Leo 2022)

comes to learning the nerves, it seems easier to put in the superficial compartment for the simple fact that if you place your palm on medial epicondyle and flair out your fingers you have the five superficial flexors – four doesn't work quite as well with this scheme. Repetitive injuries to the medial epicondyle, or *medial epicondylitis* come from continuous flexion of the forearm. This is sometimes referred to as *Golfer's Elbow* (Figs. 6.18 and 6.19).

## Deep Forearm Compartment

In the deep forearm there are three muscles, all of which are innervated by the anterior interosseus nerve:

1. The *flexor digitorum profundus* arises from the ulna and the interosseus membrane and inserts into the distal phalanges of the fingers. It flexes all the joints it crosses: the wrist, metacarpophalangeal, proximal interphalangeal, and distal interphalangeal.
2. The *flexor pollicis longus* arises from the radius and interosseus membrane and inserts into the distal phalanx of the thumb.
3. The *pronator quadratus* runs from ulna to radius and is a pronator (Fig. 6.19).

## Flexor Digitorum and Flexor Digitorum Profundus Insertions

As the four tendons of *flexor digitorum superficialis* approach the proximal phalanges each tendon splits into two bands that attach to the sides of the middle

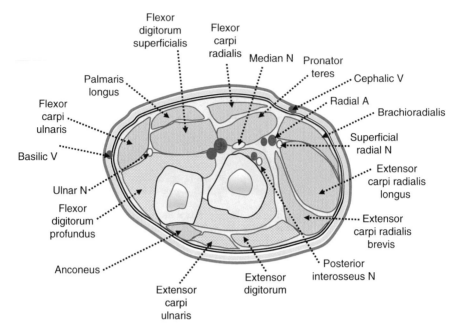

**Fig. 6.19** Cross section through the superior forearm. In the anterior forearm, arising from the medial epicondyle is the flexor carpi ulnaris, palmaris longus, flexor digitorum superficialis, pronator teres, and flexor carpi radialis. Deep to these superficial muscles note the flexor digitorum profundus arising from the ulna. Arising from the lateral epicondyle is the extensor carpi ulnaris, extensor digitorum, and extensor carpi radialis longus and brevis. The supinator runs from the ulna to the radius on the posterior side. (Leo 2022)

phalanges. This split allows the tendon of *flexor digitorum profundus* of each finger to travel through the split and continue to the distal phalanges. The tendons of both muscles are held down close to the fingers by fibrous flexor sheaths. The sheaths are composed of a combination of ligaments, some that encircle the bone and others that form a crisscross pattern enclosing the tendons. A *trigger finger* refers to a sharp sound that comes from the finger when it is flexed and extended. The sound comes from a growth on the tendon which makes a snapping noise as it moves through the ligaments around the finger.

## Dupuytren's Contracture

Just under the skin of the palm is a strong tough fibrous membrane, the palmar fascia. In some cases, this fascia becomes thick and tight which leads to flexion of the fingers. This closely resembles claw hand in appearance, but it is not a nerve injury. The symptoms are more severe in the fourth and fifth digits.

## Neurovascular Compartment in Forearm

The brachial artery enters the forearm and divides into the radial and ulnar arteries. The ulnar artery continues medially and lies beneath the flexor carpi ulnaris. It runs with the ulnar nerve. The ulnar artery gives off the common interosseus artery which quickly divides into anterior and posterior interosseus arteries. The *posterior interosseus artery* gains access to the posterior forearm by traveling over the interosseus membrane, moving from the anterior to posterior compartment, and then traveling down the posterior surface of the interosseus membrane where it runs with the *posterior interosseus nerve* which is a branch of the radial nerve.

The *anterior interosseus artery* runs in front of the interosseus membrane with the anterior interosseus nerve which is a branch of the median nerve.

The *radial artery* travels from the cubital fossa down to the wrist between the brachioradialis and the flexor carpi radialis tendons, where its pulse can be felt. Just below the elbow, the radial artery gives off the radial recurrent artery which meets up with the radial collateral artery.

The *radial nerve* enters the forearm in the lateral region of the cubital fossa. It splits into the superficial and deep branches. The deep branch becomes the *posterior interosseus nerve,* while the superficial branch travels down towards the anatomical snuff box. Wartenberg's syndrome refers to constriction of the superficial radial nerve in the forearm, typically between the brachioradialis and the extensor carpi radialis longus.

The *median nerve* enters the cubital fossa medial to the brachial artery and then travels between the two heads of the pronator teres. In the forearm it gives off two branches the anterior interosseus nerve and the palmar cutaneous branch (Figs. 6.20 and 6.21).

The median nerve continues down the forearm between the flexor digitorum superficialis and the flexor digitorum profundus. The anterior interosseus nerve travels down the forearm between the flexor digitorum profundus and the flexor pollicis longus to reach the pronator quadratus. A test for the anterior interosseus is to ask the patient to make an "Ok" sign. The successful move is based on the flexor digitorum profundus tendon to the second digit, and the flexor pollicis longus

**Fig. 6.20** Radial nerve. The radial nerve enters the elbow region and divides into a superficial and deep branch. The deep branch pierces the supinator muscle and enters the posterior forearm as the posterior interosseus nerve. The superficial branch continues to the hand and crosses the snuff box. (Leo 2022)

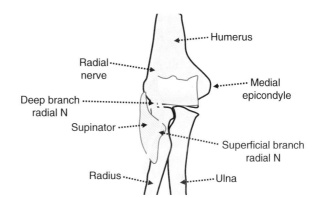

**Fig. 6.21** The median nerve. The median nerve enters the elbow region between the two heads of the pronator teres. At this point the nerve can be become entrapped. The anterior interosseus nerve branches off the median nerve between the two heads of pronator teres. (Leo 2022)

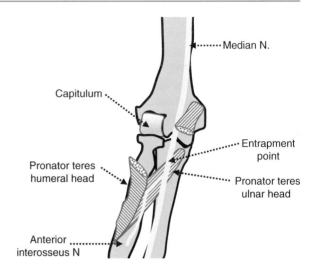

**Fig. 6.22** Anterior interosseus nerve. Panel (**a**) shows normal anterior interosseus nerve function. Panel (**b**) shows the fingers of a patient with anterior interosseus nerve palsy. (Leo 2022)

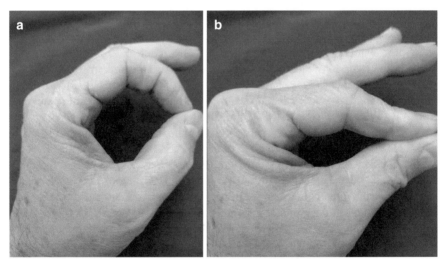

tendon going to the thumb, both of which are innervated by the anterior interosseus nerve. Damage to the nerve will result in more of a pinch than an "Ok" sign (Fig. 6.22).

## Posterior Forearm

The muscles of the posterior forearm are all innervated by the radial nerve. Many of them are involved in extension of the wrist and fingers.

1. The *extensor carpi radialis longus* runs from the lateral supracondylar ridge of the humerus to the second metacarpal.
2. The *extensor carpi radialis brevis* runs from the lateral supracondylar ridge to the third metacarpal. The muscle lies deep to the extensor carpi radialis longus. The two of them together extend and abduct at the wrist.
3. The *extensor digitorum* arises from the lateral supracondylar ridge and inserts into the extensor expansion. It is an extensor of the wrist and digits.
4. The *extensor digiti minimi* is an extension of the extensor digitorum that sends a tendon to the fifth digit. It extends the wrist and the fifth digit.
5. The *extensor carpi* ulnaris runs from the lateral epicondyle to the fifth metacarpal.
6. The *anconeus* is a small triangular shaped muscle in the superior portion of the posterior forearm that blends in with the triceps.
7. Last but not least is the *brachioradialis*. The brachioradialis is somewhat of an outlier. It arises from lateral side of the humerus in close proximity to the other extensors, however it is a flexor. It runs down the forearm and attaches to the radial tuberosity. When the arm is in the neutral position, the brachioradialis is a flexor at the elbow. Imagine you have just picked up a can of soda from a table. At this point your hand is in the neutral position. When you move your hand towards your mouth it is the brachioradialis that is responsible for this movement. Think of it as your soda drinking muscle.

These muscles that arise from the lateral elbow can become aggravated in overuse scenarios what involve continuous extension of your elbow such as playing tennis, thus the term "tennis elbow" or *lateral epicondylitis*. *Ganglion cysts* are fluid filled sacs that can appear on tendons anywhere in the body, however they are usually found on the hand, and most of these occur on the extensor tendons on the posterior wrist.

## Posterior Forearm Muscles to Thumb

There are three muscles that originate in the forearm and travel through the forearm on their way to the thumb. As they cross the wrist, they form the anatomical snuff box. They are all innervated by the radial nerve.

1. The *extensor pollicis longus* arises from the ulna and inserts on the distal phalanx of the thumb. As it crosses the distal radius it makes a turn around the *dorsal tubercle* (Lister's tubercle). The tubercle acts like a pulley to increase the leverage for the muscle. A hyperextension injury can fracture the tubercle leaving a sharp edge which can tear the tendon. A *mallet finger* refers to an injury that tears the distal end of either the extensor pollicis longus or extensor digitorum tendon with a transverse tear just before its insertion onto the distal phalange. A baseball player sliding into the base with their upper limb extended such that the distal phalanges can strike the base with a hard impact. With the tendon torn, the fingertip will be stuck in a flexed position.

2. The *extensor pollicis brevis* arises from the radius and inserts onto the distal phalanx of the thumb.
3. The *abductor pollicis longus* arises from the ulna and the radius and inserts onto the first metacarpal bone.

The *snuff box* is bounded by the extensor pollicis longus and the extensor pollicis brevis. The floor of the snuff box is the *scaphoid and trapezium*. Crossing deep to the tendons in the snuff box is the radial artery where the pulse can be felt. Crossing superficially above the tendons is the superficial branch of the radial nerve and the cephalic vein (Fig. 6.23).

The tendons of the abductor pollicis longus and the extensor pollicis brevis pass in a fibrous tunnel along the radius and deep to the extensor retinaculum. Repetitive motion injuries can occur here leading to *De Quervain's syndrome,* which is thickening of either the tendons, the sheaths, or in some cases both. This leads to pain on flexion of the thumb and wrist (Finkelstein's test.)

## Distal Radioulnar Joint

The *distal radioulnar joint* is between the sigmoid notch of the radius and the head of the ulna. The joint allows pronation and supination of the forearm. An articular disk holds the two bones together and also separates the distal radioulnar joint from the radiocarpal joint. The *articular disk* along with several smaller ligaments from

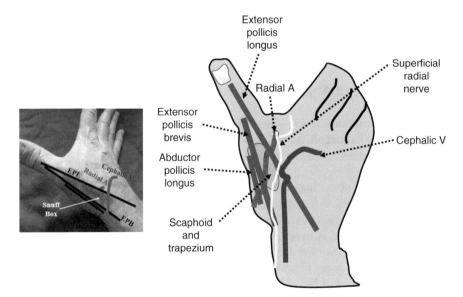

**Fig. 6.23** Snuff box. The anatomical snuff box bounded by the extensor pollicis longus and brevis. The floor is made up of the trapezium and scaphoid. The radial artery crosses deep to the tendons, while the superficial radial nerve and cephalic vein cross superficially. (Leo 2022)

the *triangular fibrocartilage complex* known as the TFCC for short. The TFCC connects the lunate, triquetrum, and ulna. The anterior and posterior distal radioulnar ligaments also contribute to joint stability. The TFCC can be injured from trauma (type I) or overuse (type II). In addition to pain and swelling of the medial wrist, patients will often report a clicking or popping feeling with wrist movement.

The *fovea* of the wrist is a point on the medial wrist between the styloid process and the tendon of flexor carpi ulnaris tendon. Remember the tendon of flexor carpi ulnaris passes over the pisiform. If the examiner can elicit pain by pressing on this region, it suggests damage to the TFCC and the distal radioulnar joint.

## The Hand

The palm of the hand is organized around three compartments: the thenar compartment containing the small muscles of the thumb, the hypothenar compartment containing the small muscles of the fifth digit, and the medial compartment situated between the thenar and hypothenar compartments. The short version of the motor nerve supply to the hand is that the median nerve innervates three and half muscles and the ulnar innervates the rest. The median nerve innervates the 3 thenar muscles and two of the four lumbricals (1/2 of the lumbricals). The ulnar nerve innervates everything else. Note that the "everything else" includes the muscles in the hypothenar compartment, the interossei, two of the four lumbricals, and the adductor pollicis.

## Carpal Bones

There are eight carpal bones arranged in two rows of four each. The first row, moving lateral to medial is the *scaphoid, lunate, triquetrum, and pisiform* (Fig. 6.24)

The radius articulates with the scaphoid and lunate. Falls on the outstretched hand typically result in a fracture of either the scaphoid, the distal radius, or the clavicle. Which bone is fractured is typically a result of the patient's age. In a teenager the clavicle is the most often fractured bone, in an elderly person the most common fracture occurs at the distal radius (Colle's fracture). In a middle-aged person, the most common fracture is to the scaphoid.

The danger of a scaphoid fracture is that because the blood supply is to the distal segment of the bone, the proximal segment will undergo avascular necrosis. The scaphoid, along with the trapezium, makes up the floor of the snuff box thus, scaphoid fractures will lead to pain in the snuff box. Scaphoid fractures can take up to two-weeks to appear in an x-ray. The scaphoid tubercle can be found just distal (on centimeter) to the wrist folds. The tendon of flexor carpi radialis passes over it (Fig. 6.15).

In addition to the scaphoid fracture, another common injury following a fall on the outstretched hand is an anterior dislocation of the lunate which on a radiograph appears as a triangular shaped piece of bone pushed anterior. Anterior dislocations

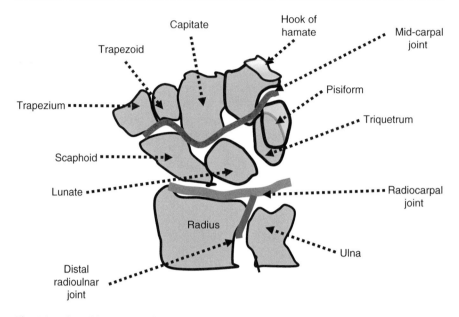

**Fig. 6.24**  Carpal bones. (Leo 2022)

**Table 6.2**  Origin of names of carpal bones

| Carpal bone | Meaning |
|---|---|
| Scaphoid | Canoe |
| Lunate | Moon |
| Triquetrum | Three sided |
| Pisiform | Pea |
| Trapezium | Quadrilateral |
| Trapezoid | Quadrilateral |
| Capitate | Compact head |
| Hamate | Hook |

of the lunate often compress the median nerve leading to the same symptoms as carpal tunnel syndrome.

The second row of carpal bones contains the *trapezium, trapezoid, capitate, and hamate*. The hook of the hamate and the pisiform protect the ulnar nerve. The hamate and pisiform also serve as an attachment for several muscles and ligaments. The carpal bones all have interesting names (Table 6.2).

## Metacarpals

The metacarpals connect the carpal bones to the phalanges forming the scaffold for the intermediate compartment. The interossei muscles also attach to these bones. The axis for abduction and adduction is through the third finger. The palmar interossei are responsible for <u>add</u>uction, and the dorsal interossei for <u>ab</u>duction. A *boxer's fracture* is to the distal metacarpals, usually of digits 2 and 3. A *Bennett's fracture* is to the base of the first metacarpal (the thumb).

## Thenar Compartment

The thenar compartment contains three muscles all of which are innervated by the recurrent branch of the median nerve which passes between the two heads of the flexor pollicis brevis

1. The *flexor pollicis brevis* has a superficial and a deep head. It arises from the flexor retinaculum and the trapezium, and it inserts onto the proximal phalanx of the thumb. It is a flexor of the thumb at the metacarpophalangeal joint
2. The *abductor pollicis brevis* arises from the scaphoid and trapezium, and it inserts onto the proximal phalanx of the thumb.
3. The *opponens pollicis* arises from the trapezium and inserts onto the proximal phalanx of the thumb.

The recurrent branch of the median nerve is sometimes referred to as "the million-dollar nerve." The reference to how much a physician could be held liable if it is cut during a surgical procedure highlights the importance of this nerve. Shortly after the median nerve passes though the carpal tunnel it gives off the recurrent branch which travels between the two heads of the flexor pollicis brevis. At this point the nerve is just under the skin and can easily be injured in lacerations of the thenar compartment. In this scenario, the patient would lose the function of the three thenar muscles. If this patient is in your office and you want to test whether the nerve is damaged, you test opposition. This is because, although the patient would lose the flexor pollicis brevis, they would still be able to flex their thumb because the flexor pollicis longus is intact. Likewise, although the patient would lose the abductor pollicis brevis, they would still have function of their abductor pollicis longus. In other words, keep in mind that for flexion and abduction of the thumb there is both a longus and a brevis, but for opposition there is no longus or brevis, just a single opponens pollicis – for the opponens there is no redundancy.

## The Hypothenar Compartment

There are three muscles in the hypothenar compartment. They all act on the fifth digit and are innervated by the deep branch of the ulnar nerve.

1. The *flexor digiti minimi* arises from the hamate and inserts into the proximal phalanx of the fifth digit.
2. The *abductor digiti minimi brevis* arises from the pisiform and inserts into the base of proximal phalanx of fifth digit.
3. The *opponens digiti minimi* arises from the hamate and inserts into the metacarpal of the fifth digit.

## Intermediate Compartment

Between the hypothenar and thenar compartments is the adductor pollicis. It has an *oblique head* arising from the second and third metacarpal, and a *transverse head* arising from the third metacarpal. The two heads merge to insert onto the proximal phalanx of the thumb. Note that it is a thenar muscle, meaning that it acts on the thumb, but it is not *located* in the thenar compartment. It is located in the intermediate compartment. It brings the abducted thumb back towards the second digit. It is innervated by the deep branch of the ulnar nerve which can be seen coming the ulnar nerve medially and going laterally to go between the two heads of the muscle.

## Palmar and Dorsal Interossei

There are four *palmar and four dorsal interossei*. To test the interossei you can ask the patient to abduct and adduct the fingers. The palmar interossei are responsible for adduction (PAD). The dorsal interossei are responsible for abduction (DAB). The axis for these movements is through the third digit, meaning that when the other fingers are brought towards the third finger this is adduction, while movement away from the third digit is abduction. Because the third digit is the axis, whichever way it moves is away from the axis and considered abduction. All of the interossei are innervated by the T1 level traveling via the ulnar nerve.

## Lumbricals

The lumbricals are unique in that they do not attach to bone, but instead run from one tendon to another. On the palmar side they are attached to the tendon of the flexor digitorum profundus, and on the dorsal side they are attached to the extensor digitorum. When they contract, they flex the metacarpophalangeal joint and extend the interphalangeal joints. The two lumbricals on the medial or ulnar side are innervated by the ulnar nerve, and the two lumbricals on the lateral or radial side are innervated by the median nerve.

## Ulnar Nerve at the Wrist

At the wrist the ulnar nerve enters *Guyon's canal* which is above the transverse carpal ligament medial to the pisiform bone – it is not in the carpal tunnel. It travels with the ulnar artery at this point and is covered by the palmar carpal ligament. Impingement at this point can occur in bike riders or office workers, who rest their hand on their bike handles or desk. As the ulnar nerve continues into the hand it splits into a superficial branch, which is sensory, and a deep branch which supplies the muscles. The motor branch travels into a second opening referred to as the pisohamate hiatus which is just a bit distal to Guyon's canal. The floor of the pisohamate

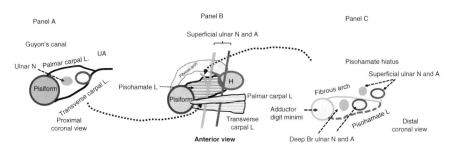

**Fig. 6.25** Pathway of ulnar nerve. Panel (**a**), a coronal proximal view of ulnar nerve in wrist, shows the boundaries of triangular shaped Guyon's canal: Roof border is palmar carpal L, floor is the transverse carpal L., and medial border is pisiform. Panel (**b**) shows the palmar view with the ulnar nerve and artery passing deep to the palmar carpal ligament (anterior boundary) in Guyon's canal, emerging from the canal and passing over the pisohamate L., and then splitting into superficial deep and deep branches to pass on either side of the fibrous arch from hypothenar muscles. Panel (**c**) is a distal coronal view, showing the deep branches passing under the fibrous arch to enter the pisohamate hiatus, while the superficial branches pass superficial to the arch. (Leo 2022)

hiatus is the pisohamate ligament, and the roof is made up by the fibrous arch. Besides the deep branch of the ulnar nerve, the deep branch of the ulnar artery runs through the *pisohamate hiatus* (Fig. 6.25).

## Froment's Sign

In a healthy individual when you place a piece of paper between their thumb and second digit, they can hold the piece of paper firmly in place with their entire thumb fully adducted against the finger by using their adductor pollicis. In a patient with an ulnar nerve palsy, they can hold the paper in place, but the thumb is held in a slightly different position. Because they have lost the adductor pollicis they use their flexor pollicis longus muscle which is innervated by the median nerve to flex the distal phalangeal joint of the thumb. Thus, instead of using the surface of the entire medial thumb they are only using the tip of the thumb to hold the paper (Fig. 6.26).

## Claw Hand

In a healthy individual the lumbricals and interossei muscles are involved with flexion of the metacarpal phalangeal joints and extension of the interphalangeal joints. With an injury to the ulnar nerve, all the interossei and the medial two lumbricals are lost. Thus, the metacarpal phalangeal joint is now extended, and the interphalangeal joints are flexed. The fingers assume a claw like position, and the clawing will be more severe in the medial two fingers because the interossei are lost in those fingers, but they are intact in the lateral two fingers.

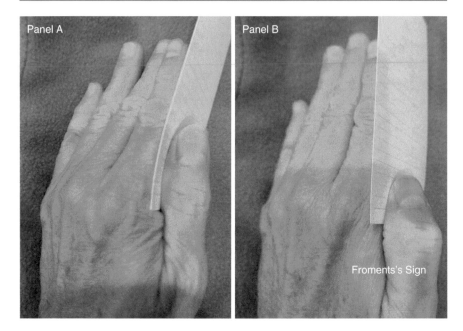

**Fig. 6.26** Froment's Sign. Panel (**a**) shows normal ulnar function when holding the piece of paper. The person is adducting the thumb with adductor pollicis. In Panel (**b**), the patient has an ulnar nerve palsy and instead of using their adductor pollicus they hold the paper by flexing the metacarpal phalangeal joint of the thumb with their flexor pollicis longus which is innervated by the median nerve. The bump at the metacarpal phalangeal joint is Froment's sign. (Leo 2022)

Claw hand can result from an injury to the ulnar nerve at either the elbow or the wrist. Interestingly, the claw hand will be more severe if the ulnar nerve is compromised at the wrist as compared to an injury at the elbow. At first glance this seems counterintuitive since usually, the closer the injury is to the midline the more severe the symptoms. However, when the ulnar nerve is cut at the wrist, this leaves the flexor digitorum profundus intact. Since this muscle is involved in flexion this will contribute to the claw hand appearance. If the nerve is cut at the elbow, then the patient loses the flexor digitorum profundus and the fingers will open up a bit.

One point to emphasize about claw hand: If the ulnar nerve is damaged the patient will have a claw hand at rest. In other words, they will probably walk into your office with an obvious claw hand. If you are walking down the street behind them, you can probably observe the claw hand. You do not need to conduct a motor test to observe the claw hand. In fact, if they have a claw hand and you suspect ulnar nerve pathology, the motor task you would check is abduction/ adduction of the fingers. The patient with ulnar palsy would lose this ability since they have lost the interossei.

## The Median Nerve at the Hand and Wrist

The median nerve enters the wrist between the palmaris longus and flexor carpi radialis, deep to the transverse carpal ligament in the carpal tunnel. The floor of the carpal tunnel is the *palmar carpal ligament*. There are ten structures in the carpal tunnel – nine tendons and a nerve. There are the four tendons of the profundus (FDP), the four tendons of superficialis (FDS), one tendon of flexor pollicis longus, and the one median nerve.

Note that back in the forearm, the median nerve gives off the *palmar cutaneous branch of the median nerve* which carries sensation from the proximal palm. This cutaneous branch passes superficial to the carpal tunnel. With compression of the median nerve in the carpal tunnel the patient will have reduced function of the thenar muscles along with pins and tingling sensation along digits 1–3 and the lateral half of digit 4. Sensation from the proximal palm will be intact because the palmar cutaneous nerve is spared because of its location over the carpal tunnel.

Just past the carpal tunnel the nerve gives off two motor branches: the recurrent branch, and the palmar digital branch which innervates the lateral two lumbricals. It also gives off a palmar digital cutaneous branch which carries sensation from digits 1–3 and the lateral half of digit 4. In addition to the motor and sensory deficits in a carpal tunnel patient, there are two tests to aid in the diagnosis (Fig. 6.27):

1. *Tinel's sign* is elicited by tapping on the anterior forearm in the vicinity of the median nerve. In a carpal tunnel patient, pins and needle sensations will be felt in the hand.

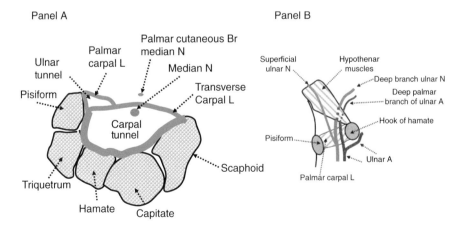

**Fig. 6.27** Carpal bones. Panel (**a**) The proximal carpal bones showing the carpal tunnel with the transverse carpal ligament (roof). The ulnar tunnel is also seen on the medial side with the palmar carpal ligament forming the roof. Panel (**b**) is distal to Guyon's canal and shows the ulnar nerve superficial to the pisohamate ligament where it splits into two branches. The ulnar artery runs lateral to the hamate. (Leo 2022)

2. In *Phalen's test,* both hands are flexed at the wrist with the dorsal surfaces placed again each other. This puts pressure on the carpal tunnel. Pain felt in the hand is considered a positive test for carpal tunnel compression. Phalen's test is sometimes referred to as the reverse prayer test.

Of note is that carpal tunnel symptoms are similar to the symptoms seen in thoracic outlet syndrome – both patients will complain of problems with their hand. However, a physical exam should reveal the differences. Thoracic outlet compression will affect both median and ulnar nerve, while carpal tunnel only affects median nerve territory.

## Nerves and Arteries on Palmar Wrist

The ulnar nerve enters the wrist just lateral to the flexor carpi ulnaris. And right next to the ulnar nerve is the ulnar artery. They are both superficial to the flexor retinaculum. The radial artery enters the wrist just lateral to the flexor carpi radialis. The median nerve enters the wrist deep to the flexor retinaculum. The main source of the *superficial palmar arch* is the ulnar artery, the main source of the *deep palmar arch* is the radial artery, however, both the radial and ulnar arteries each contribute to both arches. *Allen's test* involves compressing the two arteries and then releasing the pressure on either one. If there is sufficient patency of the arteries, then blood traveling on either artery should be sufficient to fill the entire hand (Fig. 6.28).

**Fig. 6.28**  Wrist relationships. Note the ulnar nerve and artery are lateral to the flexor carpi ulnaris. The radial artery is lateral to the flexor carpi radialis. The median nerve goes deep to the flexor retinaculum, while the ulnar nerve goes superficial. (Leo 2022)

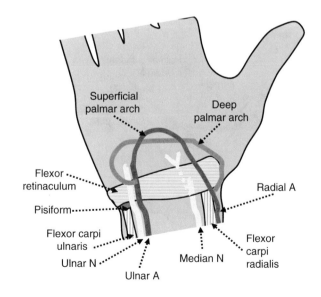

## Median Nerve Palsy

A patient with median nerve palsy is sometimes said to have an "ape hand." Over time the thenar muscles will atrophy. These patients will often be said to have "the pope's blessing" sign, or the "sign of benediction." This is easily confused with the claw hand which is seen with an ulnar palsy. If you look at a picture of the two, they look very similar, but there is a major difference.

As mentioned before, a patient with claw hand walks around with the claw hand. When they walk into your office you can see the claw hand. However, the patient with the sign of benediction does not walk around with this appearance. The sign of benediction refers to a motor test and the patient does not exhibit this sign until you test them. To explain this, we need to focus on the eight long tendons going to the four fingers. Each finger has two tendons running down the palmar side – one tendon of FDP and one tendon of FDS. If you ask a healthy person to flex their fingers, they are using all eight tendons. In a patient with a median nerve palsy, only two tendons are functioning - the two tendons of FDP going to digits 4 and 5. So, when you ask this person to flex their fingers, they can only flex digits 4 and 5, resulting in a claw appearance (Fig. 6.29).

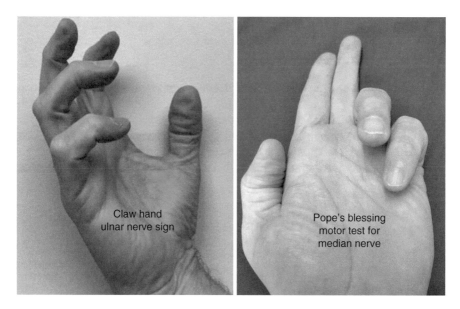

Claw hand
ulnar nerve sign

Pope's blessing
motor test for
median nerve

**Fig. 6.29** Claw hand and Pope's blessing. Claw hand is a sign for ulnar nerve palsy. Pope's blessing is what happens in a patient with a median nerve palsy on attempted finger flexion. The only two tendons working are the two tendons of flexor digitorum profundus on the ulnar side. (Leo 2022)

## Ulnar Collateral Ligament and Gamekeeper's Thumb

The metacarpophalangeal joint of the thumb is supported by the *ulnar collateral ligament*. The ligament is prone to hyperextension injuries, such as a skier falling and landing on their outstretched thumb. A high incidence was also seen in Scottish gamekeepers who killed their prey such as rabbits by pushing down on their necks with an outstretched thumb.

## Nerves to Fingers

In the hand, on the palmar side, both the median and ulnar nerves give rise to *common palmar digital nerves*. As these nerves approach the metacarpal phalangeal joints, they split into *proper palmar digital nerves* which travel down and innervate the palmar side of the digits. However, the proper palmar digital nerves also give rise to the dorsal branches of the palmar digital nerves which cross the fingers from anterior to posterior to innervate the distal fingertips (nailbeds) on the dorsal side of the hand. Keep in mind that on the dorsal side of the hand, the skin above the proximal and middle phalanges is innervated by the nerves on the dorsal side of the hand which come from the radial and ulnar nerves (Fig. 6.30).

## Upper and Lower Tunk Injuries

Two other injuries that can result in nerve deficits are upper and lower trunk injuries. These injuries occur following strain on the shoulder which can damage the roots emerging from the spinal cord. To think about these injuries, you can mimic this on yourself. If you are standing with your left upper limb hanging down by your side, take your right hand and push down on your left shoulder. You should feel it get tighter in your neck area. Injuries that push down on your shoulder will damage the

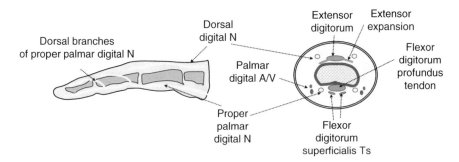

**Fig. 6.30** Nerves to fingers. The proper digital nerves are on the palmar side with the palmar digital artery and vein. The proper palmar digital nerves send dorsal branches from the palmar side to the dorsal side to innervate the nail beds. The dorsal digital branches are only on the proximal dorsal side of the fingers. (Leo 2022)

superior part of the plexus which is C5-C6, while the lower part of the plexus is relaxed. *These are superior trunk injuries.*

To mimic *lower trunk injuries*, if you fully abduct your left upper limb, with your hand and fingers trying to touch the ceiling, you should feel tightness in your armpit (the upper thoracic region in the mid axillary line), while the upper part of your shoulder relaxes. Thus, it is the lower part of the brachial plexus, C6-T1, that is injured.

1. *Lower trunk injuries* that damage C8-T1 will lead to weakness in the hand in both median and ulnar nerve territories. In addition, the patient may present with Horner's syndrome resulting from damage to the preganglionic sympathetic fibers that emerge at the T1 level to jump on the ascending sympathetic trunk on their way to the head. Lower trunk injuries can occur during a delivery when the upper limb is pulled, or when a child is playing on a jungle gym and hangs by their hand on the bars, etc.
2. *Upper trunk injuries* that damage C5–6 roots will lead to damage in the shoulder and arm regions. If we look at what nerves are affected, what these nerves normally do, and what happens when they are damaged, we can think through the symptoms. C5 roots get into the musculocutaneous nerve, which is involved in supination and flexion. Without this nerve, the upper limb will be extended at the elbow and pronated. Likewise, C5–6 roots also go to the axillary nerve which will normally abduct the shoulder. Without the deltoid, the lower limb will be adducted. Thus, the lower limb will hang by the side, and will be pronated. This is sometimes referred to as "waiter's tip" sign which refers to the waiter walking by the table with their hand out subtly waiting for a tip.

## Distal Fractures of the Radius

Falling on the outstretched extended hand can lead to a fracture of the distal tibia (transverse fracture) known as *Colle's fracture* - or a "Dinner Fork Deformity." Looking at the radius from the side it resembles a dinner fork with a bump on it. The bump is made by the proximal segment pushed anteriorly, and the distal segment pushed posteriorly.

A *Smith's fracture* most likely occurs from a fall on the flexed hand. In contrast to Colle's fracture, the distal segment of the radius will be displaced towards the palmar side.

## Fractures of the Humerus

There are four common fractures that can damage associated arteries and nerves (Fig. 6.31):

**Fig. 6.31** Humerus
fractures. There are four
common fractures to the
humerus, all of which can
damage a different nerve.
(1) Surgical neck: Axillary
nerve, (2) Midshaft: Radial
nerve, (3) Supracondylar:
Median nerve, (4) Medial
epicondyle: Ulnar nerve.
(Leo 2022)

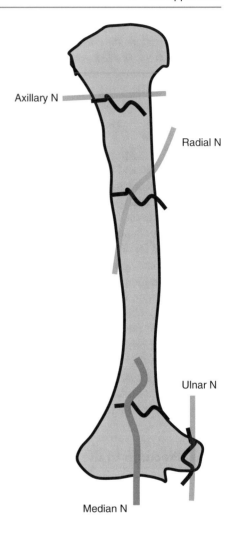

1. A fracture of the *surgical neck* can damage the axillary nerve and posterior humeral circumflex artery
2. *A mid-shaft* humeral fracture can damage the radial nerve and the profunda brachii artery. Keep in mind that compartments are usually innervated at the superior portion of the compartment. When it comes to a radial nerve fracture this means that the triceps is intact, so the patient would still be able to extend at the elbow, but they would have a deficit of wrist and finger extension. The patient would have "wrist drop" meaning that without extension of the wrist, the wrist would be stuck in flexion. Besides a fracture at this point, Saturday night palsy refers to compression of the radial nerve along the humerus which leads to loss of extension of the wrist and fingers. The term *Saturday night palsy* is named for the person who came home from the bar on Saturday night and fell asleep in a chair with their arm resting all night on the top of the chair. This leads to a

temporary compression of the radial nerve and subsequent radial nerve palsy signs. Poorly fitting crutches can also aggravate the radial nerve here.

3. A supra*condylar fracture* is to the distal humerus which can damage several different nerves, but the median nerve is most likely nerve to be affected. In addition, the brachial artery can be compressed which leads to a loss of blood flow to the forearm. This can lead to a shortening the muscles of the forearm which results in the hand, wrist, and fingers being flexed into a claw-like position. This is referred to as *Volkmann's contracture.*

4. A fracture of the *medial epicondyle* can damage the ulnar nerve and the superior ulnar collateral artery.

## Peripheral Nerve Map of the Hand

In addition to the motor deficits in the hand following injuries, patients will often have sensory deficits, which especially when talking about the hand and fingers are quite detrimental. On the palm of the hand, the median nerve supplies the thumb and digits 1–3, and the lateral half of 4. The ulnar nerve carries sensation from the hypothenar region and the medial half of digit 4 and all of the palmar surface of digit 5 (Fig. 6.32).

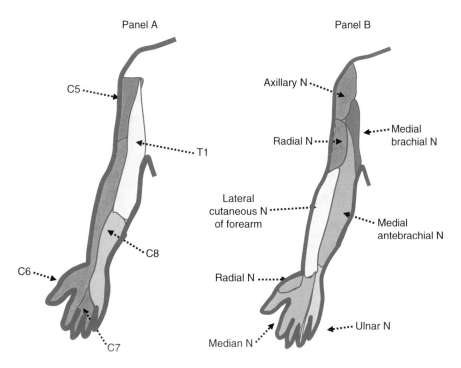

**Fig. 6.32** Roots vs peripheral nerves. Panel (**a**) shows the dermatomes of the upper limb. The thumb is C6, middle fingers are C7, and pinky is C8. Panel (**b**) shows the peripheral nerve map of the upper limb. (Leo 2022)

On the dorsum of the hand, the radial nerve is responsible for a patch of skin centered around the first dorsal webspace. In addition, the proximal dorsal side of the digits are innervated by the radial and ulnar nerves (Fig. 6.32).

## Dermatomes of Upper Limb

Note that the thumb is C6, middle fingers are C7, pinky is C8, and the armpit is T1. With radiculopathies you want to think about the *dermatome map*, with peripheral nerve injuries you want to think about the *peripheral nerve map*. For a more in-depth discussion see the chapter on the back. If you think of making a "6" by pinching your thumb and second digit it can be reminder that the thumb dermatome is C6 (Fig. 6.32).

## Myotomes of the Upper Limb

When it comes to the nerve root levels of the upper limb, the shoulder is C 4, 5. The elbow is C 5, 6, 7, and 8. The wrist is C 6, 7, 8, and T1. When it comes to hand flexion of the fingers is C 8. An easy way to remember this is to interlock your flexed fingers together and see that you are making an "8." Abduction and adduction of your fingers is a test for T1 (Fig. 6.33, Table 6.3).

Panel A                                    Panel B

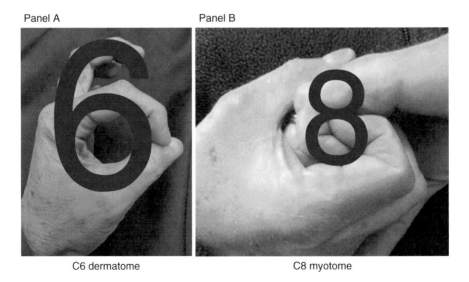

C6 dermatome                              C8 myotome

**Fig. 6.33** Tricks to remember root levels. Panel (**a**) If you make a pinching motion with your thumb and second digit, you are making what looks like a "6." The thumb is the C6 dermatome. Panel (**b**) If you put your fingers together and make a "figure 8" it should help you remember that flexion of the fingers, the myotome, is C8. (Leo 2022)

**Table 6.3** Upper limb nerve roots and motor function

| Shoulder | |
| --- | --- |
| Abduction | C5 |
| Elevation above horizontal | C4 |
| Elbow | |
| Flexion | C5, 6 |
| Extension | C7, 8 |
| Wrist | |
| Extension | C6, 7 |
| Flexion | C6, 7 |
| Radial deviation | C7, 8 |
| Ulnar deviation | C 6 |
| Fingers | |
| Flexion | C8 |
| Extension | C7, 8 |
| Abd/adduction | T1 |

# Further Reading

D'Arcy CA, McGee S. Does this patient have carpel tunnel syndrome? JAMA. 2000;283(23):3110–7.

Chidgey LK. The distal radioulnar joint: problems and solutions. J Am Acad Orthop Surg. 1995;3(2):95–109.

Moore K, Dalley AF, Agur A. Clinically oriented anatomy. 7th ed. Baltimore: Lippincott Williams and Wilkins; 2014.

Razak L. Pathophysiology of pelvic organ prolapse. In: Rizvi RM, editor. Pelvic floor disorders. IntechOpen; 2018. https://doi.org/10.5772/intechopen.76629. Available from: https://www.intechopen.com/chapters/60935.

Rosse C, Gaddum-Rosse P. Hollinshead's textbook of anatomy. 5th ed. New York: Lippincott-Raven; 1997.

Tay SC, Tomita K, Berger RA. The "ulnar fovea sign" for defining ulnar wrist pain: an analysis of sensitivity and specificity. J Hand Surg Am. 2007;32(4):438–44.

Standring S. Gray's anatomy: the anatomical basis of clinical practice. London: Elsevier; 2005.

Umar M, Qadir I, Azam M. Subacromial impingement syndrome. Orthop Rev. 2012;4(2):e18.

Xiao K, Zhang J, Li T, Dong YL, Weng XS. Anatomy, definition, and treatment of the "terrible triad of the elbow" and contemplation of the rationality of this designation. Orthop Surg. 2015;7:13–8.

# The Back

7

## Occipital Bone

Along the back of the occipital bone, there are several important landmarks. The bump that you can feel on the back of your skull is the *external occipital protuberance*. The point of the external occipital protuberance is the *inion*. Running laterally from the external occipital protuberance is the *superior nuchal line*. And then inferior and parallel to it is the *inferior nuchal line*.

## Atlas (C1)

The *atlas* or C1 sits right below the skull. It does not have a vertebral body or a intervertebral disk. Laterally are the two lateral masses with their *superior articular facets* and *inferior articular facets*. The superior articular facets articulate with the occipital condyles to form the *alanto-occipital joint*. The main movements at this joint are flexion and extension – think of a person nodding "yes." The atlas also has an anterior and posterior arch to complete its ring structure. On the superior surface of the posterior arch, on each side, there is a groove for the vertebral artery as it passes from lateral to medial on its way to the foramen magnum. The atlas does not have a spinous process but instead has a posterior tubercle. On its anterior arch there is an articular surface on the posterior side for the articulation with the dens.

## Axis (C2)

The most prominent feature of the *axis* (C2) is the superioraly projecting dens (or odontoid process) that lies against the posterior surface of anterior arch of the atlas. The superior articular facets of the axis meet the inferior facets of the axis (C2) to form the *lateral atlantoaxial joints*. Movement at the atlantoaxial joints mainly

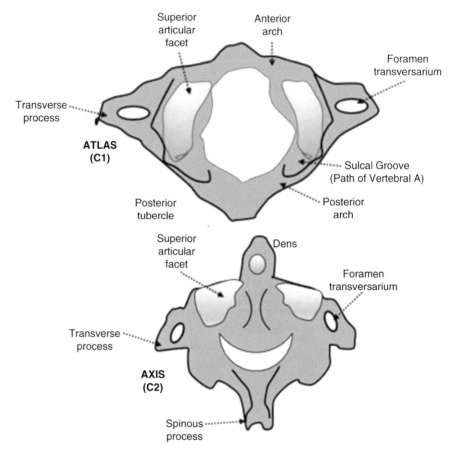

**Fig. 7.1** The atlas and axis. (Leo 2022)

involves side-to-side movement – think of person nodding "no." The articulation of the dens with the axis in the midline forms the single *medial atlantoaxial joint* (Fig. 7.1).

## Cruciate and Alar Ligaments

The dens is held in place by several ligaments. The most prominent is the cruciate ligament with its four bands resembling a cross. Running horizontally across the dens and holding it in place is the transverse ligament. The superior and inferior bands run vertically to aid in support. Besides the cruciate ligment there is the odontoid ligament made up of apical and alar ligaments. The apical ligament runs from the top of the dens to the occiptal bone, and the alar ligament projects superiorly and diagonally from the dens to the occipital condyles. The *tectorial membrane* is the extension of the posterior longitudinal ligament from C2 to the skull (Fig. 7.2).

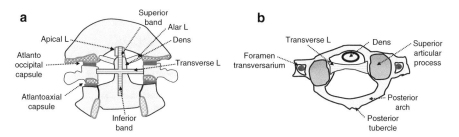

**Fig. 7.2** Atlas and axis. Panel (**a**) is a posterior view of the cruciform ligament – shaped like a cross. The alar ligament attaches to the den. It has a superior and inferior band, plus a transverse ligament. Panel (**b**) is a superior view of the atlas showing the dens held in place against the atlas by the transverse ligament. (Leo 2022)

## Cervical Fractures

The atlas is a ring, and when rings are fractured, just like the pelvis, there are typically multiple fracture lines. A *Jefferson fracture* is a burst fracture to the atlas (C1) following severe trauma – such as diving into the shallow end of the pool or a lake. It usually results in four fracture lines forming a square with a fracture at each corner of the square: two to the anterior arch, and two to the posterior arch. If the patient survives the trauma they will typically recover and have no long term deficits.

A hangman's fracture is a burst fracture that involves the axis (C2). It often occurs when there is significant whiplash with the head being rocked back and forth resulting in a bilateral fractures of the pedicles or pars interarticularis.

Another common fracture of the axis is to the dens. With a dens fracture the bone typically looses its blood supply resulting in avacular necrosis. There is typically enough space within the canal to accommodate the displaced dens so that the spinal cord is not necessarily compromised. Compression fractures can damage the C3-C7 vertebrae. The most common cervical fracture is to C5.

Injuries to cervical fractures are life-altering events. The phrenic nerve comes from C3-C5 which means that patients with complete transections of the cord at C3 or higher will need permanent ventialation to live. If the lesion is below C8 the patient will be able to use crutches. Remember C8 is important for the hands. If the lesion is below C6 they will not be able to use crutches but the will be able to use a wheelchair. They will need assistance getting into and out of the chair but once they are in it they will have some mobility.

## Suboccipital Triangle

The suboccipital triangle sits between the base of the skull and the top of the vertebral column. Its scaffold consists of a series of strap-like muscles that need to balance two different jobs. On one hand they must be strong enough to protect the head, brain and spinal cord, but they also need to allow a certain amount of

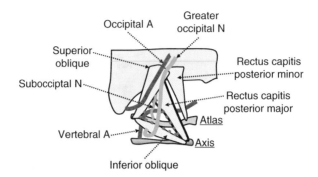

**Fig. 7.3** Suboccipital triangle. The suboccipital triangle is bounded by the dotted blue line. In the floor of the triangle is vertebral artery. Below the inferior oblique muscle is the greater occipital nerve (dorsal ramus C2). The suboccipital nerve (dorsal ramus C1) is found within the suboccipital triangle. (Leo 2022)

flexibility for the head to move. To understand the suboccipital triangle you need to discuss the bones, ligaments, nerves, and arteries just inferior to the base of the skull.

The borders of the suboccipital triangle are composed of three muscles: (1) the rectus capitus posterior major, (2) the obliquus capitus inferior, and the (3) obliquus capitus superior. In the floor of the triangle, running from lateral to medial, is the vertebral artery. Emerging from the triangle is the suboccipital nerve which is the dorsal ramus of C1. Emerging below the triangle is the greater occipital nerve (Fig. 7.3).

The rectus capitis posterior minor runs from the posterior tubercle of the atlas to the inferior nuchal line of the skull. The rectus capitis posterior major lies lateral and runs from the spinous process of the axis to the skull. The obliquus capitis inferior (inferior oblique) runs from the spinous process of the axis (C2) to the transverse process of the atlas (C1). The obliguus capitus superior (superior oblique) runs from the transverse process of the atlas to the skull.

## Back Ligaments

The ligaments of the back surround the vertebral bodies and the vertebral canal. Knowledge of these ligaments can be tested by asking about lumbar punctures and which structures a needle will move through – and which structures it will not move through in various scenarios.

## Anterior and Posterior Longitudinal Ligaments

The *anterior* and *posterior longitudinal ligaments* lie on either side of the vertebral bodies. The anterior ligament is in front (anterior) of the vertebral bodies and resists hyperextension of the neck, and the posterior ligaments are behind (posterior) the vertebral bodies and resist hyperflexion. The posterior longitudinal ligament forms the anterior boundary of the vertebral canal.

The *ligmentum flavum* forms the posterior surface of the vertebral canal and runs from C2 to S1. It is a thick, tough ligament connecting the anterior lamina of the vertebra. It blends in with and contributes to the articular capsule of the facet joints. In elderly individuals the ligament can become ossified, which can in turn lead to spinal stenosis. Running between the spinous process of each vertebra is the *interspinous ligament*, and then running like a ribbon or a strap from one spinous process to another is the *supraspinous ligament*.

Note that the spinal canal is bounded anteriorly by the posterior longitudinal ligament, and posteriorly by the ligamentum flava. During a laminectomy to relieve the pressure on the spinal cord, with a posterior approach, the surgeon removes the spinous process and then the lamina in the appropriate region. At this point, the surgeon is looking at the ligamentum flava – remember the ligamentum flava is the posterior border of the spinal canal.

## Spinal Meninges

In the cranium the dura is tightly adherent to the skull. The *thecal sac* is the space enclosed by the dura. Outside of the thecal sac is the *epidural space*. Normally there is no epidural space in the cranium, however in some conditions, such as trauma to the pterion, fluid can drain between the skull and dura and create a space – an epidural hemotoma. Thus in the cranium there is a potential space. However in the spinal column there is a true space between the vertebra and the dura. The spinal nerves and venous plexuses travel through this space. This allows anesthesia to be placed into the epidural space to regionally block pain sensation. The anesthesia can be adminstered in several different locations; either directly in the midline or slightly off the midline at the L2 vertebra. Another location is in the midline just below the S4 spinous process of the sacrum. If you place your finger just below the S4 spinous process it will be bound on either side by the right and left sacral cornua. This marks the *sacral hiatus* through which you can gain access to the epidural space.

In the epidural space around the spinal cord there is a valveless *internal vertebral plexus* which carries blood back to the heart from regions such as the pelvis. It can also serve as a conduit for malignant cells which can lead to cancer of the pelvic organs spreading to the lungs, and eventually to the brain. Deep to the dura is the arachnoid, and then the subarachnoid space.

A needle destined for the epidural space will not go as deep as one destined for the subarachnoid space. It will go through the skin, supraspinous ligament, interspinous ligament, and then the ligamentum flava (Fig. 7.4).

Lumbar punctures are usually performed between L3 and L4, or L4 and L5 vertebrae. The L4 vertebrae is horizontally across from the highest point of the iliac crest. A needle inserted in the midline to gain access to the subarachnoid space will go through the: supraspinous ligament, interspinous ligament, ligamentum flava, the dura mater, and finally the arachnoid, As the needle moves into the space it will

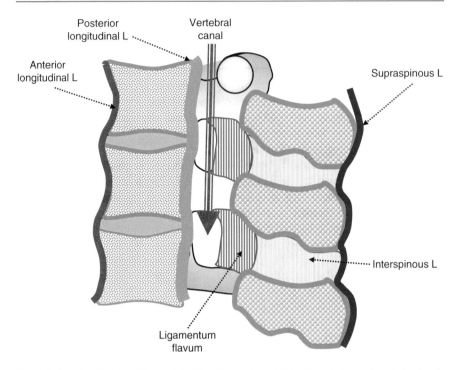

**Fig. 7.4** Lumbar Vertebra. The vertebral bodies are bounded by the anterior and posterior longitudinal ligaments. The red arrow is running down the vertebral canal, which is bounded by the posterior longitudinal ligament and the ligamentum flavum. (Leo 2022)

encounter resistance at both the ligamentum flavum, and the dura mater. Note that the needle should not go through the posterior longitudinal ligament, and clearly not through the anterior longitudinal ligament (Fig. 7.5).

## Cervical Vertebrae

The cervical vertebrae going from C3 to C7 all have openings in the transverse processes. These *foramen transversarium* transmit the vertebral artery. The spinous processes of C3-C6 are notched or bifed. The C7 vertebra has an elarged spinous process refered to as the *vertebral prominens,* but it is flat instead of notched. The *nuchal ligament* runs from the skull to the C7 spinous process. The superior facet faces backward, upward, and slightly medially. The inferior facet faces forward, downward, and laterally (Fig. 7.6).

The *carotid tubercle* is the anterior tubercle of the C6 transverse process which is a bony prominence that separates the carotid artery from the vertebral artery. The common carotid artery runs anterior to the tubercle and its pulse can be felt here. Posterior to the tubercle is the vertebral artery crossing to enter into the foramen transversarium of C6.

**Fig. 7.5** The spinal cord is bounded by the dura. The needle in the subarachnoid space had to travel through the ligament flavum and the dura. The needle in the epidural space is between the ligamentum flavum and the dura mater. (Leo 2022)

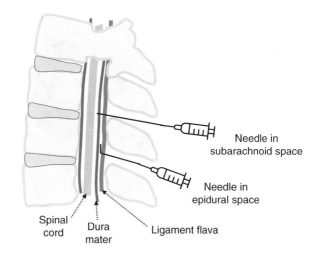

Needle in subarachnoid space

Needle in epidural space

Spinal cord

Dura mater

Ligament flava

**Fig. 7.6** Cervical vertebra. The transverse processes have anterior and posterior tubercles. The spinal nerve travels between the anterior and posterior tubercles. Note the bifid spinous process. (Leo 2022)

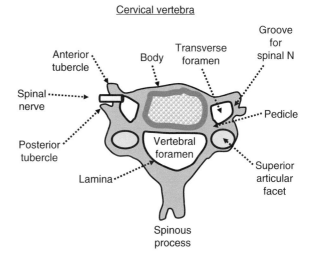

Cervical vertebra

Anterior tubercle

Body

Transverse foramen

Groove for spinal N

Spinal nerve

Pedicle

Posterior tubercle

Vertebral foramen

Lamina

Superior articular facet

Spinous process

## Thoracic Vertebrae

There are 12 thoracic vertebrae. The T1 vertebra resembles the cervical vertebrae but as you proceed down the column they become larger, with T12 being the largest. T1-T9 all have a demifacet where each rib articulates with two vertebral bodies. T10–12 all have full facets. The facet joints of the thoracic vertebrae are oriented in superior inferior direction. The superior articular facet faces anteriorly and meets up with an inferior articular facet facing posteriorly. The vertebral artery runs anterior to the thoracic vertebral bodies. Aneurysms of the thoracic aorta can erode the anterior left lateral edges of the vertebral bodies from T5 to T8. Jumped Facets refers to the facet joints becoming locked together following trauma. It most often occurs in the lower cervical in the region of C4 and C6 (Fig. 7.7).

**Fig. 7.7** Thoracic vertebra. The superior articular facet will meet the inferior articular facet from the body superior to the vertebra shown. The inferior articular facet will meet the superior facet from the vertebra below. There is a costal facet on the transverse process for meeting the tubercle of a rib. The Superior and inferior costal facets on the body join with the head of the rib. (Leo 2022)

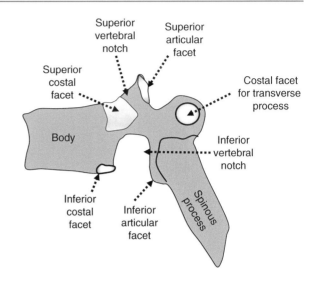

## Lumbar Vertebrae

The five lumbar vertebrae are the largest vertebral bodies with L5 being the largest. On the lumbar vertebra the superior articular facets face posteromedial. The inferior facet faces anterolateral. The joints are thus in a sagittal plane to resist axial rotation. The spinous processes are flat.

## Ribs

The *costovertebral joint* is between the head of a rib and the vertebral bodies. There are two articular facets on the head of each rib. One facet articulates with the rib above it and one with the same numbered vertebral body. For instance, rib 5 articulates with T5 and T6. The radiate ligament sits between the head of the rib and the vertebral body. Note that ribs 10, 11, and 12 only articulate with one rib thus they only have one facet (Figs. 7.8 and 7.9).

There is also a tubercle on each rib that articulates with the transverse process of the same numbered rib forming the *costotransverse joint* which is covered by the ligament of the head of the tubercle.

## Disk Herniations

The spinal cord ends at the L1 (or L2) vertebral body. Thus, in the anatomy lab when you do a laminectomy of L1 and expose the spinal cord you are looking at the end of the cord (conus medullaris), which is the S 2, 3, 4 spinal cord level. You will also see the cauda equina at this point which is the collection of nerve roots from the lumbar and sacral regions traveling down in the vertebral canal alongside the spinal

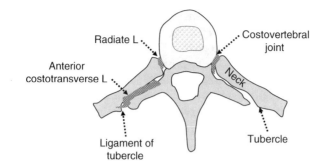

**Fig. 7.8** The T6 Vertebral Body and its Connection with the 6th Rib. Note the costovertebral joint where the head of the rib meets the vertebra. The tubercle of the rib meets the transverse process which is covered by the ligament of the tubercle which continues anterior as the anterior costotransverse ligament. The radiate ligament attaches the head of the rib to the vertebra. (Leo 2022)

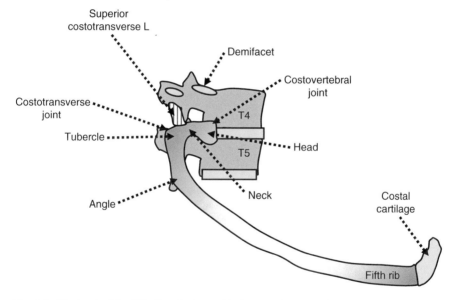

**Fig. 7.9** The head of the fifth rib articulates with the superior costal facet of T4 and the inferior costal facet of T5 to form the costovertebral joint. The transverse costal facets articulate with the tubercle to form the costotransverse joint. (Leo 2022)

cord to eventually exit via their respective intervertebral foramen, In the cervical region, the spinal nerves exit above the equivalent vertebral body. So, the C1 nerve exits above the C1 level (the atlas) and the C2 nerve exits above C2 (the axis). This pattern continues down to the level of the C7 vertebra where the C7 nerve exits above the C7 vertebral body, and the C8 nerve between C8 and the T1 vertebra. And then starting with the thoracic vertebra the nerve exists below the equivalent vertebral body, with the T1 nerve exiting below T1 vertebral body.

The disks located between the vertebral bodies are composed of a tough circumferential outer layer – the *annulus fibrosus* – and a jelly like soft inside – the *nucleus pulposus* (a remanent of the notochord). The disks are kept between the vertebral bodies by the *anterior and posterior longitudinal ligaments*. However, as we age, the ligaments can become weak. This usually happens at the lateral portion of the posterior longitudinal ligament, so that herniated disks usually herniate posterolateral. The disk then hits the spinal nerve which is passing right beside it.

In the cervical region the nerves travel at right angles to exit the spinal cord. If there is a disk herniation between C3 and C4 it will hit the C4 nerve. However, in the lumbar region because the nerves have to travel down to exit at their appropriate level, a disk herniation say between L4 and L5 will hit the L5 nerve. In most cases, especially on exams, the disk herniation in this example will spare S1. But keep in mind that in the real world if the disk herniation is large enough it could hit the S1 nerve (Fig. 7.10).

Looking at the vertebra from a posterior view, imagine we have cut the pedicle of each vertebra with a bone saw. We can see the pedicles are at the top of each vertebra. The intervertebral foramen is between the pedicles of two adjacent vertebra. If we focus on the L4 and L5 vertebra, we see a disk between the two, and exiting at the top of the foramen is the L4 nerve. If this disk herniates then it will not hit the L4 root, which is exiting above the disk, but will hit the L5 root as it passes by the disk to exit one level down. In other words, a disk herniation between L4 and L5 will hit the nerve exiting one level down, which is L5.

## Spondylolisthesis Versus Spondylolysis

The pars interarticularis is the small piece of bone between the superior and inferior articular facets. *Spondylolysis is* a stress fracture along the lytic line in the pars interarticularis - at the collar in the scotty dog picture. The most common site is L5.

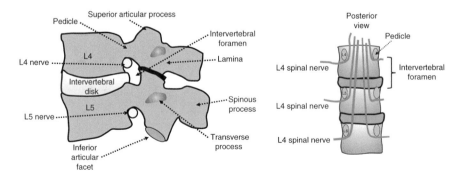

**Fig. 7.10** Two views of the nerves and vertebral body relationships. Note the L4 spinal nerve exits at the superior margin of the intervertebral foramen. If the disk between L4 and L5 herniates it will hit the L5 nerve. (Leo 2022)

**Fig. 7.11** Scotty dog and spondylolysis. The dog's collar is the pars interarticularis which is the site of spondylolysis. The facet joint is between the superior articular facet (the dog's head) and the inferior articular process (the dog's front foot) of vertebra above it. (Leo 2022)

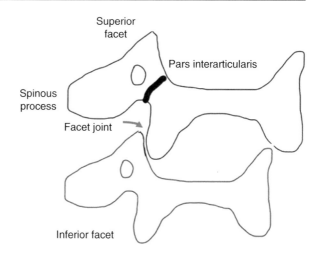

Superior facet

Pars interarticularis

Spinous process

Facet joint

Inferior facet

*Spondylolisthesis* is when one vertebra slides forward over the vertebra below it (listhesis = to slip). *Ankylosing spondylitis* refers to fused vertebra. The patient will have a hunched forward position.

On a radiograph a straightforward way to picture a spondylolysis is to think of a picture of a scotty dog. The fracture of the pars interarticularis occurs at the dog's collar (Fig. 7.11).

## Disk Herniations Versus Peripheral Nerve Trauma

It is important to understand the difference between cutting a peripheral nerve versus cutting a root (a radiculopathy). Keep in mind that any individual root goes to several different levels, and every nerve receives contributions from more than one level. As an example, take the femoral nerve, it receives contributions from L2, L3, and L4 (Fig. 7.10).

If the femoral nerve is cut, then the muscles supplied by the femoral nerve – the quadriceps – will be completely paralyzed. Conversely, if the L4 root is damaged then the femoral nerve still gets a contribution from L2 and L3 so the quadriceps will not be paralyzed but will be weak. In addition, with femoral nerve damage you want to think about the peripheral nerve map, and with a root compromised you want to think about the dermatome map (Figs. 7.12 and 7.13).

However, if you cut a peripheral nerve the muscles innervated by that nerve will exhibit complete flaccid paralysis. Note that in the case of a muscle that is innervated by two nerves (not very common), that the second nerve can send a signal to the muscle (Fig. 7.13).

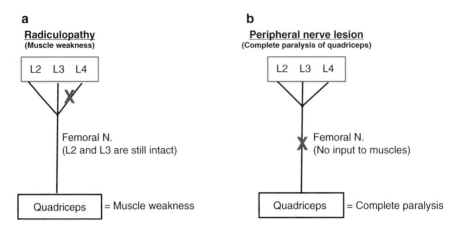

**Fig. 7.12** Radiculopathy versus peripheral nerve lesion. Panel (**a**) The femoral nerve receives contributions from L 2, 3, and 4. If the L4 root is damaged then the quadriceps will be weak because L2 and 3 are still intact. Panel (**b**) If the femoral nerve is severed then the quadriceps will be completely (100%) paralyzed. (Leo 2022)

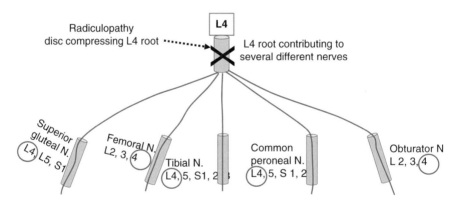

**Fig. 7.13** Root damage. The L4 root travels into several different nerves. And any given nerve receives contributions from several different levels. Each nerve that gets a branch from L4 will be compromised but because each nerve receives contributions from other levels their muscle groups will not be completely paralyzed. The question for the clinician then is what nerve gets most of its supply from L4. For the femoral nerve, the most important root is L4 which is why with a radiculopathy of L4, the quadriceps will be noticeably weak. (Leo 2022)

## Abormal Curves of Spine

Kyphosis is an exaggeration of the thoracic curvature, usually resulting from osteoporosis. Lordosis is an exaggeration of the lumbar curvature usually resulting from a spondylolisthesis or pregnancy. Scoliosis is a lateral curvature (Table 7.1).

**Table 7.1** Summary of the relationship of structures to vertebral body levels. (Leo 2022)

| Vertebrae level | Structures |
| --- | --- |
| C4 | Bifurcation of common carotid |
| C6 | Start of esophagus and trachea |
| C7 | Vertebral prominens |
| T2 | Superior border of scapula |
| T2/3 | Suprasternal notch, Top of aortic arch and the origin of three main branches off aorta. Left Brachiocephalic vein crossing from left to right in front of these three branches |
| T4 | Aortic arch ends |
| T4 | Sternal angle |
| T7 | Inferior angle of scapula |
| T8 | Caval opening. IVC and right phrenic nerve |
| T10 | Esophageal hiatus, R/L vagus nerves |
| T12 | Aortic hiatus, Azygous vein, Thoracic duct, Celiac trunk |
| L1 | Superior mesenteric artery, renal veins, end of spinal cord |
| L3 | Inferior mesenteric artery |
| L4 | Abdominal aorta bifurcation |
| L5 | Start of IVC |
| S2 | End of dural sac |

# Further Reading

Boone JM, Abrahams PH, Meiring JH, Welch T. Lumbar Puncture for the Generalist; South African Family Practice. 2004;46(2):38–42.

Drake RL, Vogl W, Mitchell AW. Gray's anatomy for medical students. New York: Elsevier; 2005.

Hoppenfeld JD, Hoppenfeld S. Orthopaedic neurology: a diagnostic guide to neurologic levels. Philadelphia: Wolters Kluwer; 2018.

Moore K, Dalley AF, Agur A. Clinically oriented anatomy. 7th ed. Baltimore: Lippincott Williams and Wilkin; 2014.

Razak L. Pathophysiology of pelvic organ prolapse. In: Rizvi RM, editor. Pelvic floor disorders. IntechOpen; 2018. https://doi.org/10.5772/intechopen.76629. Available from: https://www.intechopen.com/chapters/60935.

Riascos R, Bonfante A, Cotes A, Guirguis M, Hakimelahi R, West C, editors. Imaging of atlanto-occipital and atlantoaxial traumatic injuries: what the radiologist needs to know. Radiographics. 2015;35(7):2121–34. Available at: Imaging of Atlanto-Occipital and Atlantoaxial Traumatic Injuries: What the Radiologist Needs to Know | RadioGraphics (rsna.org)

Rosse C, Gaddum-Rosse P. Hollinshead's textbook of anatomy. 5th ed. New York: Lippincott-Raven; 1997.

Standring S. Gray's anatomy: the anatomical basis of clinical practice. London: Elsevier; 2005.

Westbrook JL. Anatomy of the epidural space. Anaesth Intensive Care Med. 2012;13(11):551–4.

# The First Three Weeks

## 8

When it comes to the first three weeks there is a simple rule to follow. At the end of week one, there is one germ layer, and one supporting membrane; at the end of week two, there are two germ layers and two supporting membranes; and at the end of week three, there are three germ layers and three supporting structures. Before looking at the specifics, consider the following from the view of the *tissue types*:

1. There are four types of tissue in the adult: Muscle, Connective, Nervous and Epithelial. Muscle tissue comes from mesoderm; Nervous tissue comes from ectoderm; Connective tissue comes from mesoderm, and Epithelia tissue comes from endoderm, mesoderm, and ectoderm.

And from a different point of view, the view of the *three germ layers*:

2. There are three germ layers: endoderm, ectoderm, and mesoderm. All three germ layers will give rise to epithelial tissue: Endoderm will give rise to epithelial; Ectoderm will give rise to nervous tissue and some epithelial; and Mesoderm will give rise to connective tissue, and some epithelial tissue. For instance, mesoderm gives rise to the epithelial tissue that lines some of the structures of the heart, kidney, and reproductive systems (Fig. 8.1).

## Ovulation and Fertilization

Week one starts at fertilization and ends at implantation. Therefore, ovulation occurs right before week one. At ovulation the ovary ejects a secondary oocyte arrested in *metaphase II*. At this point the oocyte is surrounded by a thick barrier – the *zona pellucida*. And outside the zona pellucida are several layers of cells – *the corona radiata*. At ovulation, the secondary oocyte crosses the peritoneal cavity and is swept up by the fimbria to enter the fallopian tube. In some cases, the ovary is fertilized while it is in the peritoneal cavity, which leads to an ectopic pregnancy.

© The Author(s), under exclusive license to Springer Nature Switzerland AG 2022    259
J. Leo, *Clinical Anatomy and Embryology*,
https://doi.org/10.1007/978-3-031-03807-5_8

**Fig. 8.1** Overview of embryology. (Leo 2022)

Big Picture

**All three germ layers give rise to some epithelia:**
**Endoderm:** Epithelium
**Mesoderm:** Connective, Muscle, Some Epithelia
**Ectoderm:** All Nervous Tissue, Some epithelia
Note that mesoderm lines some organs of cardiovascular, reproductive and urinary systems

*or look at it another way,*

***There are four kinds of tissue that come from*:**
1) **Nervous**: Ectoderm
2) **Connective**: Mesoderm (and Neural crest in the head)
3) **Muscle**: Mesoderm
4) **Epithelia**: Endoderm, Ectoderm, Mesoderm

After being swept up by the fimbria, as the oocyte travels along the fallopian tube it moves into the ampulla. If a spermatocyte is present, then it will attach to the oocyte, typically in the ampulla. For the sperm to attach to the oocyte it has to travel through the corona radiata, and then reach the zona pellucida. On the head of the sperm the acrosome will release its hydrolytic enzymes and burrow through the zona pellucida. The membranes of the spermatocyte and oocyte fuse, and the oocyte then completes meiosis II. This is followed by the intermingling of the chromosomes from the male and female pronuclei to form the zygote. The mitochondria from the sperm does not enter the secondary oocyte, so an individual's mitochondria is derived from the maternal side. In addition, once the DNA from the sperm enters the oocyte, the cortical reaction occurs and there is an electrical depolarization of the egg's membrane which prevents any subsequent sperm from entering the oocyte. This is day one, the starting line.

## Week One

The zygote will now start to divide. As the developing fetus divides into a 2-cell, 4-cell, 8-cell stage, etc. this is referred to as cleavage, and during these divisions the fetus does not get any larger. Instead, each cell gets smaller and smaller to fit into the same sized space. This makes sense on at least one level because during cleavage the fetus is still in the fallopian tube on its trip to the uterus. If it kept growing with each division it would soon be too large for the fallopian tube (Fig. 8.2).

While it is still in the fallopian tube it will enter the 16-cell stage where it is referred to as a morula. At day three the fetus is in the early morula stage, and by day 4 it is in the later morula stage – 32 cell stage. The morula, at least to outward appearance is an undifferentiated mass of cells. In Latin, morula means a cluster of grapes.

At day 5, as the morula approaches the uterus the cells will start to differentiate. A portion of the cells of the morula will migrate towards one end forming the inner cell mass. The remaining cells will form the outer cell mass, which will become the trophoblast. Between the inner cell mass and the outer cell mass is the blastocyst

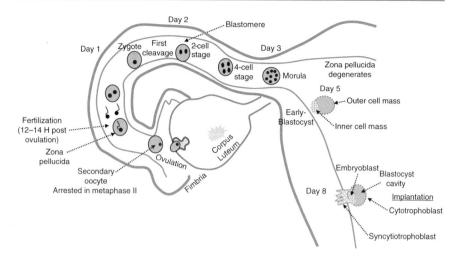

**Fig. 8.2** First week. The secondary oocyte stuck in metaphase II is ovulated. Fertilization occurs in the ampulla of the uterine tube. The zygote is formed and starts dividing. Just prior to implantation, the zona pellucida degenerates. At this point the inner cell mass and the outer cell mass have formed with the blastocyst cavity between them. Note that implantation occurs at Day 8 which is the start of the second week. (Leo 2022)

cavity (blastocoele). The morula has now become the blastula. At this point, the zona pellucida is degenerating and being sloughed off so that the blastula can implant in the uterine wall. The inner cell mass is a source of undifferentiated embryonic stem cells which is now referred to as the embryoblast. At day 7 the blastula is ready to implant into the uterine endometrium.

In summary, remember that at the end of week one, we have one germ layer– the embryoblast; there is one extraembryonic support structure- the trophoblast, and there is one cavity – the blastocyst. At this point the trophoblast starts secreting human chorionic gonadotropin (B-HCG) which will instruct the corpus luteum to secrete progesterone. Think of HCG as the signal for the mother that she is pregnant. It is also the basis for several of the pregnancy tests as it is present in blood and urine.

## Clinical Scenarios

### Hydatidiform Mole

In normal conception, a sperm, either a haploid 23X or 23Y is injected into the oocyte to meet with a maternal 23X to form the full diploid complement of 46XX or 46XY. A molar pregnancy refers to a noncancerous tumor that develops in this early stage when the sperm and ovary first meet. Instead of the normal joining of the maternal and paternal DNA, the embryo only contains paternal DNA, at least in the case of a complete mole. Moles can be categorized as complete or incomplete moles. A complete mole consists of abnormal placental tissue and fluid filled cysts. An incomplete mole has a combination of normal and abnormal placental tissue

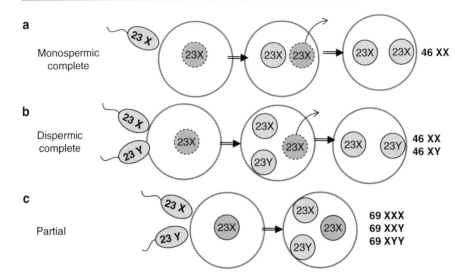

**Fig. 8.3** Hydatidiform Mole. Panels (**a**) and (**b**) are complete moles where the maternal DNA has been ejected from the egg and replaced with paternal DNA. Panel (**c**) is a partial mole where some maternal DNA remains. (Leo 2022)

along with fluid filled cysts. *Choriocarcinomas* can happen after any pregnancy but are more likely to occur with hydatidiform moles.

There are several variations on the formation of a hydatidiform mole (Fig. 8.3):

1. *Monospermic Complete Mole.* The DNA from the male (23X) enters the oocyte and the 23X from the female is ejected from the oocyte. The 23X from the male then replicates to from 46 XX but all the DNA is from the male. There is no fetal tissue present.
2. *Dispermic Complete Mole.* Two sperm attach to the egg and inject their DNA– either a 23X a 23Y or a combination – into the oocyte. The maternal DNA is ejected resulting in a 46 XX or 46 XY which all come from the father. There is no fetal tissue present in this type of mole.
3. *Partial Mole.* Unlike the examples above, with a partial mole there will still be some maternal DNA. Two sperm inject their DNA -either a 23X or a 23 Y-which meets with the 23X from the mother resulting in a 69 XXX, 69 XXY, or 69 XYY. There will be some fetal tissue present.

## Twins

Twins can be classified according to the type of *zygosity* and *chorionicity*. Zygosity refers to the type of conception:

1. *Dizygotic (fraternal or non-identical twins)* are formed by two different sperm and two different eggs (multiple ovulation). They account for approximately

70% of twins. In this scenario, there will be two amniotic cavities, and two chorionic cavities – diamniotic and dichorionic. The twins will develop independent of each other and have the same genetic relationship as developing siblings. Thus, they share on average 50% of genes (range between 38–61%).

2. *Monozygotic (identical twins)* come from the splitting of a zygote and share 100% of their genes. The later the zygote splits, the more embryonic structures they share.

*Chorionicity* refers to the type of placenta. The key to examining the different scenarios is to look at the normal timing of the development of the chorion and amnion. The chorion normally develops at day 3 so if the split occurs before day 3, typically at the 2-cell stage, then two separate chorions and amnions will develop. If the split is after day 3 then there will only be one chorion. The amnion on the other hand does not develop until day 8 (just before primitive streak develops) so if the split occurs before day 8 then two amnions will develop, and if it occurs after day 8 then one amnion develops. Twin formation (the splitting of zygote) after day 8 is rare. If it does occur, there is a strong chance of twin-twin transfusion, with the likely scenario that both fetuses do not develop and there is a spontaneous abortion (Fig. 8.4).

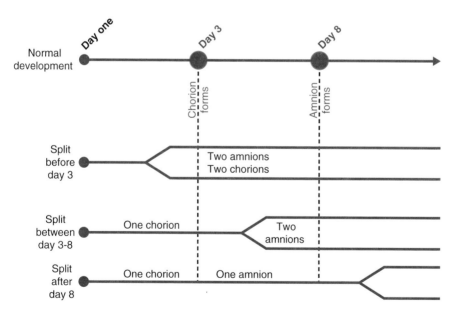

**Fig. 8.4** Twins and Supporting Structures. The chorion develops at Day 3, and the amnion develops at day 8. If the split occurs before day 3 there will be two chorions and two amnions. If it occurs between day 3 and 8, then there will be one chorion and two amnions. If it occurs after day 8 there will be one amnion and one chorion. (Leo 2022)

## Heteropaternal Superfecundation

*Heteropaternal superfecundation* is the rare scenario where a woman gives birth to twins, but the twins are from two fathers. Two events must occur for this to happen. First, the woman must ovulate at least two eggs in a single cycle, and second, the woman must have sex with two different men during this time period. This creates the scenario where two eggs are fertilized at the same time by the sperm from two different fathers and the woman gives birth to twins with different paternal DNA. Besides this scenario, it can also occur as an accident with invitro fertility equipment, where the sperm from two fathers is mixed together. On average, these types of twins will share 25% of their DNA. Also, as an aside, this is fairly common in dogs or cats, where half a litter can come from one male and the other half of the litter from another male. Again, in humans this is extremely rare, and I have only mentioned it because I think it aides in understanding the nature of the process of how twins are formed.

## Stem Cells: Totipotent. Pluripotent, Oligopotent

The critical issue with stem cells is the timing of when the cells are harvested – undifferentiated cells have the most potential to differentiate into other cells. For a researcher when it comes to harvesting stem cells, the earlier the better, because as time goes on the cells become more differentiated. At the zygote stage there is no differentiation. At the morula, there is some differentiation, and by the time the fetus reaches the week three, with three germ layers, there is even more differentiation. The term *totipotent* refers to an undifferentiated cell that technically has the potential to give rise to all the future cells of an embryo along with the extraembryonic supporting structures. A zygote is considered a totipotent cell. A *pluripotent* cell has the potential to give rise to all the future cells of the embryo but not to the extraembryonic supporting structures. The inner cell mass of a morula is considered a pluripotent cell. As development proceeds, and the cells become more differentiated, the stem cells are considered *oligopotent.* For instance, a lymphoid cell can give rise to T-cells and B-cells but not to red blood cells.

## Week Two and Differentiation of Trophoblast and Embryoblast

In short, during the second week of development the embryoblast will give rise to two germ layers: the epiblast and hypoblast; the trophoblast will give rise to two layers: the cytotrophoblast and syncytiotrophoblast; and two supporting structures develop: the amnion and the chorion. Think of "The Rule of Twos."

As the blastula attaches to the uterine wall, the inner cell mass is facing the uterine wall and will burrow into the endometrial layer of the uterus. Implantation typically occurs on the posterior superior portion of the uterus. *Placenta previa* is when the placenta covers the cervix. Vaginal bleeding during the second or third trimester is one sign of placenta previa.

The trophoblast now differentiates into the *cytotrophoblast* and *syncytiotrophoblast*. Both of these structures plus the extraembryonic somatic mesoderm will become part of the chorion. The chorion is the fetal contribution to the placenta:

1. The *cytotrophoblast* is the site of mitotic activity.
2. The *syncytiotrophoblast* is the structure that burrows into the uterine wall. It also produces HCG which doubles every 24 hours during early pregnancy. Alterations in HCG levels serve as an indicator of pathology. High levels of HCG are associated with a hydatidiform mole, and low levels are associated with an ectopic pregnancy. The syncytiotrophoblast will come into contact with the maternal blood system.

The decidua is the maternal contribution to the placenta which comes from the uterine endometrium which is referred to as the *functionalis layer*.

## Epiblast and Hypoblast

The inner cell mass will now form the bilaminar disk composed of: (1) the epiblast and (2) the hypoblast. The epiblast is a cuboidal layer of cells that will eventually give rise to all three germ layers. However, at this point, it will also give rise to cells that move laterally and surround the future amniotic cavity sitting just above the epiblast. Below the epiblast, is the hypoblast which are tall columnar cells that surround the developing yolk sac.

The epiblast also gives rise to the extraembryonic mesoderm which in the early stages surround the developing embryo. By the end of the second week, this extra-embryonic mesoderm will split into two layers:

1. The *extraembryonic somatic mesoderm* surrounds the cytotrophoblast. The connecting stalk is where the visceral and somatic layers meet.
2. The *extraembryonic visceral mesoderm* surrounds the yolk sac and developing embryo. Note that the extraembryonic coelom now lies between the extraembryonic somatic and visceral mesoderm. The visceral layer of mesoderm is also the site of early hematopoiesis.

At this point the placenta is more prominent. Note that the placenta is a joint production of the mother and the fetus (Fig. 8.5).

**Fig. 8.5** Gastrulation. The epiblast cells migrate towards the midline located primitive groove. When they reach the midline, they drop down to the hypoblast where they push the hypoblast cells off to the sides. This becomes endoderm. Some cells from epiblast land in the middle layer and become mesoderm. The cells that stay in the epiblast become ectoderm. (Leo 2022)

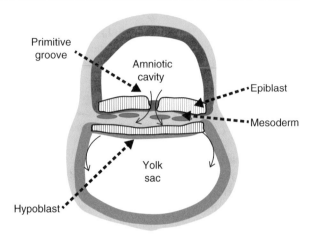

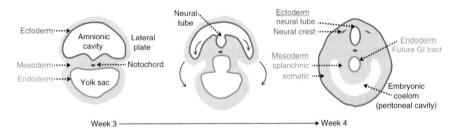

**Fig. 8.6** Body Folding. Starting at week three, the amniotic cavity and mesoderm start curling around to pinch off the yolk sac. At the same time the neural tube is forming. At the end of week four, you can see three tubes: the yolk sac, the neural tube, and the coelom. Red = ectoderm, Blue = mesoderm, and Green = endoderm. (Leo 2022)

## Week Three and Gastrulation

In week three, the two germ layers will differentiate into three germ layers via gastrulation. This process starts with the development of the primitive streak in the midline. The epiblast cells will give rise to all three germ layers.

1. *Endoderm.* The epiblast cells migrate towards the primitive streak. At the primitive streak they will then migrate down towards the hypoblast cells and displace them by pushing them off laterally. Thus, the original hypoblast calls are pushed aside by the epiblast cells which now become the endoderm.
2. *Mesoderm.* In some cases, the epiblast cells that migrate towards the primitive streak also come to land between the epiblast and hypoblast and become the mesoderm. This is a mesenchymal layer meaning that in contrast to the cells lined up in rows like the endoderm, these mesoderm cells are secreting substances that will surround them and separate them from their neighbors.
3. *Ectoderm.* Not all the epiblast cells will migrate down at the primitive streak. Those that stay will and become the ectoderm (Figs. 8.5 and 8.6).

# Body Folding

## Further Reading

Carlson B. Human embryology and developmental biology. 6th ed. New York: Elsevier; 2018.

Graham A, Richards J. Development and evolutionary origins of the pharyngeal apparatus. Evol Develop. 2012;3:24.

Moore KL, Persaud TVN. The developing human: clinically oriented embryology. 11th ed. New York: Saunders; 2019.

Sadler TW. Langman's medical embryology. 14th ed. New York: Lippincott Williams and Wilkins; 2018.

Sweeney L. Basic concepts in embryology: a student's survival guide. New York: McGraw-Hill; 1997.

# Development of the Major Organs

**9**

## Neurulation: Plate, to Groove, to Tube

The nervous system starts to develop in the third week of development with the formation of the notochord in the mesoderm. The ectoderm above the notochord will condense into the *neural plate* – at this point just a flat piece of tissue. The edges of the neural plates then rise up, and in the process form the *neural groove*. The edges of the groove then start to come together forming the *neural tube*. The neural tube will drop down to become surrounded by mesoderm. The ventral surface of the neural plate also gives rise to neural crest cells which migrate down towards the notochord. The *neural crest* cells give rise to numerous cell types, one of which is the dorsal root ganglia cells lying alongside the neural tube. As the neural tube is closing, the ends, referred to as *neuropores*, are the last structures to close – think of two zippers starting in the midline and moving towards the ends to close the tube. The rostral neuropore closes at day 25, and the caudal neuropore closes at day 27 (Fig. 9.1).

## Neural Tube Defects

Failure of the neuropores or the neural tube to close leads to congenital defects. The defects below are listed below going from least severe to most severe (Fig. 9.2).

1. *Spina bifida occulta* is a failure of the vertebrae around the spinal cord to develop. It can go undetected for years as it is often asymptomatic. Other than a tuft of hair over the defect there may be no obvious symptoms. Because the meninges are intact, there is no alteration in alpha fetoprotein (AFP) levels. The word "occulta" means hidden.
2. *Spina bifida with meningocele* is a failure of the vertebrae and the meninges to develop in the region of the defect. The meninges typically protrude through the defect. There is an increase in AFP.

© The Author(s), under exclusive license to Springer Nature Switzerland AG 2022
J. Leo, *Clinical Anatomy and Embryology*,
https://doi.org/10.1007/978-3-031-03807-5_9

**Fig. 9.1** Neurulation. (**a**) Ectoderm cells migrating towards the midline. (**b**) Neural folds forming. (**c**) Neural Tube has formed. Neural crest cells dropping down into mesoderm to form ganglia and other cells. (Leo 2022)

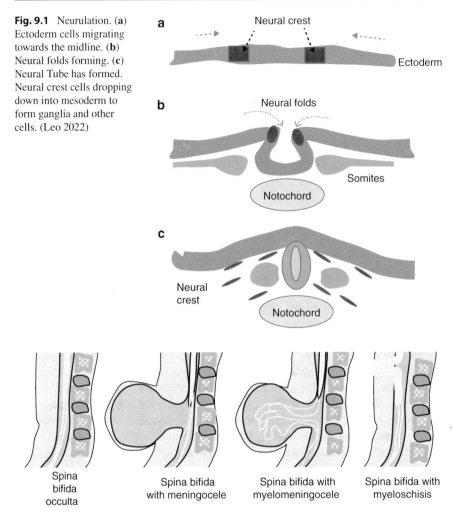

**Fig. 9.2** Neural Tube Defects. (Leo 2022)

3. *Spina bifida with meningomyelocele* is a failure of the vertebrae, meninges, and spinal cord to develop. The spinal cord can protrude through the defect. It often occurs with Arnold-Chiari type 2.
4. *Spina bifida with myeloschisis* is the most severe of the spina bifidas and leads to the spinal cord being present on the back. There will be an increase in AFP.
5. *Anencephaly* is a failure of the anterior neuropore to close resulting in failure of the cerebral hemispheres to develop. There will an increase of AFP.

You can see in the table above that AFP is increased in some of the conditions but not all. AFP is normally present around the fetal spinal cord. Only small amounts of AFP will be found in the amniotic cavity of a healthy embryo. With open neural tube defects, the AFP leaks out of the defect and into the amniotic cavity. This is why in spina bifida occulta there is no increase in AFP, but in the other neural tube defects there is an increase in AFP.

The term *spina bifida cystica*, encompasses the neural tube defects with a cyst on the back. Thus, spina bifida with either a meningocele, a meningomyelocele, or a myeloschisis are considered types of spina bifida cystica.

## Pituitary Development

The pituitary gland develops from two different regions of ectoderm. The posterior pituitary arises from an out pocketing of neural tube forming the third ventricle. The anterior pituitary comes from Rathke's pouch which is an outpocketing of ectoderm from the roof of the mouth. Rathke's pouch normally closes. In some cases, it fails to close and a craniopharyngeal canal remains as a small connection between the sphenoid bone and the sella turcica. The adult pituitary comes to lie inferior to the optic chiasm. Pituitary adenomas and craniopharyngiomas both aggravate the optic chiasm.

## Heart Development

The heart starts as a simple tube. It is best to follow the flow of blood through the tube. The blood first comes into the tube at the sinus venosus (venous pole). From here it goes to the primitive atrium, then the primitive ventricle, then the bulbus cordis, and finally the truncus arteriosus. The simple tube then starts rotating to the right and ventrally. At the end of its rotation the ventricles lie mostly ventral and caudal to the atria. The outflow tracts end up in the midline (Fig. 9.3).

## Fetal Circulation

Blood from the placenta enters the fetus via the umbilical veins. There are three bypasses in fetal circulation:

1. The first bypass is at the *ductus venosus*. Since the blood does not need to go through the fetal liver, it bypasses it and goes into the inferior vena cava. In the adult, the ductus venosus becomes the *ligament venosum*.
2. As the blood continues in the inferior vena cava past the liver it enters the right atrium and moves superiorly towards the *foramen ovale* to bypass the lungs. The foramen ovale is an opening between the right and left atria. In the adult the foramen ovale becomes the *fossa ovalis*.
3. Since some blood from the right atrium gets into the right ventricle it moves through the *ductus arteriosus* which is a connection between the pulmonary trunk and the aorta. In the adult, the ductus venosus becomes the *ligamentum arteriosum*.

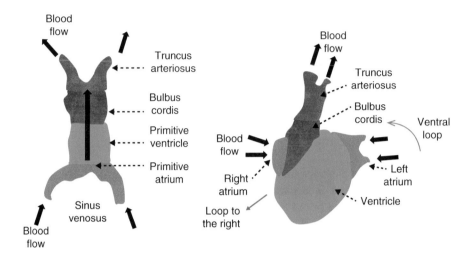

**Fig. 9.3** Heart Development. The early heart is a tube. Blood enters at the sinus venosus, then moves through the primitive atrium, primitive ventricle, bulbus cordis, and truncus arteriosus. The tube rotates to the right and ventrally. In the adult, for the most part, the ventricles become mostly ventral and caudal to the atria, with the outflow tracts ending in the midline. (Leo 2022)

The blood coming from the placenta is high in $O^2$ (80%) but it meets with the fetal blood coming from the inferior vena cava (IVC). Past the liver, the $O^2$ concentration is now at 65% which is right before the IVC enters the right atrium, Meanwhile the blood from the superior vena cava (SVC) is descending from the head to also enter the right atrium. Note that the $O^2$ concentration is lower in the SVC than the IVC as the two channels enter the right atrium. And in the right atrium, we have a crossing over of the two channels. The blood from the IVC heads towards the foramen ovale, while the blood from the SVC is channeled towards the tricuspid valve to go into the right ventricle. Thus, the blood coming into the right atrium has two channels to exit:

1. The blood coming from the IVC enters the inferior portion of the right atrium and then travels through the foramen ovale to enter the left atrium, then goes to the left ventricle to go out the aorta.
2. The blood coming down from the SVC goes into the right ventricle, then heads out the pulmonary trunk. At this point, since the blood does not need to go into the lungs, it bypasses the lungs by going through the ductus venosus to enter the aorta.

Also note that the $O^2$ concentration in the proximal aortic arch is different than the distal portion. Coming out of the heart the blood in the first part of the aorta is high in $O^2$ at about 65%. The advantage of this, is that the brain via the common carotid arteries is getting blood with a high concentration of $O^2$ to feed the brain's high metabolic rate. Note that the ductus venosus joins the aortic arch just distal to the first three branches of the aorta, which dilutes the $O^2$ concentration in the blood going down the descending aorta to approximately 60% (Fig. 9.4).

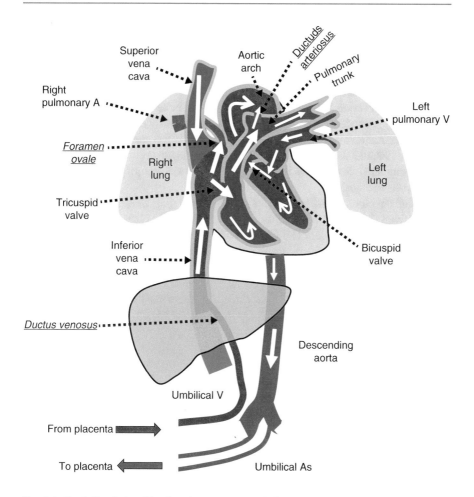

**Fig. 9.4** Fetal Circulation. The three bypasses are underlined and italicized. Blood from the placenta Bypasses the liver via ductus venosus. It then joins the inferior vena cava and enters the right atrium. From here it crosses foramen ovale to enter the left atrium and travel to the left ventricle. From left ventricle it passes via aortic arch to descending aorta. However, some of the blood entering the right atrium will pass to the right ventricle and go out the ductus arteriosum to bypass the lungs. (Leo 2022)

## Development of the Atrial Septum

The primitive atrium is open between the right and left sides. During week 3 the septum primum starts as an outgrowth of the superior portion of the atrium. It is a wall that descends towards the center of the heart to the endocardial cushions. The endocardial cushions will go from a round mass to form the cross shaped valves in the center of the heart. As the septum primum descends towards the endocardial cushions there is still an opening between the right and left atria which is the foramen primum. The developing heart needs this communication between the two atria.

Eventually the septum primum will reach the endocardial cushions to seal off the communication between the two sides. Fortunately, just as the septum primum reaches the endocardial cushions, along the superior portion of the septum primum, small openings start to appear which soon come together to form one larger opening – the foramen secundum. Without the foramen secundum forming there would be no communication between right and left atria. Note that the foramen primum and foramen secundum are both openings in the septum primum. The presence of foramen secundum allows the right and left atria to still communicate. At this point the septum secundum now forms. It is another wall (the second wall) that is in the right atrium, and it now moves inferiorly, parallel to the septum primum, to close off the foramen secundum.

During development this opening is a one-way flap that allows blood to be shunted from the right atrium across to the left atrium. At birth as pressure rises on the left side, the flap closes. The *fossa ovalis* is where the septum primum and septum secundum meet. In the adult, if you are in the right atrium, you will see the fossa ovalis which is a thin sheet, like a door, and on the superior surface of the door is a ridge – the limbus of the fossa ovalis. If you are in the left atrium, you are looking at the valve of the foramen ovale which is the remanent of the septum primum (Fig. 9.5).

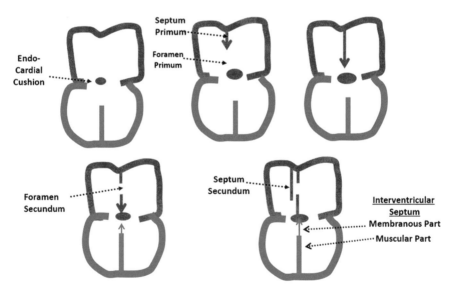

**Fig. 9.5** Septal Development. The septum primum grows towards the endocardial cushions. The opening between the two atria is the foramen primum at this point. As septum primum and endocardial cushions fuse, the foramen secundum then opens in the septum primum. The septum secundum then grows down to cover the foramen secundum. (Leo 2022)

## Development of the Ventricular Septum

At the same time the atrial septum is forming, the ventricular septum is forming. There is a larger muscular portion which ascends from the apex to divide the ventricle into right and left sides. In addition, descending from the endocardial cushions is the membranous portion if the interventricular septum. The muscular portion and the membranous portions fuse to form the wall between the right and left ventricles.

## Left-to-Right Shunts

The most common heart defect is a membranous interventricular septal defect, which will lead to a left-to-right shunt. Atrial defects are also common and there are various types of atrial septal defects. Because the interatrial septum starts superiorly and moves inferiorly towards the endocardial cushions there are opportunities for defects along the wall, either superiorly or inferiorly. Primum defects are down low by the endocardial cushions, while the secundum defects are higher on the wall:

1. If the septum primum fails to meet up and fuse with the endocardial cushions, there is an *ostium primum defect*. These occur in the inferior portion of the wall.
2. If there is excessive resorption of the septum primum, or a failure of the septum secundum then this is an *ostium secundum defect*. These occur on the superior portion of the wall.
3. A *patent foramen ovale* is a failure of the foramen ovale to close which allows blood to be shunted from left to right.

Septal defects will result in left-to-right shunts because the pressure is higher on the left side of the heart. In many cases, over time, this increased pressure will lead to pulmonary hypertension. As the pressure on the right side goes up, eventually the shunt will reverse and turn into a right-to-left shunt. This is referred to *Eisenmenger's complex*.

A *patent ductus arteriosus* (PDA) occurs when the ductus arteriosus does not close at birth. When this happens blood will be shunted from the aorta to the pulmonary trunk because of the higher pressures in the aorta. Maternal rubella infections are a predisposing factor to development of a PDA. PDA is also more common in babies born at high altitudes (above 8000 feet). Patients will have a machine-like diastolic murmur heard at the left upper chest.

## Right-to-Left Shunts

There are several right-to-left shunts. Because the blood is shunted away from the liver, these patients will be cyanotic.

*Tetralogy of Fallot* results from an abnormal migration of neural crest cells which leads to failure of the truncus and conus to separate which results in an anterior placed aorticopulmonary septum leading to the following defects (think IHOP).

1. **I**nterventricular septal defect
2. **H**ypertrophied right ventricle
3. **O**verriding Aorta
4. **P**ulmonary Hypertension

The patient will have a boot shaped heart. At birth, the babies will often have a bluish tint to their skin. They will also have rounded nail beds (clubbing of the fingers). As they reach 2–4 months of age, they will often TET spells, which typically occur after eating. They will turn blue, become agitated, and cry. They will often assume a squatting position to increase the blood flow to the lungs. Surgery can repair the defect.

*Persistent truncus arteriosus* occurs when the truncus arteriosus fails to separate into the aorta and pulmonary trunks which allows oxygenated and deoxygenated blood to mix which leads to cyanosis.

*Transposition of the great vessels* occurs when the aorta and pulmonary trunk come from the wrong sides. The blood going out the aorta will then not be carrying oxygen to the body. Surgery must be performed immediately. It is often associated with maternal diabetes, rubella, and viral illnesses.

## Coarctation of the Aorta

The closing of the ductus arteriosus involves a complicated signaling pathway, in some cases, a small portion of the aortic arch can get caught up in this process and become constricted. It can happen either just proximal or just distal to the ductus arteriosum. In can lead to increased blood pressure in the head and upper limb regions, but a reduced pulse in the lower limbs (Fig. 9.6).

**Fig. 9.6** Coarctation of the Aorta. With the preductal version the constriction is proximal to the ductus arteriosus which remains patent. In a post ductal version the ductus closes. (Leo 2022)

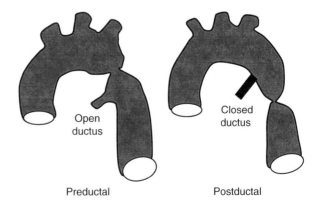

Open ductus

Closed ductus

Preductal                    Postductal

1. With a *preductal coarctation*, which is seen in infants, the ductus remains open which means blood can still get down to the lower body, but this blood will have lower than normal $O^2$ levels.
2. With a *postductal coarctation*, which is seen in adults, because of the various anastomoses, the blood will travel down the internal thoracic arteries, to the anterior intercostal arteries, to the posterior intercostal arteries and then into the descending aorta. With time the intercostal arteries will become large and burrow into the inferior borders of the ribs which can be seen as *rib notching* on images.

## Development of the GI Tract and Associated Organs

The GI tract starts as a tube of endoderm which can be divided into foregut, midgut, and hindgut endoderm. The tube becomes suspended by dorsal and ventral mesentery which is attached to the ventral and dorsal walls. During week 4 the stomach becomes dilated, and its differential growth rates leads to the tract rotating. The dorsal side rotates to the left and the ventral side rotates to the right. By week 5 the midgut has also elongated to the point where it has to leave the abdominal cavity and move into the yolk stalk. At the point where the midgut makes a U-turn and comes back into the abdominal cavity the vitelline duct which opens into the yolk sac is present.

Within the ventral mesentery the liver starts to form as a liver diverticulum. The ligament between the anterior body wall and the liver is the falciform ligament. The ligament between the liver, the stomach, and the duodenum is the lesser omentum (hepatogastric and hepatoduodenal ligaments). These ligaments are discussed in detail in Chapter Three (Fig. 9.7).

Within the dorsal mesentery, the spleen and kidney start to develop. The splenorenal ligament connects the spleen and the kidney, while the gastrosplenic ligament connects the stomach and spleen. Here is a way to think about these ligaments and determine if the adult ligament is a remnant of either the dorsal or ventral

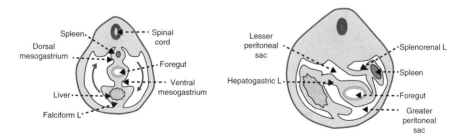

**Fig. 9.7** Development of Mesenteries. The liver develops in the ventral mesentery as an outgrowth of foregut endoderm. The falciform ligament runs from liver to anterior abdominal wall. The spleen develops in the dorsal mesentery from mesoderm. The splenorenal ligament connects the spleen to the posterior wall. (Leo 2022)

mesentery. If you look at an adult ligament, ask yourself if it is attached to the liver. If it is attached to the liver in the adult, that means it came from the ventral mesentery. For instance, the falciform ligament is attached to the liver, so it came from ventral mesentery. But the splenorenal ligament is not attached to the liver so it came from dorsal mesentery.

## Development of the Pancreas and Liver

At the start of week 5 the ventral and dorsal pancreatic buds (endoderm) appear on the right and left sides of the foregut just distal to the stomach. The ventral bud gives rise to the uncinate process of the pancreas. The dorsal bud gives rise to the head, the neck, body, and tail of the pancreas. As the gut rotates, the ventral bud rotates posteriorly, while the dorsal bud rotates anteriorly. If the pancreas does not rotate correctly, it can form a loop around the intestine. This *annular pancreas* can block the GI tract (Fig. 9.8).

As the pancreas is developing, the small intestine is also changing. At the start of week 4 the duodenum has a patent lumen. The duodenum grows so quickly that at the start of week 6 its lumen closes, and it says closed for several days. It eventually recanalizes. Duodenal atresia refers to a failure of the duodenum to recanalize. Stomach contents will then back up in the stomach and the proximal duodenum which can be seen as a double bubble sign on radiographs. Jejunal atresia results in a triple bubble sign.

## Clinical Scenarios

A *Meckel's diverticulum* results from a failure of the vitelline duct to close. What remains is a short piece of tissue projecting from the ileum. Think of the Rule-of-Two's. The diverticulum is found 2 feet from the ileocecal junction, it is typically 2

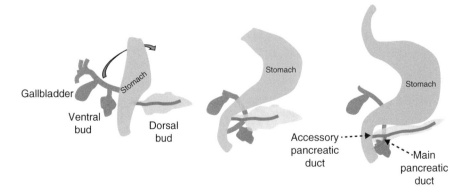

**Fig. 9.8** Pancreas Development. The pancreas develops from the ventral and dorsal pancreatic buds. (Leo 2022)

inches long, there are two types of tissue – gastric and pancreatic, and 2% of those with the diverticulum develop complications.

A herniation on the right side at the site of the umbilical vein is a *gastroschisis*. It herniates directly into the amniotic cavity.

An *omphalocele* is a failure of the normally herniated midgut to come back into the abdominal cavity. It occurs in the midline at the yolk stalk and is covered by amnion. In most cases there are other congenital anomalies.

*Hirschsprung's disease* is caused by a failure of neural crest cells to migrate into the descending colon. Normally this neural crest tissue will give rise to the postganglionic parasympathetic ganglia. Without the ganglia and the parasympathetic nerves, there is no peristalsis. The affected tract will tightly constrict so fecal material cannot move through it. This will lead to a build-up of material in the proximal bowel (megacolon) usually in the transverse colon.

Malrotation of the midgut involves a failure of the gut to rotate leading to misplacement of the gut.

## The Kidney

Think of kidney development as a movie with three episodes. Episode one, or the first stage of kidney development, involves the formation of the pronephros. The pronephros is short lived and degenerates by the end of week four.

Episode two involves the formation of the mesonephric ducts and mesonephric tubules during week four. The *mesonephric tubules* are derived from mesoderm and take the place of the pronephros. Also forming from the mesoderm are the *mesonephric ducts* that grow and descend to meet up with the urogenital sinus. By the end of week 8 the mesonephric tubules degenerate, however the mesonephric ducts remain to eventually go on to become part of the male reproductive tract.

Episode three involves the interaction of two pieces of mesoderm. The *ureteric bud* is an outgrowth of the mesonephric duct, so it arises from mesoderm. Meanwhile, along the posterior abdominal wall the *metanephric blastema* is being formed from mesoderm. The ureteric bud and the metanephric blastema then form the adult kidney. The metanephric blastema will form the nephrons and the tract up to where the collecting ducts start. The ureteric bud will form the outflow tract from the collecting ducts on out (Fig. 9.9).

In some cases, the kidneys do not form – *renal agenesis*. As long as one kidney is present there will not be an issue, however if neither kidney develops this is incompatible with life. During the pregnancy there will be an oligohydramnios. Normally, the kidneys produce amniotic fluid. Without them, there will be a lack of fluid. Without the protective function of the amniotic fluid, increased pressure on the fetus will lead to a flattened face. The amniotic fluid is also essential for normal lung development so without the fluid there will be *pulmonary hypoplasia* – reduction in the size of the lung. The patient will typically have clubbed fingers. The combination of all these symptoms together is referred to as *Potter's sequence*.

**Fig. 9.9**  Development of Kidney. The kidney arises from the (1) ureteric bud which is an outgrowth of the mesonephric duct, and (2) the metanephric blastema which arises from mesoderm. The cloaca is the common opening for the bladder and the hindgut. Note the urorectal septum is growing down the urogenital sinus to divide it into the bladder and anal canal. (Leo 2022)

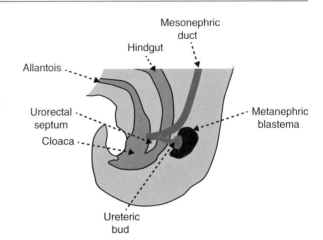

A *horseshoe kidney* refers to a failure of the kidney to ascend because it gets caught up around the inferior mesenteric artery. Instead of two kidneys there is one horseshoe shaped kidney.

## Urogenital Sinus

Think of the urogenital sinus as a warehouse sending out parts to various different regions of the body. The urogenital sinus is an out pocketing of endoderm from the cloaca. The upper part of the sinus gives rise to the epithelial lining of the bladder. During development, the mesonephric ducts form the muscular wall of trigone of the bladder and the ejaculatory ducts. The detrusor muscle which forms the wall of the bladder comes from mesoderm.

In the male the urogenital sinus also gives rise to the prostatic and membranous urethra. The prostatic urethra in turn, gives rise to the prostate gland.

Also emerging from the urogenital sinus is the *allantois*. In birds, it is used to process waste products. In humans, the blood vessels in the allantois are taken over by the embryo and used as the umbilical blood vessels. The umbilical veins carry oxygen rich blood from the placenta to the fetus, and the umbilical arteries carry oxygen poor blood from the fetus back to the placenta. In the adult, the *medial umbilical ligaments* are from the obliterated umbilical arteries; the median *umbilical ligaments* is from the obliterated *urachus* – the connection between bladder and allantois; and the *lateral umbilical ligaments* house the inferior epigastric arteries and veins.

If the urachus does not close off, and instead remains patent, then urine can drain at the umbilicus. This is referred to as a patent or persistent urachus.

## Development of Vagina and Uterus

The adult vagina is derived from both endoderm and mesoderm. During week 9 of development the paramesonephric ducts, which are mesoderm, attach to the sino-vaginal sinuses at the sinovaginal bulb, which is endoderm. As development proceeds the paramesonephric ducts and sinovaginal bulbs pull away from the urogenital sinus to form the vagina. The uterus also develops from the fusion of the paramesonephric ducts. The prostatic utricle in the male is the remanent of the paramesonephric ducts and thus homologous to the uterus. If the paramesonephric ducts fail to fuse correctly this can result in a bicornuate uterus (sometimes referred to as a heart shaped uterus). There are typically no symptoms with a bicornuate uterus, and the woman will most likely be unaware of it unless she becomes pregnant. It does increase the chance of a miscarriage (Figs. 9.9 and 9.10).

## Mesonephric and Paramesonephric Ducts (Fig. 9.11)

## Head and Neck Region

During the third week of development, neural crest cells migrate into the head to form the pharyngeal arches. At this early stage there are six arches. The arches form a tube with the inside of the tube coming from endoderm and forming pouches, while the outside of the tube comes from ectoderm and forms the pharyngeal grooves (or clefts). Pharyngeal groove one forms the epithelium of the external auditory tube, and pharyngeal pouch one forms the middle ear canal and auditory

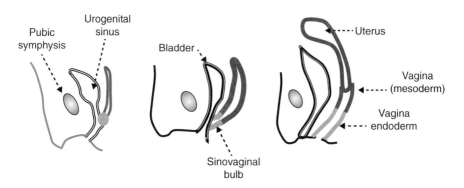

**Fig. 9.10** Development of Vagina. The uterus come from the paramesonephric ducts which fuse in the midline. The ducts are connected to the bladder wall at the sinovaginal bulb. The sinovaginal bulb pulls away from the bladder to give rise to lower 2/3rds of the vagina. The upper 1/3 of the vagina comes from the mesoderm of the paramesonephric ducts. (Leo 2022)

**Fig. 9.11** Development of Male/Female Reproductive Tracts. In females the paramesonephric ducts give rise to the fallopian tube, cervix, and upper part of the vagina. In males the mesonephric ducts give rise to the seminal vesicle, epididymis, ejaculatory duct, and ductus deferens. (Leo 2022)

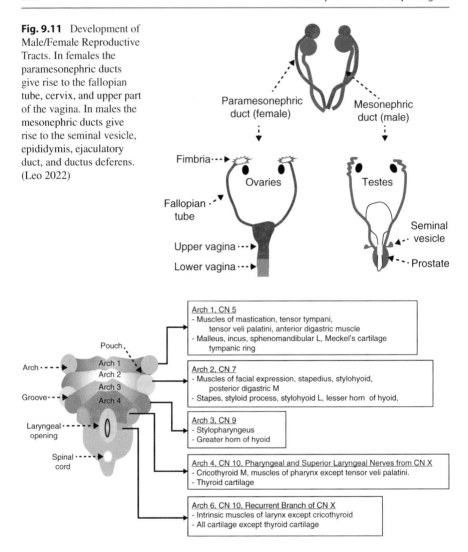

**Fig. 9.12** Pharyngeal Arches. (Leo 2022)

tube. Pharyngeal pouch two forms the epithelium of the palatine tonsil. Pharyngeal pouch three gives rise to the inferior parathyroid and thymus. Pharyngeal groove four gives rise to the superior parathyroid and ultimobranchial body (Fig. 9.12).

To organize the arches, you want to think of the nerves. Arch 1 is CN V, arch 2 is CN 7, arch 3 is CN IX, arch 4 is part of CN X, specifically the pharyngeal and superior laryngeal branches, arch 5 is going to disappear, and arch 6 is the recurrent laryngeal nerve a branch of CN X (Fig. 9.13).

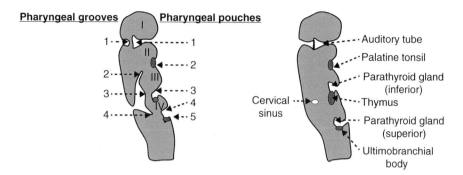

**Fig. 9.13** Pharyngeal Pouches and Grooves. Pharyngeal *groove* 1 forms the external ear canal. Pharyngeal *pouch* 1 forms the epithelial lining of the auditory tube and middle ear. Pharyngeal *arch* 2 overgrows grooves 2, 3, and 4. Sometimes a cervical cyst remains. Pharyngeal *pouch* two forms the epithelial lining of the palatine tonsil, *pouch* 3 forms the inferior parathyroid gland and thymus. Pharyngeal *pouch* 4 forms the superior parathyroid gland and the C-cells of the thyroid. (Leo 2022)

There are issues that can occur due to disruptions with the arches, grooves, and pouches:

First arch syndromes involve faulty development of the first arch which leads to facial anomalies. *Treacher Collins Syndrome* includes agenesis of the mandible, poorly developed eyelashes of the lower medial lid, abnormalities of the external and middle ear, deafness, and a drooping of the outer angle of the eye. *Pierre-Robbins Sequence* involves a sequence of events, meaning that each event causes the next event. It starts with a small mandible, which in turn leads to downward displacement of the tongue, which in turn leads to obstruction of the airway, all of which leads to a failure of the palate to form – *a cleft palate.*

Normally arch 2 grows over clefts 2, 3, and 4. When it does this, it will leave behind an ectodermal covered sinus, which will eventually be absorbed. In some instances, this structure remains which can lead to sinuses, cysts, or fistulas in the neck, usually parallel to the sternocleidomastoid muscle.

DiGeorge Syndrome arises from a microdeletion on the long arm of chromosome 22 and leads to defects with the arches and pouches of 3 and 4. Symptoms vary from one patient to another but often include heart defects, a cleft palate, a high face, small teeth, low set ears, and immune deficiencies.

The thyroid gland does not develop from the pharyngeal arches, but instead arises from foregut endoderm at the back of the tongue at the foramen cecum. The tissue then migrates inferior through the neck to end in the adult position. Along its migratory pathway it leaves a trail called the thyroglossal duct which is eventually reabsorbed. If this duct persists the patient will have a thyroglossal cyst that can be found along this pathway.

## Development of the Facial Bones

The face starts development in week four by a combination of the neural crest cells and mesoderm from the first arch. Specifically, the frontonasal prominence comes from neural crest cells, and the maxillary and mandibular prominences come from the mesoderm. The maxillary prominences start laterally and then expand medially to fuse with the midline located nasal prominence. Coming off the maxillary prominences are the palatal shelves which both expand medially to fuse in the midline. A cleft lip is the result of a failure of the medial nasal prominences to fuse with the maxillary prominence. A cleft palate is a failure of the two palatine shelves to fuse (Fig. 9.14).

## Polyhydramnios Versus Oligohydramnios

Amniotic fluid is produced by the kidneys and excreted into the amniotic cavity. The fetus then swallows the amniotic fluid. Congenital anomalies that result in a blockage of the intestinal tract will cause an increase in the amniotic fluid since the fetus cannot swallow it – polyhydramnios. If the kidneys do not develop then there will be no amniotic fluid – oligohydramnios.

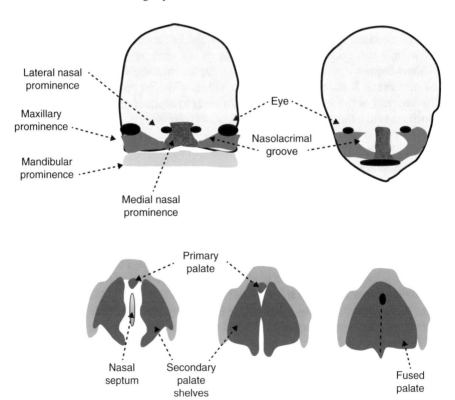

**Fig. 9.14**  Development of Facial bones and Palate. (Leo 2022)

## Development of the Trachea

At week 4 the developing lung arises as the respiratory diverticula from the foregut endoderm which results in one tube going to both esophagus and future lung. The respiratory diverticula will then divide into two bronchial buds to form the lungs The trachea eventually separates from the esophagus to form its own tube. In some instances, this separation leads to defects. The most common one being a *tracheo-esophageal fistula* with esophageal atresia. In this case the esophagus ends as a blind tube, usually along the distal 1/3rd of the esophagus, while the terminal esophagus maintains its connection with the trachea. This results in symptoms such as: polyhydramnios, cyanosis after eating, and reflux of stomach contents into the lungs (Fig. 9.15).

## Ectoderm

The ectoderm gives rise to two divisions, (1) *surface ectoderm*, which gives rise to the skin of the body and (2) *neural ectoderm*, which forms the neural tube and the neural crest tissue:

1. The *neural ectoderm* arises in the midline over the notochord. The neural tube gives rise to the CNS which includes the brain, spinal cord, optic nerve, and retina. This also includes the neurohypophysis, the pineal gland, astrocytes, oligodendrocytes.
2. The *neural crest cells* are mesenchymal cells that migrate to several different regions. They give rise to all the ganglia in the PNS, which includes the dorsal root ganglia, the postganglionic autonomic ganglia, and the adrenal medulla. But they also migrate to several other body regions. In the head they migrate into the

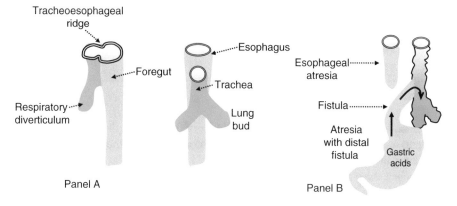

**Fig. 9.15** (**a, b**) Development of Lungs and Trachea. The lungs start as a respiratory diverticulum, an outgrowth of foregut endoderm. As it separates from the foregut, the tracheoesophageal ridge separates the trachea from the foregut. In some cases, there is an esophageal atresia with a tracheo-esophageal fistula between the distal esophagus and trachea. (Leo 2022)

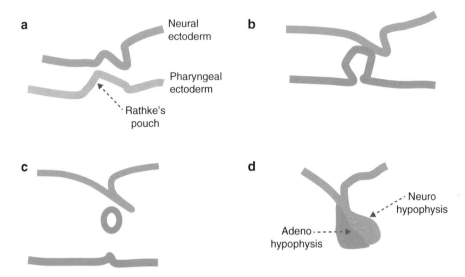

**Fig. 9.16** (**a–d**) Development of the Pituitary. The pituitary comes from two different sources of ectoderm. One is pharyngeal ectoderm, Rathke's pouch. The second source is neural ectoderm. (Leo 2022)

pharyngeal arches to give rise to some of the bones and cartilage of the skull. They also give rise to the parafollicular cells of the thyroid gland. Around the brain they become the pia and arachnoid. They also migrates into the skin to give rise to melanocytes. And they migrate to the heart to give rise to the atrioventricular septum. The *surface ectoderm* gives rise to the hypodermis (not the dermis) and the hair, nails, enamel of the teeth, and Rathke's pouch. Remember from the discussion on the development of the face, that the first groove gives rise to the epithelium of the external ear, and the first pouch gives rise to the epithelium of the inner ear. Note that parotid gland comes from ectoderm. Also note that the entire pituitary comes from ectoderm, but that the anterior pituitary comes from Rathke's pouch, while the posterior pituitary comes from the neural tube (Fig. 9.16).

## Endoderm

The endoderm gives rise to the epithelial lining of the GI tract, divided into foregut, midgut, and hindgut. And from the foregut endoderm comes the respiratory diverticulum which gives rise to the parenchyma of the lungs and the epithelium lining the trachea. Also from the foregut endoderm are the submandibular and sublingual glands, plus the thyroid gland. Remember the thyroid gland arises at the back of the tongue at the foramen cecum. In the ventral mesentery the liver starts as a diverticulum from the midgut, and this liver diverticula also gives rise to the gallbladder, biliary system, and pancreas. The spleen starts off in the dorsal mesentery, but it comes from mesoderm. Another way to look at it, or word it, is that the artery of the midgut is the celiac trunk which goes to all midgut structures except the spleen – which comes from mesoderm.

Moving down to the hindgut, the urogenital sinus comes from hindgut endoderm, and it in turn gives rise to the epithelium of the bladder, which in turn gives rise to the pancreas, the urethra, and lower vagina.

Note that organs whose epithelium comes from endoderm are surrounded by tissue that comes from mesoderm.

## Mesoderm

During early development the mesoderm forms the nucleus pulposus of the notochord. The mesoderm gives rise to all the muscle tissue, including, smooth, skeletal, and cardiac muscle. It also gives rise to all the connective tissue, bone, serous membranes, blood, cartilage, lymph, gonads, spleen, adrenal cortex, kidneys, and ureters. Remember the ureter arises from the mesonephric duct, a mesoderm structure that also give rise to the vas deferens, and seminal vesicles, epididymis, and ejaculatory ducts. As mentioned above, the pancreas comes from the urogenital sinus which is endoderm. In the heart the mesoderm gives rise to epithelium.

In females, the paramesonephric ducts, a mesoderm structure, gives rise to the uterus, fallopian tube, cervix, and upper part of the vagina.

## Mesoderm Divisions

During week three, the mesoderm divides into three sections: (1) paraxial mesoderm, (2) intermediate mesoderm, and (3) lateral plate mesoderm. Their names give away their locations. The paraxial mesoderm is just lateral to the notochord, the lateral plate mesoderm is the most lateral of the three divisions, and between the two is the intermediate mesoderm (Fig. 9.17).

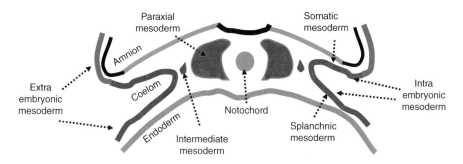

**Fig. 9.17** Mesoderm and its Derivatives. The mesoderm has three divisions: (1) paraxial, (2) intermediate, and (3) lateral plate. The lateral plate, in turn, divides into two layers: the somatic and splanchnic layers. (Leo, 2022)

The lateral plate mesoderm is shaped like a "Y" with one arm becoming the somatic layer of lateral plate mesoderm, or *somatopleure,* and the second arm becoming the splanchnic layer of the lateral plate mesoderm, also known as *splanchnopleure.* Located at the junction of the "Y" is the intraembryonic coelom, which is continuous with the extraembryonic coelom early in development. At the end of the lateral body wall folding, these two cavities will be separated.

1. The somatopleure layer of mesoderm is originally adjacent to the ectoderm which surrounds the amniotic cavity. It will go on and form the body wall and the parietal layers of the pleura, peritoneal cavity, and the pericardial cavity
2. The splanchnopleure layer is adjacent to the endoderm. With the lateral folding of the body wall, the splanchnic layer will become the visceral layers of the three cavities, pericardium, pleura, and peritoneal.

As the somatopleure layer of mesoderm folds, it eventually meets in the mid-line and closes the peritoneal and pericardial cavities. In the abdomen, the meeting of the two layers in the midline gives rise to the ventral and dorsal mesentery. The ventral mesentery eventually degenerates, except for the falciform ligament and the lesser omentum. The dorsal mesentery remains to allow blood vessels to travel from the posterior wall to the various intraperitoneal organs. An *omphalocele* results from a failure of the two sides to fuse in the midline in the lumbar region. An *ectopia cordis* results from failure of the two sides to fuse in the midline in the thoracic region.

The intermediate mesoderm will give rise to the kidneys, ureter, vas deferens, and gonads. The paraxial mesoderm resembles a cord on the sides of the notochord which eventually differentiates into segmented blocks of tissue referred to as somites. The somites in turn give rise to the dermatomes (dermis and associated structures), myotomes (axial and appendicular skeletons), and sclerotomes (cartilage, tendons, bone).

## Early Venous Drainage

Initially in early heart development there are two sinus horns (right and left) draining into the sinus venosus. And draining into each horn are three veins:

1. The vitelline veins drain the yolk sac. They form a plexus around the duodenum (portal vein). The left vitelline vein regresses while the right becomes the hepatic portion of the inferior vena cava.
2. The right and left common cardinal veins receive blood from the anterior and posterior cardinal veins and in turn drain into the sinus venosus. During the second month of development, the right and left anterior cardinal veins form an anastomosis which becomes the left brachiocephalic vein. The inferior portion of the right anterior cardinal vein becomes the superior vena cava. The proximal portion of the left anterior cardinal vein normally regresses. If it does not regress,

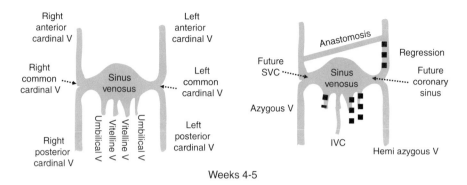

**Fig. 9.18** Early Venous Drainage. The sinus venosus receives blood from the common cardinal, umbilical, and vitelline veins. An anastomosis forms between the right and left anterior cardinal veins which will become the left brachiocephalic vein. (Leo 2022)

then the patient will have a double superior vena cava. On the other hand, if the right side regresses, the patient's superior vena cava will be on the left side. The right posterior cardinal vein forms the proximal portion of the azygous vein.

3. The umbilical veins carry oxygen rich blood from the placenta to the fetus. The right umbilical vein regresses by day 44. From day 44 onward, the left umbilical vein is responsible for delivering blood to the liver (Fig. 9.18).

## Further Reading

Carlson B. Human embryology and developmental biology. 6th ed. New York: Elsevier; 2018.

Gittenberger-De Groot AC, Bartelings MM, Deruiter MC, Poelmann RE. Basics of cardiac development for the understanding of congenital heart malformations. Pediatr Res. 2005;57(2):169–76.

Graham A, Richards J. Development and evolutionary origins of the pharyngeal apparatus. Evol Develop. 2012;3:24.

McKenzie J. The first arch syndrome. Arch Dis Child. 1958;8(1):477–86.

Moore KL, Persaud TVN. The developing human: clinically oriented embryology. 11th ed. New York: Saunders; 2019.

Sadler TW. Langman's medical embryology. 14th ed. New York: Lippincott Williams and Wilkins; 2018.

Sweeney L. Basic concepts in embryology: a student's survival guide. New York: McGraw-Hill; 1997.

# 100 Key Anatomy Words

| | | |
|---|---|---|
| 1 | Infratemporal fossa nerve | V3 |
| 2 | Pterygopalatine fossa nerve | V2 |
| 3 | Bell's palsy, where is lesion? | Facial canal |
| 4 | Claw hand | Ulnar nerve |
| 5 | Pope's blessing | Median nerve |
| 6 | Mallet finger | Tear of extensor digitorum longus |
| 7 | Callot's triangle, what artery? | Cystic artery |
| 8 | Most posterior structure in hepatoduodenal ligament | Portal vein |
| 9 | Trauma, lower limb laterally rotated | Femoral neck fracture |
| 10 | Dashboard injury, lower limb medially rotated | Posterior hip dislocation |
| 11 | Anterior layer rectus sheath Above pectinate line | Ext Abd Obl, Int Abd Obl, transversus abdominus muscles |
| 12 | Lesser omentum subdivisions | Hepatoduodenal, hepatogastric ligaments |
| 13 | Ulcer of the first part of duodenum | Gastroduodenal artery and hepatic duct. |
| 14 | Between SMA and aorta | Left renal vein, uncinate process, duodenum |
| 15 | Jugular foramen syndrome | CN 9, 10, and 11 |
| 16 | Otic ganglia | Parasympathetics to parotid |
| 17 | Running with superficial temporal artery | Auriculotemporal nerve |
| 18 | Landmark for inguinal hernias | Inferior epigastric artery |
| 19 | SLAP tear, tendon? | Glenoid labrum near where long head of the biceps inserts |
| 20 | First 10–15% of shoulder abduction | Supraspinatus |
| 21 | Cavernous sinus nerves? | CNs 3, 4, 6, and V1 and V2, not V3 |
| 22 | Medial strabismus, nerve damaged? | CN 6 |
| 23 | Jefferson fracture | C1 |
| 24 | Dislocated lunate, symptoms? | Mimics carpal tunnel |
| 25 | Handlebar palsy | Ulnar nerve |
| 26 | DeQuervain syndrome | Extensor pollicis brevis and abductor pollicis longus |
| 27 | Pope's blessing | Motor test for median nerve |
| 28 | Claw hand | Ulnar nerve sign |
| 29 | Right to left shunts | Transposition of great vessels, persistent truncus arteriosus, tetralogy of Fallot |

J. Leo, *Clinical Anatomy and Embryology*,
https://doi.org/10.1007/978-3-031-03807-5

| 30 | Tetralogy of Fallot | Interventricular septal defect, hypertrophied right ventricle, overriding aorta, pulmonary hypertension |
|----|---------------------|------------------------------------------------------------------|
| 31 | Base of heart | Left atrium |
| 32 | Dermatome of thumb | C6 |
| 33 | Unhappy triad | Medial collateral, medial meniscus, ACL |
| 34 | Tarsal tunnel nerve | Tibial nerve |
| 35 | Pott's fracture | Medial malleolus and distal fibula |
| 36 | Fracture of femoral neck | Lower limb laterally rotated |
| 37 | Posterior hip dislocation | Lower limb medially rotated |
| 38 | Pes anserinus | Sartorius, gracilis, semitendinosus |
| 39 | Subclavian steal syndrome | Blockage of subclavian artery proximal to vertebral A |
| 40 | Carotid tubercle | Anterior tubercle of C6. Common carotid is anterior, vertebral is posterior |
| 41 | Posterior humeral circumflex A | Runs with axillary nerve |
| 42 | Posterior superior iliac spine | End of dura, S2 vertebra, middle of sacroiliac joint, dimples of Venus |
| 43 | Pudendal nerve block | Ischial spine, sacrospinous ligament |
| 44 | Pulse in snuff box | Radial artery |
| 45 | Gamekeeper's thumb | Ulnar collateral ligament |
| 46 | Froment's sign | Ulnar nerve |
| 47 | Pronator teres syndrome | Median nerve |
| 48 | Midshaft humeral fracture | Radial nerve, wrist drop |
| 49 | Supracondylar fracture | Median nerve |
| 50 | Emergency airway opening | Cricothyrotomy |
| 51 | Piriform recess | Internal laryngeal nerve |
| 52 | Posterior Cricoarytenoid | Only muscle that opens the glottis |
| 53 | Aortic aneurysm, horse voice | Left recurrent laryngeal nerve |
| 54 | Esophageal hiatus | T10, esophagus and right and left vagus nerves |
| 55 | Duodenal ulcer | Gastroduodenal artery |
| 56 | Arteries to terminal esophagus | Left gastric artery |
| 57 | Lesser sac | Between stomach/lesser omentum and pancreas |
| 58 | Nutcracker syndrome | SMA and aorta sandwiching the left renal vein |
| 59 | Lienorenal ligament: dorsal or ventral mesentery? | Dorsal mesentery |
| 60 | Scalene triangle boundaries | Anterior and middle scalenes and first rib |
| 62 | Beginning of portal vein behind what organ? | Pancreas |
| 63 | Femoral hernia and pubic tubercle | Femoral hernia lateral to PT |
| 64 | Adductor hiatus | Femoral A becomes popliteal artery. Opening in adductor magnus |
| 65 | Most important ligament for medial arch in foot | Plantar calcaneonavicular (Spring) L |
| 66 | Subtalar joint | Talus and calcaneus |
| 67 | Chopart joint | Talonavicular and calcaneocuboid ligaments |
| 68 | Bunion | Hallux valgus |
| 69 | Nerves traveling through tendinous ring in orbit | CNs 3, 6, and nasociliary |
| 70 | Gag reflex | CN 9 afferent, CN 10 efferent |
| 71 | Pott's fracture | Tibia (med malleolus) and fibula |
| 72 | Dorsalis pedis pulse, where? | Lateral to extensor hallucis longus. |
| 73 | Posterior rectus sheath, superior to arcuate line | Internal abdominal oblique and transversus abdominus |

| 74 | Trachea ends | T6 |
|---|---|---|
| 75 | Rib notching | Coarctation of aorta |
| 76 | Gastrosplenic ligament: dorsal or ventral mesentery? | Dorsal |
| 77 | Machine-like murmur | PDA |
| 78 | Cremaster muscle: what layer? | Internal abdominal oblique muscle |
| 79 | Lowest point peritoneal cavity in females | Rectouterine pouch |
| 80 | Supracondylar fracture | Median nerve |
| 81 | Whiplash injury | Anterior longitudinal ligament |
| 82 | Waiter's tip | Upper trunk injury |
| 83 | Spondylosis | Pars interarticularis |
| 84 | Deep fibular nerve sign | Foot drop |
| 85 | Foramen spinosum | Middle meningeal artery |
| 86 | Amnion, what layer | Ectoderm |
| 87 | Deep inguinal ring | Fascia transversalis |
| 88 | Pelvic diaphragm muscles? | Levator ani and coccygeus |
| 89 | Membranous urethra, what space? | Deep perineal space |
| 90 | CN 4 palsy, head tilt? | Head tilt away from the side of lesion |
| 91 | Prostate: endo, ecto, or meso? | Endo |
| 92 | Superior part of vagina: endo, ecto, or meso | Endo |
| 93 | Stab wound to the right of sternum at rib 4 | Right atrium |
| 94 | Stab wound to left of sternum, rib 4 | Right ventricle |
| 95 | Loop of Henle: In medulla or cortex of kidney? | Cortex |
| 96 | Left to right shunts | ASD, VSD, PDA |
| 97 | Radial head dislocation | Annular ligament |
| 98 | Sensation to first dorsal web space | Radial nerve |
| 99 | Abduction/adduction of fingers | Ulnar nerve |
| 100 | Sensation between 1st and 2nd toes | Deep fibular nerve |

# Index

© The Editor(s) (if applicable) and The Author(s), under exclusive license to Springer
Nature Switzerland AG 2022
J. Leo, *Clinical Anatomy and Embryology*,
https://doi.org/10.1007/978-3-031-03807-5

Printed in the United States
by Baker & Taylor Publisher Services